3D Bioprinting

Dedication

The author dedicates this book to his parents Guluzar and Suleyman

3D Bioprinting

Fundamentals, Principles and Applications

Ibrahim T. Ozbolat

ELSEVIER

AMSTERDAM • BOSTON • HEIDELBERG • LONDON
NEW YORK • OXFORD • PARIS • SAN DIEGO
SAN FRANCISCO • SINGAPORE • SYDNEY • TOKYO
Academic Press is an imprint of Elsevier

Academic Press is an imprint of Elsevier
125 London Wall, London EC2Y 5AS, United Kingdom
525 B Street, Suite 1800, San Diego, CA 92101-4495, United States
50 Hampshire Street, 5th Floor, Cambridge, MA 02139, United States
The Boulevard, Langford Lane, Kidlington, Oxford OX5 1GB, United Kingdom

Library of Congress Cataloging-in-Publication Data
A catalog record for this book is available from the Library of Congress

British Library Cataloguing-in-Publication Data
A catalogue record for this book is available from the British Library

ISBN: 978-0-12-803010-3

For information on all Academic Press publications
visit our website at https://www.elsevier.com/

Publisher: Joe Hayton
Acquisition Editor: Fiona Geraghty
Editorial Project Manager: Naomi Robertson
Production Project Manager: Jason Mitchell
Designer: Victoria Pearson

Typeset by TNQ Books and Journals

Contents

About the Author

Ibrahim Tarik Ozbolat is an associate professor of Engineering Science and Mechanics Department, Biomedical Engineering Department, the Huck Institutes of the Life Sciences, and the Materials Research Institute at The Pennsylvania State University, University Park, Pennsylvania, USA. Previously, he was a faculty member of The University of Iowa, Iowa City, Iowa, USA, and spearheaded Advanced Manufacturing Technology Group and the Biomanufacturing Laboratory. He received his PhD in tissue engineering from the Industrial and Systems Engineering Department at the University at Buffalo (SUNY) in Buffalo, New York, USA, and dual BS degrees in Mechanical Engineering and in Industrial Engineering from Middle East Technical University, Ankara, Turkey. Dr. Ozbolat is an internationally recognized expert in the area of 3D bioprinting. His research on bioprinting for tissue and organ fabrication has been published in several high quality of venues, received numerous national and international awards, and featured in national and international media, broadcast TVs, and press numerous times. He frequently gives invited talks at national and international forums, conferences, and seminars and organizes demonstrations and events to public and youth to encourage participation of future's engineers in medicine, engineering, and science.

Preface

Bioprinting is an emerging field that makes a revolutionary impact on medical sciences. It has attracted numerous researchers from various academic disciplines as well as the public. Bioprinting offers great precision on spatial placement of cells, proteins, DNA, drugs, and biologically active particles to better guide tissue generation and formation. This emerging technology appears to be more promising for advancing tissue engineering toward functional tissue and organ fabrication for transplantation, ultimately mitigating organ shortage and saving lives.

In this regard, development of a very comprehensive book covering all aspects of bioprinting is highly useful for the academic and educational circles, public, and the emerging bioprinting industry. The benefits of this book to the readership are in threefolds. First of all, the book is *a unique source* for academicians and researchers covering almost all aspects of bioprinting spanning raw materials, processes, machine technology, products, applications, limitations, and future perspectives. The growing research interest and the market in this field will make this book highly demandable. Secondly, it helps the bioengineers, tissue and manufacturing engineers as well as medical doctors to understand features of each bioprinting processes, the bioink and bioprinter type, and select the appropriate process for a given application such as tissue engineering and regenerative medicine, transplantation, clinics, or pharmaceutics. Thirdly, it is a *great source* for upper undergraduate- and graduate-level courses in the area of bioprinting, biofabrication, and tissue engineering considering the great worldwide interest on new undergraduate and graduate programs in biofabrication.

The book is outlined in 10 chapters including Introduction, Design for Bioprinting, The Bioink, Extrusion-Based Bioprinting, Droplet-Based Bioprinting, Laser-Based Bioprinting, Bioprinter Technologies, Roadmap to Organ Printing, Applications of 3D Bioprinting, and Future Trends.

Chapter 1 introduces tissue engineering, 3D printing in tissue engineering, principles of bioprinting and its components, and historical evaluation and classification of bioprinting processes. Chapter 2 discusses design for bioprinting covering the steps taken from medical imaging to bioprinting. Chapter 3 covers the bioink materials; their physical, chemical, and biological properties; compatible bioprinting techniques; and the comparison of bioink types.

In Chapters 4–6, the author discusses three major groups of bioprinting modalities including extrusion-, droplet-, and laser-based bioprinting, respectively. In each modality, the process and its characteristics and main components are described, the underlying physics is presented in addition to suitable bioink and cell types printed, and major accomplishments achieved so far.

In Chapter 7, bioprinter technologies are highlighted covering the components of bioprinters as well as the commercially available bioprinters in the market along with a detailed discussion on the limitations of bioprinter technologies. Chapter 8 covers the organ printing topic, introduces the state-of-the-art followed by the roadmap for organ printing with a step-by-step description. Chapter 9 presents the application areas of bioprinting, including tissue engineering and regenerative medicine, clinics and transplantation, pharmaceutics, and cancer research. Finally, Chapter 10 discusses the future trends in bioprinting that will revolutionize the organ transplantation technology in the next couple of decades.

Acknowledgments

The author extends his gratitude and deep appreciation to all his students, staff, and visiting faculty who have worked in his laboratory over the last 5 years at The University of Iowa from 2011 to 2015 and at the Pennsylvania State University since 2015. The author is grateful to the many funding agencies that have funded the bioprinting work in this laboratory.

The author wishes to thank the following agencies and institutions for sponsoring the bioprinting-related research projects over the past 5 years:

- National Science Foundation, USA
- National Institutes of Health, USA
- The Institute for Clinical and Translational Science at The University of Iowa, USA
- Osteology Foundation, Switzerland
- Diabetes in Action Research and Education Foundation, USA
- The University of Iowa, USA
- The State of Iowa, USA
- The Pennsylvania State University, USA
- The Huck Institutes of the Life Sciences, USA
- The Materials Research Institute, USA
- Center for Computer Aided Design, USA
- Ministry of National Education, Turkey

The author thanks Dr. Aleksandr Ovsianikov from TU Wien for his suggestions in Chapter 6. The author particularly wishes to acknowledge the following visiting faculty, scientists, staff, students, and interns for their contributions to this book. It would not be in print today without your personal contributions...

Thank you!

Current visiting faculty, staff, students, and interns
Alyssa Sipos
Ashley Leberfinger, MD
Bugra Ayan
Dino Ravnic, MD
Donna Sosnoski
Elias Rizk, MD
Fisayo Olashore
Hemanth Gudupati
Kazim Kerim Moncal
Madhuri Dey
Merve Buluk
Monika Hospodiuk

Ryan McFadden
Srinivas Koduru
Veli Ozbolat, PhD
Weijie Peng, PhD

Former staff and students
Amer Dababneh (McLaughlin Body Company)
Eric Warren (University of Colorado Anschutz Medical Campus)
Farzaneh Dolati (The Whirlpool Corporation)
Howard Chen (The University of Iowa)
Laura L. Hupp (Shook, Hardy & Bacon L.L.P.)
Melanie Laverman (The University of Iowa)
Ning Peng, PhD (The University of Iowa)
Rebecca Barrett (The University of Iowa)
Yahui Zhang, PhD (Micro Medical Solutions Inc.)
Yang Wu (The University of Iowa)
Yin Yu, PhD (Harvard Medical School)

1

Introduction

CHAPTER OUTLINE

All truths are easy to understand once they are discovered; the point is to discover them
Galileo Galilei

1.1 Tissue Engineering

Since the first successful kidney transplant in 1954 was performed between two identical twins (Merrill et al., 1956), organ transplantation has become a life-saving procedure for many disease conditions that hitherto were considered incurable. In the United States of America (USA), an average of 79 people receive transplants every day; however, the number of donors is much less than the number of patients waiting for a transplant (Ozbolat and Chen, 2013). Moreover, infections and rejection of the tissue by the host often make the transplantation process more challenging (Desmet et al., 2008). The solution to this problem, as with the solutions to other grand engineering challenges, requires long-term solutions by building or manufacturing healthy living organs from a person's own cells, which would relieve suffering and save lives.

Current medical procedures aim to restore tissue function to patients with diseased or damaged tissues through tissue transplantation and implants. Tissue engineering has grown as a multidisciplinary scientific field of biology, biomaterials, and engineering that has rapidly emerged and combines engineering principles with life sciences to replace damaged tissues or restore malfunctioning organs by mimicking native tissue (Langer and Vacanti, 1993). One of the common strategies in tissue engineering is to develop engineered scaffolds that provide an optimum environment or housing for cell attachment and growth, tissue regeneration, fluid movement, and structural integrity. The main reason for the scaffolding approach is the need to maintain the shape and mechanical properties of the mimicked tissue engineered, to assist in cell attachment, and to provide a substrate for cell proliferation into three-dimensional (3D) functioning tissues (Hutmacher et al., 2004). Developed 3D porous engineered constructs enable cell attachment, proliferation, and regeneration. Upon implantation, scaffold material starts degrading, and cells grow and proliferate through pores. Eventually, degraded sites constitute new tissue and restore the functionality of the diseased or damaged tissue.

Several traditional fabrication techniques have been used for tissue scaffolds, including phase separation, membrane lamination, melt molding, fiber bonding, molding, gas foaming, solvent casting, freeze drying, and particulate leaching (Leong et al., 2003). Most of the abovementioned techniques are, however, limited in terms of manufacturing reproducibility and flexibility. Building patient-specific anatomically correct shapes with well-controlled internal geometry, including pore size and pore distribution, is highly challenging. In addition, they include manual interventions and inconsistent and inflexible processing procedures with the use of toxic solvents and porogens that limits the inclusion of cell and protein impregnation. 3D printing, also known as additive manufacturing, has been a game-changing technology in the rapid manufacturing of complex products and has been adopted in tissue engineering for biofabrication of 3D scaffolds (Hamid et al., 2011).

1.2 Three-Dimensional Printing in Tissue Engineering

3D printing opens a revolutionary era in medical product design and development and is widely used to fabricate 3D scaffolds by layer-by-layer deposition. In general, biomaterials are deposited through a dispensing unit to specific points on the space to create a scaffold with well-controlled geometry. Three-dimensional bioprinting has been extensively used for building tissue-engineered constructs due its repeatability and high accuracy in microscale fabrication resolution (Sachlos et al., 2003). 3D printing techniques such as fused deposition modeling, precision-extrusion deposition, selective laser sintering, three-dimensional printing, and stereolithography (SLA) have been used to fabricate biologically active tissue constructs by replacing the materials being processed with biocompatible materials such as synthetic and natural polymers, natural and inorganic ceramic materials, or recently developed biodegradable metals (Ozbolat and Hospodiuk, 2016). Adaptation of 3D printing into tissue engineering brings unique capabilities in rapid fabrication of tissue scaffolds with controlled porosity and internal architecture, tunable mechanical and structural properties, and the ability to load drug or protein molecules for enhanced cellular response and customized/multifunctional characteristics, which can guide the cellular environment for enhanced tissue regeneration. To achieve a truly interconnected internal architecture for cell growth and proliferation, an internal structure is formed by depositing cylindrical microfilaments parallel to each other in every layer using a certain lay-down pattern.

Despite its great benefits in the biofabrication of anatomically correct tissue scaffolds, 3D printing in tissue engineering faces several limitations in the generation of complex tissues and organs for transplantation or other uses. First of all, there is a lack of precision in cell placement due to manually driven seeding and placement of cells on the scaffold microarchitecture. It is highly challenging to manually seed, place, and pattern cells precisely in a scaffold construct; however, several cell type groups are organized and interact in very complex patterns in natural tissues and organs. In addition, seeding cells in high cell density is very limited because cells can only attach on the surface of the scaffold and cannot penetrate into the biomaterial in the scaffold. Scaffold biomaterials also occupy a significant volume of space in the scaffold, which do not let the cells grow into sufficient cell numbers. In addition, the need for a vascular network is essential to develop thick tissues and organs to facilitate an efficient exchange of media to keep the cells oxygenized, viable and functional, and it is very difficult to create such a network using 3D printing technologies alone. These difficulties have led many researchers toward the development of bioprinting technologies, where cells can be encapsulated in high cell density and printed and patterned into desired spaces to obtain anatomically correct tissue constructs with patterned cells interacting as in native tissue and organs.

1.3 Three-Dimensional Bioprinting

Three-dimensional bioprinting is an emerging field that makes a revolutionary impact on medical sciences. It has gained significant attention from numerous researchers from various academic disciplines as well as the general public. Bioprinting could be defined as a computer-aided transfer process for simultaneous writing of living cells and biomaterials with a prescribed layer-by-layer stacking organization to fabricate bioengineered constructs for tissue engineering, regenerative medicine, or other biological studies (Mironov et al., 2009; Ozbolat, 2015). The major difference between 3D printing for tissue engineering and 3D bioprinting is that bioprinting involves the printing of living cells and other biologics. It offers great precision on spatial placement of cells, proteins, DNA, drug particles, grow factors, and biologically active particles to better guide tissue generation and formation. This emerging technology appears to be more promising for advancing tissue engineering toward functional tissue and organ fabrication for transplantation, ultimately mitigating organ shortage and saving lives.

The 3D bioprinting process can be divided into three crucial technological steps: preprocessing, processing (actual printing), and postprocessing (Mironov et al., 2006). Preprocessing is a blueprint of tissue or organ design using imaging and computer-aided

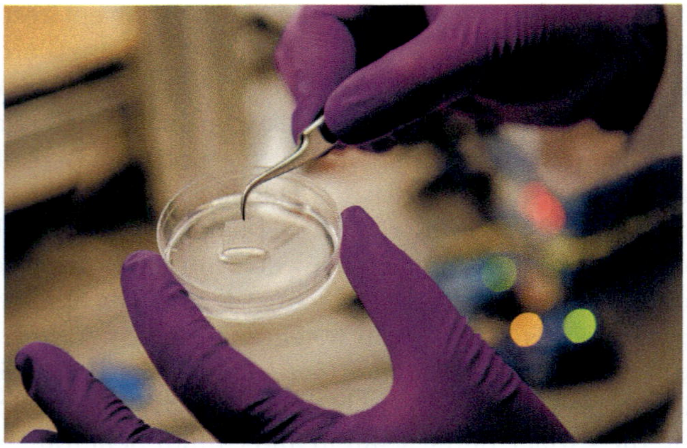

FIGURE 1.1 Bioprinting of cell-laden porous tissue scaffolds *(Courtesy of The University of Iowa, Iowa City, Iowa, USA).*

design (CAD) techniques. Accordingly, after the blueprint is designed, the actual printing is processed through a bioprinter. Fig. 1.1 shows a bioprinted cell-laden tissue construct printed rapidly, where cells are encapsulated inside the bioprinted construct. As the third step, the bioprinted construct must then undergo the process of cell proliferation, tissue remodeling, and maturation in a specially designed chamber "bioreactor" that accelerates tissue maturation. The bioreactor device is used when the printed tissue construct is grown in laboratory settings for different purposes, such as research studies or drug testing; however, the tissue construct is implanted in a living body if the ultimate goal is to regenerate the diseased or damaged tissue. The living body can still be considered as a bioreactor, where the abovementioned tissue remodeling and generation takes place.

1.3.1 Principles of Three-Dimensional Bioprinting and Its Components

Bioprinting or direct cell printing is an extension of tissue engineering, as it intends to create de novo organs. Bioprinting offers a controllable fabrication process, which allows precise placement of various biomaterial and/or cell types simultaneously according to the natural compartments of the target tissue or organs. A bioprinting system consists of three major components: (1) hardware system, (2) software system, and (3) the transferring medium to deliver the cells. The hardware system is made of a robotics printing system that can move in a minimum of three axes in the space and a deposition system to deliver cells to the printing stage. Both hardware components are controlled by a software system. Fig. 1.2 shows the Fabion bioprinter developed by Bioprinting Solutions (Moscow, Russia) with five deposition heads, where motion system and the deposition system are controlled in tandem to fabricate hybrid vascularized tissue constructs. Each deposition head is capable of bioprinting different cell types and has a different z-axis motion system to independently control the associated print head. The deposition on the three heads is mechanically controlled, and the rest are controlled numerically.

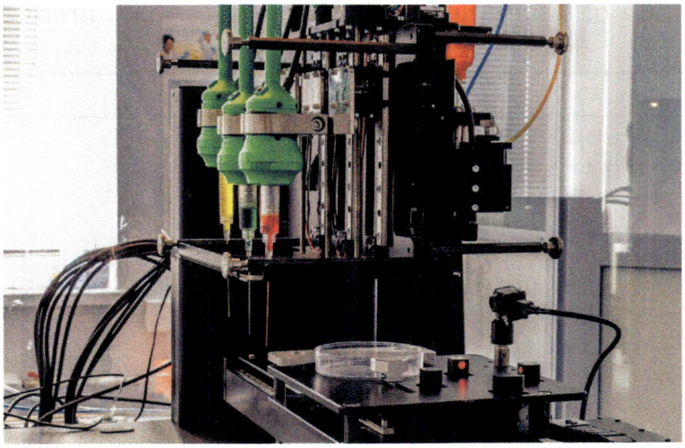

FIGURE 1.2 The Fabion bioprinter with a five-nozzle dispensing system enabling hybrid fabrication of tissue constructs *(Courtesy of Bioprinting Solutions, Russia).*

The software system uses the input data and control motion of a robotics system as well as the deposition of cells simultaneously to print and locate them at predefined positions in the space. The software system can use user-provided printing directions or generate these instructions directly through medical CAD models, which can be obtained via processing of medical images such as magnetic resonance imaging or computed tomography scan data. These CAD models are further processed to generate a toolpath plan with deposition instructions to the robotic system. Deposition of cells is carried out in a medium using an external source of energy such as laser, mechanical, thermal, or pneumatic potential energy. The medium, which is called the bioink, enables the transfer of cells to the printing stage. The bioink is made of aqueous biocompatible materials that allow cells to grow and oxygenize sufficiently to keep them viable. Printing of cells in the transferring medium is performed using a robotics system, where the bioink (homocellular or heterocellular) is deposited, solidified, and stacked layer-by-layer in 3D.

1.3.2 Historical Evolution

For now, bioprinting of 3D fully functional solid organs for transplantation remains elusive; however, the field is moving forward. Currently, there is a plethora of research being done on bioprinting technology and its potential as a source for tissue grafts and organ transplants. A timeline for the evolution of bioprinting technology up to the current state of the art is illustrated in Table 1.1.

Bioprinting was first demonstrated by Klebe in 1998 as cytoscribing technology, a method of micropositioning cells and constructing two-dimensional (2D) synthetic tissues (Klebe, 1988). In that study, cytoscribing was carried out using a Hewlett Packard (HP) inkjet printer and a graphics plotter for high positioning of cells. With the first attempt of generating cartilage tissue in the shape of an ear on the dorsa of a mouse in 1996, Vacanti and Langer opened up a great venue, where tissue engineering started to

Table 1.1 A Timeline for the Evolution of Bioprinting Technology up to the Current State of the Art

Year	Development
1988	2D micropositioning of cells using cytoscribing technology
1996	Observation that cells stick together and move together in clumps
1996	First use of natural biomaterial in human for tissue regeneration
1998	Invention of cell sheet technology
1999	Laser direct write (LDW)
2001	First tissue-engineered bladder (using synthetic scaffold seeded with patient's own cells)
2002	Bioprinting using inkjet technology is enabled
2003	Inkjet printing generates viable cells
2004	A modified inkjet printer dispenses cells
2004	3D tissue with only cells (no scaffold) is developed
2006	3D cellular assembly of bovine aortal is fabricated
2007	Digital printing
2008	Concept of tissue spheroids as building blocks
2009	First commercial bioprinter (Novogen MMX)
2009	Scaffold-free vascular constructs
2010	Hepatocytes are patterned in collagen using LDW successfully
2012	In situ skin printing
2012	Application of inkjet printing to repair human articular cartilage
2012	Bipolar wave-based drop-on-demand jetting
2012	Engineering of an artificial liver using extrusion-based (syringe) bioprinting
2014	Integration of tissue fabrication with printed vasculature using a multiarm bioprinter
2016	Bioprinting of larger-scale perfusable tissue constructs

emerge in generating tissues in 3D. Later attempts in 3D scaffolding technologies by several researchers in addition to cell sheet technology rely on manual interventions of the biomaterials in 3D with randomly controlled architecture. In 1999, printing of cells using laser-based bioprinting was demonstrated for the first time by Odde and Renn (1999), revealing that cells could be patterned in 3D to biomimetically develop tissue analogs with complex anatomy. In 2003, Boland and his coworkers started inkjet-based bioprinting by modifying an HP inkjet printer, and cells were successfully printed and patterned. Several researchers then attempted 3D printing of tissue scaffolds using extrusion-based techniques with or without cells (Ozbolat and Hospodiuk, 2016). In 2009, Forgacs and his coworkers demonstrated the first bioprinted tissue using the concept of tissue spheroids as building blocks without a need for a scaffold (Norotte et al., 2009); the technology later translated into the market, and the first bioprinter was commercialized. Next, an in situ bioprinting concept envisioned by Campbell and Weiss (2007)was attempted by researchers at the Wake Forest Regenerative Medicine Institute by inkjet bioprinting of skin on an animal model (Skardal et al., 2012). With the announcement of the first manufacturing institute in the United States in the area of 3D printing and additive manufacturing, 3D printing was boosted; enormous progress has been made in the last four years, which has affected bioprinting technology positively as well. Since then, bioprinting has been widely used in tissue engineering and regenerative medicine and has resulted in several spin-offs to commercialize breakthrough technologies worldwide. Recent approaches in hybrid vascularized tissue printing with next-generation bioprinters and perfusable vascularized tissue models will push the technology even further to create scale-up tissues toward organ printing (Ozbolat, 2015).

1.3.3 Classification of Bioprinting Techniques

The most promising technologies in bioprinting impose the self-assembly and self-organizing capabilities of cells delivered through the application of techniques that can be categorized into three major groups according to their working principles: extrusion-, droplet-, laser-based bioprinting. The reader is referred to Fig. 1.3 for detailed classification of currently existing bioprinting techniques.

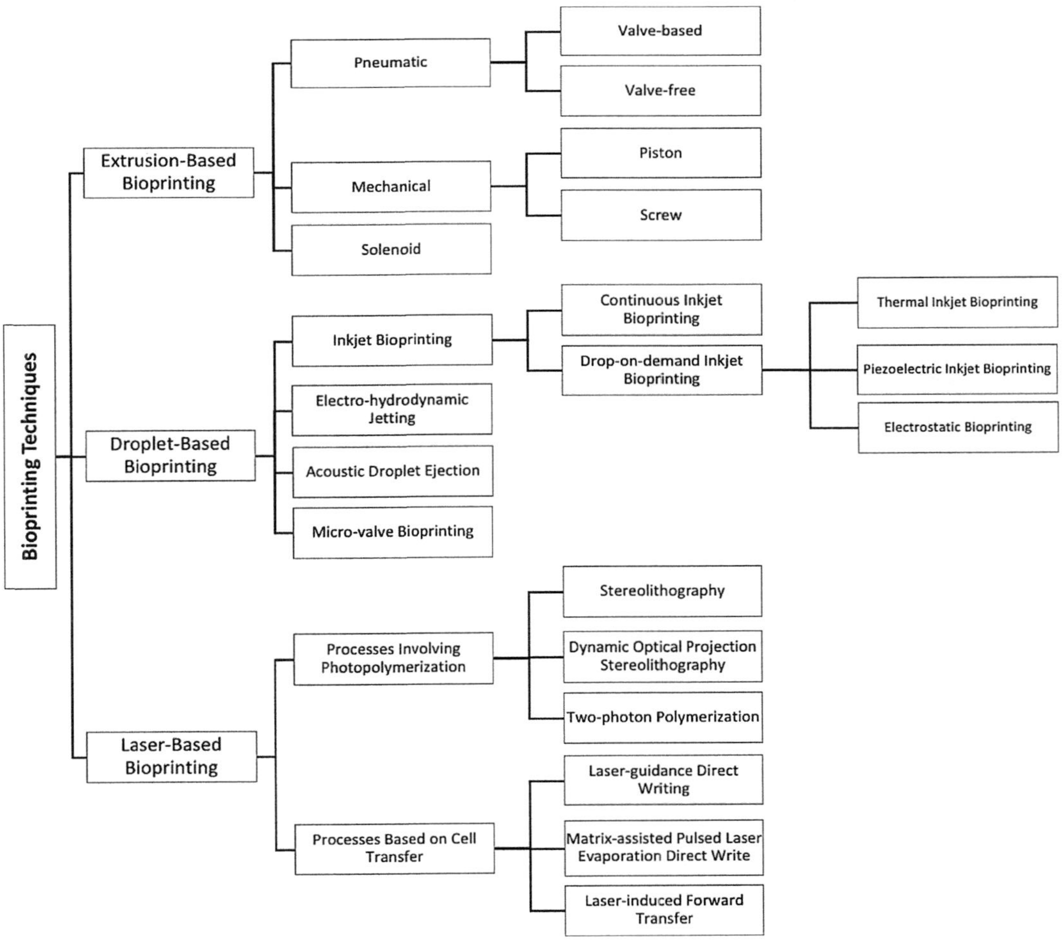

FIGURE 1.3 Classification of bioprinting techniques.

Extrusion-based bioprinting utilizes the mechanical or pneumatic potential energy to extrude the bioink, overcome surface tension-driven droplet formation, and draw the bioink in the form of cylindrical filaments. According to its working mechanism, extrusion-based bioprinting can be categorized into (1) pneumatic, (2) mechanical, or (3) solenoid microextrusion.

Droplet-based bioprinting, on the other hand, utilizes thermal, acoustic, or electric energy to print cells encapsulated in small droplets of bioink that are deposited and assembled layer-by-layer. Droplet-based bioprinting can be grouped into four technologies: (1) inkjet bioprinting, (2) electrohydrodynamic jetting, (3) acoustic droplet election, and (4) microvalve bioprinting. Inkjet bioprinting can be subclassified into continuous or drop-on-demand inkjet bioprinting. Drop-on-demand inkjet bioprinting can be further grouped into thermal, piezoelectric, and electrostatic bioprinting.

Laser-based bioprinting utilizes laser energy to selectively print and precisely pattern cells onto a substrate. It can be classified into two major categories: (1) processes involving photopolymerization and (2) processes based on cell transfer. The former can be subclassified into SLA, dynamic optical projection SLA, and two-photon polymerization, and the latter can be subclassified into laser-guidance direct writing, matrix-assisted pulsed laser evaporation direct write, and laser-induced forward transfer.

Each bioprinting technique has unique features and possesses certain advantages and disadvantages with respect to printing capabilities, resolution, deposition speed, scalability, bioink and material compatibility, ease of use, printing speed and price, and commercial availability, as well as fundamental aspects of biocompatibility. All these aspects are presented in detail throughout the book, but background information on 3D bioprinting is presented in Box 1.1 for the reader.

BOX 1.1 BACKGROUND INFORMATION ON THREE-DIMENSIONAL BIOPRINTING

Definition of bioprinting: Bioprinting can be defined as the simultaneous positioning of biomaterials and living cells in a prescribed layer-by-layer stacking organization to fabricate engineered tissues and organs (Ozbolat, 2015).

Emergence of bioprinting: Bioprinting was first demonstrated by Klebe in 1988 as cytoscribing technology, a method of micropositioning cells and constructing 2D synthetic tissues. In that study, cytoscribing was carried out using a Hewlett Packard (HP) inkjet printer and a graphics plotter for high positioning of biologics (Klebe, 1988).

Advantages of bioprinting: As listed below, bioprinting has numerous advantages over the other biofabrication techniques.

- Bioprinting enables fabrication of anatomically correct tissue constructs according to the medical image data obtained from patients.
- Bioprinting allows fabrication of porous structures with controlled architecture.
- Bioprinting has the ability to coculture multiple cell types locally.
- Bioprinting facilitates precise patterning of cells and biologics.
- Bioprinting enables controlled deliver of growth factors and genes.
- Bioprinting allows fabrication of tissue models in high-throughput manner.
- Bioprinting has the ability to integrate vascularization within engineered tissues.

BOX 1.1 BACKGROUND INFORMATION ON THREE-DIMENSIONAL BIOPRINTING—cont'd

Bioink (Chapter 3): The biomaterial solution used in bioprinting of living cells is referred to as "bioink." In bioprinting processes, there are four main types of bioink materials utilized including hydrogels, microcarriers, cell aggregates, and decellularized matrix components.

Modalities of bioprinting: Depending on their bioink deposition mechanism, bioprinting modalities can be classified into droplet-, extrusion-, and laser-based bioprinting.

- **Extrusion-based bioprinting (Chapter 4):** It is a combination of a fluid dispensing and an automated robotic system for extrusion and bioprinting, respectively. During bioprinting, bioink is dispensed by a deposition system, under the control of a computer, resulting in precise deposition of cells encapsulated in cylindrical filaments of desired 3D custom-shaped structures.
- **Droplet-based bioprinting (Chapter 5):** It is a bioprinting modality that allows patterning of living cells and other biologics using various energy sources such as sound, heat, and electric to generate droplets in a high-throughput manner. It offers greater advantages due to its simplicity and agility with precise control on deposition of biologics including cells, growth factors, genes, and drugs.
- **Laser-based bioprinting (Chapter 6):** It is a modality of bioprinting allowing high-precision patterning of biologics or fabrication of tissue constructs using laser energy. It offers greater advantages due to its precise control on deposition of biologics including cells, growth factors, genes, drugs, and biomaterials.

Bioprinter (Chapter 7): The 3D printer used in deposition of bioink solutions for fabrication of tissue and organ construct is referred to as "bioprinter." An ideal bioprinter has specific requirements including but not limited to the ability to dispense various biomaterials simultaneously, high resolution and accuracy, high-degree-of-freedom motion capability, sufficient motion speed, user-friendliness, full-automation capability, sterilibility, affordability, versatility, and compactness.

Application areas (Chapter 9): Bioprinting has a broad utility in various application areas such as tissue engineering and regenerative medicine, transplantation and clinics, drug screening and high-throughput assays, and cancer research. Bioprinting technology has been used for the fabrication of a wide variety of tissues including bone, brain, cancer, cardiac, cartilage, heart valve, liver, lung, neural, pancreas, retinal, skin, vascular, and composite tissues (Ozbolat et al., 2016).

1.4 The Organization of the Book

The specific aim of this book is to provide fundamentals, principles, physical interpretation, applications, and future perspectives of 3D bioprinting. The book instructs the reader from the basics of 3D bioprinting all the way to organ printing and future trends such as four-dimensional (4D) bioprinting and bioprinting new types of organs. It provides a thorough description of various bioprinting processes and technologies used in 3D bioprinting of tissues and organs using living cells and presents components of bioprinting in detail from the design phase to the tissue maturation and implantation phases.

The book is organized into 10 chapters: Introduction, Design for Bioprinting, The Bioink, Extrusion-Based Bioprinting, Droplet-Based Bioprinting, Laser-Based Bioprinting, Bioprinter Technologies, Roadmap to Organ Printing, Applications of 3D Bioprinting, and Future Trends.

This chapter covers tissue engineering and the use of 3D printing in tissue engineering, acquaints the reader with bioprinting and its principles and components, and presents historical evaluation and classification of bioprinting techniques.

Chapter 2, "Design for Bioprinting," presents the design phase of bioprinting, covering the steps taken from medical imaging to the physical bioprinting process. The chapter covers design consideration for bioprinting, blueprint modeling, and toolpath planning.

Chapter 3, "The Bioink," covers the bioink types and their processing and fabrication techniques and offers a comparison of bioink types, including hydrogel-based and hydrogel-free bioink materials such as cell aggregates in different forms, microcarriers or decellularized matrix components. A detailed comparison is presented on the bioprintability, mechanical integrity, ease of solidification and formability, affordability, abundance and commercial availability, appropriate regulatory for clinical use, and ability to facilitate engraftment with the endogenous tissue without generating an immune response.

Chapter 4, "Extrusion-Based Bioprinting," provides the reader with the principles, components, and physics-based process modeling of extrusion-based bioprinting. It also discusses suitable bioink, cell types printed and major accomplishments achieved in the literature. It discusses current advancements in extrusion-based bioprinting technology and highlights future directions to transform the technology to generate viable end products for tissue engineering and regenerative medicine.

Chapter 5, "Droplet-Based Bioprinting," discusses droplet-based bioprinting and its fundamentals, the main physical phenomenon behind it and its applications. The chapter covers four major droplet-based bioprinting techniques: inkjet bioprinting, electrohydrodynamic jetting, acoustic droplet ejection, and microvalve bioprinting. Current limitations and future directions are also presented for the reader.

Chapter 6, "Laser-Based Bioprinting," presents currently existing laser-involved techniques in printing living cells, including processes involving photopolymerization and processes based on cell transfer. Fundamentals, physics of laser-induced forward transfer process, and up-to-date achievements are discussed, and limitations and future directions are provided to the reader.

Chapter 7, "Bioprinter Technologies," highlights the existing bioprinter technologies classified under three major bioprinting modalities. A comparative evaluation is performed for commercially available bioprinters in the market, and a detailed discussion is made on pros and cons of bioprinter technologies in terms of the compactness, resolution, accuracy, high-degree-of-freedom motion capability and motion speed, commercial availability, full-automation capability, user-friendliness, sterilibility, affordability, and versatility of the bioprinters.

Chapter 8, "Roadmap to Organ Printing," introduces the state of the art and provides a step-by-step roadmap for organ printing, spanning differentiation of stem cells to transplantation and in vivo safety, efficacy, and monitoring of organs. Special focus is given to bioprinting of an integrated vascular network via two means: direct and indirect vasculature printing.

Chapter 9, "Applications of 3D Bioprinting," presents the current applications of bioprinting technology in areas such as basic research in tissue engineering and regenerative medicine, transplantation and clinics, drug testing and high-throughput assays, and cancer research.

Finally, Chapter 10, "Future Trends," presents future perspectives in bioprinting that will revolutionize medicine in the next couple of decades. The discussion includes biofabrication of fully functional organs for transplantation, going beyond just mimicking biology to making technologically improved humans through bioprinting new types of organs, bioprinting genes for guided-tissue response, and in situ and 4D bioprinting possibilities in the near future.

1.5 Summary

This chapter introduces 3D bioprinting technology for tissue engineering and regenerative medicine, which has a great potential in biofabrication of de novo tissues and organs for transplantation or other biological uses. Although still in its infancy, this technology appears to be promising for advancing tissue engineering toward organ fabrication, ultimately mitigating organ shortage and saving lives. With the adoption of 3D printing technology in tissue engineering, anatomically correct tissue constructs have been started to be built by controlling the position of cells in the constructs and enabling patterning and better interactions. In this chapter, principles and elements of 3D bioprinting are discussed, and evaluation of the technology is presented along with remarkable achievements during the last decade. Finally, a classification of bioprinting technologies is made under three major groups: extrusion-, droplet-, and laser-based technologies.

References

Campbell, P.G., Weiss, L.E., 2007. Tissue engineering with the aid of inkjet printers. Expert Opinion on Biological Therapy 7 (8), 1123–1127.

Desmet, T., Schacht, E., Dubruel, P., 2008. Rapid prototyping as an elegant production tool for polymeric tissue engineering scaffolds: a review. in tissue engineering: roles. Materials and Applications 141–189.

Hutmacher, D.W., Sittinger, M., Risbud, M.V., 2004. Scaffold-based tissue engineering: rationale for computer-aided design and solid free-form fabrication systems. Trends in Biotechnology 22 (7), 354–362.

Hamid, Q., Snyder, J., Wang, C., Timmer, M., Hammer, J., Guceri, S., et al., 2011. Fabrication of three-dimensional scaffolds using precision extrusion deposition with an assisted cooling device. Biofabrication 3 (3), 34109.

Klebe, R., 1988. Cytoscribing: a method for micropositioning cells and the construction of two- and three-dimensional synthetic tissues. Experimental Cell Research 179 (2), 362–373.

Langer, R., Vacanti, J.P., 1993. Tissue engineering. Science 260 (5110), 920–926.

Leong, K.F., Cheah, C.M., Chua, C.K., 2003. Solid freeform fabrication of three-dimensional scaffolds for engineering replacement tissues and organs. Biomaterials 24 (13), 2363–2378.

Merrill, J.P., et al., 1956. Successful homotransplantation of the human kidney between identical twins. Journal of the American Medical Association 160 (4), 82–277.

Mironov, V., et al., 2009. Biofabrication: a 21st century manufacturing paradigm. Biofabrication 1 (2), 022001.

Mironov, V., Reis, N., Derby, B., 2006. Bioprinting: a beginning. Tissue Engineering 12 (4), 631–634.

Norotte, C., et al., 2009. Scaffold-free vascular tissue engineering using bioprinting. Biomaterials 30 (30), 5910–5917.

Odde, D.J., Renn, M.J., 1999. Laser-guided direct writing for applications in biotechnology. Trends in Biotechnology 17 (10), 385–389.

Ozbolat, I.T., 2015. Bioprinting scale-up tissue and organ constructs for transplantation. Trends in Biotechnology 33 (7), 395–400.

Ozbolat, I.T., Chen, H., 2013. Manufacturing living things. Industrial Engineer 45, 30–34.

Ozbolat, I.T., Hospodiuk, M., 2016. Current advances and future perspectives in extrusion-based bio-printing. Biomaterials 76, 321–343.

Ozbolat, I.T., Peng, W., Ozbolat, V., August 2016. Application areas of 3D bioprinting. Drug Discovery Today 21 (8), 1257–1271.

Sachlos, E., et al., 2003. Novel collagen scaffolds with predefined internal morphology made by solid freeform fabrication. Biomaterials 24 (8), 1487–1497.

Skardal, A., et al., 2012. Bioprinted amniotic fluid-derived stem cells accelerate healing of large skin wounds. Stem Cells Translational Medicine 1 (11), 792–802.

2

Design for Bioprinting

CHAPTER OUTLINE

Simplicity is the ultimate sophistication
Leonardo da Vinci

2.1 Introduction

Tissue engineering, an interdisciplinary field of biology, biomaterials, and engineering, is seeking to restore tissue functions by developing engineered three-dimensional (3D) tissue constructs providing the optimum environment for cell attachment and growth, tissue regeneration, fluid movement, and structural integrity (Langer and Vacanti, 1993). Engineered tissue constructs attempt to mimic both the anatomical shape (external geometry) and opposite impression of internal architecture of replaced tissues. The acquisition of the external geometry of tissue constructs is critical to precisely represent anatomically correct shapes. In regenerative medicine, noninvasive medical imaging techniques including, but not limited to, computed tomography (CT), magnetic resonance imaging (MRI), and ultrasound imaging techniques are widely used for acquisition of patient-specific information. Upon acquisition of the 3D model of tissues and organs from the patient, an internal architecture needs to be designed, which includes internal channels and interconnected pores enabling cell attachment, cell proliferation, nutrient flow, and tissue regeneration (Ozbolat et al., 2012). The internal architecture and topology has a substantial influence on growth and proliferation of cells; hence, an optimum design is needed to accelerate tissue regeneration. If the designed tissue constructs are developed for transplantation purposes, they must possess the anatomically correct shapes of the tissues and organs from individual patients and they should engraft with the host.

In addition to facilitating cellular activity postbioprinting, design of tissue constructs must incorporate a tolerance of mechanical load, mechanical and biochemical stimulation as well as flexibility in shape and size to accommodate growth within the patient (i.e., tissue constructs for pediatric cases). For instance, the majority of bone tissue undergoes mechanical loading, so a bone construct must be designed to withstand mechanical stresses while the tissue is generating within the constructs. Similarly, during regeneration of articular cartilage tissue, dynamic loads are applied to the implanted constructs during tissue repair. Thus, the designed tissue construct must withstand the dynamic loads until complete regeneration takes place. Tissue constructs must also satisfy biological requirement such as cell attachment and proliferation, cell signaling, and transport of nutrients and metabolic waste products. Thus, mechanical, biological, and biochemical characteristics of the regenerating tissue environment should inform the design of tissue constructs prior to bioprinting.

Despite the wide array of biofabrication techniques used in manufacturing of tissue constructs, most do not allow generation of highly intricate geometries including the anatomical shape of the tissue as well as the complex porous internal architecture. Thus, 3D bioprinting offers several advantages over traditional scaffold fabrication techniques, such as solvent casting particulate leaching, gas foaming, and molding. A porous tissue constructs can be built in high resolution with the proper design to provide the appropriate microenvironment for cellular components for successful regeneration of tissues and organs. One of the major advantages of 3D bioprinting is that patient-specific information can be directly incorporated into the biofabrication process to generate

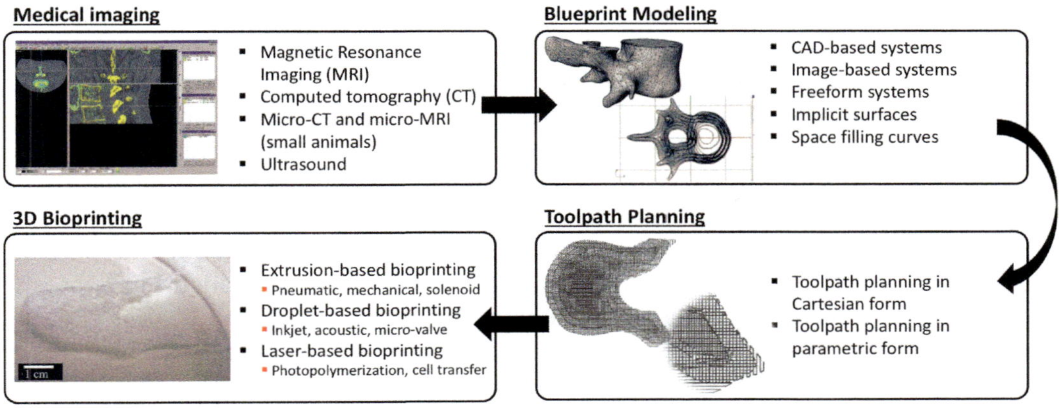

FIGURE 2.1 The major steps involved in bioprinting design including medical imaging, blueprint modeling, toolpath planning, and 3D bioprinting. *CAD*, Computer-aided designing.

anatomically correct shapes. Fig. 2.1 shows the major steps involved in design of tissue constructs for 3D bioprinting. First, medical images obtained from MRI, CT scans, ultrasound coupled with alternative approaches (i.e., reverse engineering) can be used to generate a 3D model of the tissue and organ to be replaced. Next, various blueprint modeling approaches, such as computer-aided design (CAD)–based systems, image-based systems, freeform systems, implicit surfaces, and space-filling curves, are instrumental in the design of the internal architecture of tissue constructs. Then, toolpath algorithms are used to generate path plans in Cartesian or parametric form. Finally, different 3D bioprinting modalities, such as extrusion-, droplet-, and laser-based bioprinting, can be used to fabricate tissue constructs.

This chapter discusses each of these steps in detail. In Section 2.2, design requirements for bioprinting are presented. Section 2.3 presents currently available medical imaging techniques used in tissue engineering and regenerative medicine. Section 2.4 elucidates blueprint modeling approaches used in generation of internal architecture and topology of engineered tissue and organ constructs, and Section 2.5 describes current toolpath planning approaches. Finally, design limitations and future directions are presented in Sections 2.6 and 2.7, respectively.

2.2 Design Requirements for Three-Dimensional Bioprinting

In regenerative medicine, synthetic engineered implantable tissues and organs should have functional gradients to mimic their original counterpart in addition to conformational geometries that have been extensively studied in the literature (Sun et al., 2004). Engineered tissue constructs attempt to mimic both the external geometry and opposite impression of internal architecture of replaced tissues. Cells loaded in tissue constructs need nutrients, proteins, growth factors, and waste removal, making mass and fluid transport vital to cell survival. The size, geometry, orientation, interconnectivity, and surface chemistry of pores and channels determine the nature of nutrient flow (Khoda et al., 2013a,b). Moreover, interconnectivity of pores has a direct impact on cell migration and tissue ingrowth. Thus, a well-connected internal network of channels is vital to the survival and development of the generated tissue, allowing deeper fluid and nutrient transport and release of biomaterials and biomolecules. An optimal engineered tissue design incorporates these features to accelerate cell growth and proliferation.

Determining the optimum porosity of designed constructs is crucial as the porosity mediates cell attachment and growth both in vitro and in vivo. Although high porosity supports cell growth and tissue generation, it limits the integrity and load-bearing capacity of tissue constructs; thus, the optimum porosity lies within a critical range. The porosity distribution is a multiobjective criterion to meet biological and mechanical requirements simultaneously. Therefore, internal architecture should be designed with different regions having appropriate porosity levels to meet abovementioned requirements. The majority of tissue constructs have been designed with constant porosity level throughout their structure because of design and manufacturing limitations (Khoda et al., 2011); however, the porosity level should vary spatially based on mechanical, biological, and functional requirements. For example, fabrication of vertebral bone constructs with uniform material and structural architecture is not a reasonable approach. Natural bones exhibit functional gradients throughout their structures. The load exerted on a native vertebra is distributed more to the outer regions compared to inner sites. Moreover, cell loading and proliferation starts from the exterior side of the bone construct and cell ingrowth proceeds through the core. This necessitates higher porosity in the exterior regions and lower porosity in the core. High porosity supports more cell growth and proliferation but limits integrity and load-bearing capacity of tissue constructs; thus porosity levels in distinct regions of the construct should be appropriate for the functional requirements of each region.

In this regard, Hollister and his coworkers (Hollister et al., 2002; Hollister and Lin, 2007; Lin et al., 2004) used an image-based homogenization method integrated within a topology optimization approach to design microstructural and material properties for tissue constructs, matching elastic properties and porosity of bone tissue simultaneously. Porosity and effective stiffness properties were optimized within theoretical boundaries with the objective of mimicking the properties of natural tissues. Required porosity was ensured for a wide range of permeability to enable cell/gene delivery with suitable stiffness properties to human bone tissue by choosing the true biomaterial and unit cell architecture together. Studies (Wettergreen et al., 2005b; Wettergreen et al., 2005a) addressed the porosity determination in each layer mapping from CT scan and achieving the desired porosity using unit cells from a library as building blocks. In all of the abovementioned studies, 3D printing was used to fabricate tissue constructs and achieved improved mechanical properties.

Table 2.1 presents the design factors affecting tissue construct properties such as mechanical, biological, geometric, transport, and bioprinting. All these properties affect the performance of the construct upon implantation. During scaffold design and fabrication,

Table 2.1 Tissue Construct Design Consideration and Parameter Selections Affecting Tissue Construct Properties

Properties	Design Consideration	Selections Affecting Tissue Construct Properties
Mechanical	Structural integrity, internal architecture stability, strength, and stiffness	Bioink selection, internal architecture, porosity and pore distribution, bioprinting modality
Biological	Cell loading, cell distribution, nutrition, cell attachment and growth, cell viability and differentiation, cell–cell and cell–matrix interactions, cell aggregation, and tissue formation	Layout, pore size, interconnectivity, vasculature, cell density, bioink selection, bioprinted cell types
Geometric	Anatomical fit, tissue topology	External geometry, tissue density
Transport	Nutrient and oxygen delivery, waste removal, growth factor, and drug delivery	Interconnectivity and permeability, bioink selection
Bioprinting	Environmental conditions during bioprinting, bioprinting parameters, control, and resolution	Bioink and bioprinting modality selection, bioprinter

(Modified from Gomez, 2007).

biomaterial selection, internal architecture, porosity level and interconnectivity, external geometry, permeability, and compatible bioprinting processes must be carefully considered for enhanced tissue healing to occur. In addition to design factors, fabrication of tissue constructs is also of considerable importance in tissue engineering, where operating and environmental conditions, control mechanisms, resolution, and bioink selection are key factors in the process. Three major bioprinting modalities, including extrusion-based bioprinting (EBB), droplet-based bioprinting (DBB), and laser-based bioprinting (LBB), have been used to fabricate 3D tissue constructs using a layer-by-layer deposition scheme (Ozbolat and Hospodiuk, 2016; Gudapati et al., 2016). EBB has been the most common bioprinting modality due to ease of operability, scalability, and a wide range of compatible bioink materials. In fabrication of porous tissue constructs using EBB, material deposition starts and stops periodically depending on the internal architecture, which results in nonuniformity in the deposited layer. Therefore, the total number of starts and stops during the deposition process needs to be minimized; this can be achieved by decreasing number of discontinuities. Traditional unit cell applications in computer-aided tissue engineering (Sun et al., 2004) limit the connectivity of internal network channels resulting in congestions in nutrient flow. Due to the shortcomings of current CAD technologies in representations of such microstructures or the inability to transfer microstructure information to bioprinters, enhanced pore architecture with interconnected channels needs to be addressed in the bioprinting process to provide better functionality and nutrient flow (Khoda et al., 2013a,b).

2.3 Medical Imaging

To design tissue constructs (i.e., tissue scaffolds, and tissue and organ substitutes), geometric properties of the constructs should be acquired to generate accurate and anatomically correct representation of native tissues and organs. There are currently a number of noninvasive medical imaging techniques used for imaging live tissues and organs. The most common ones include MRI, CT, and ultrasound and are used to represent a patient's anatomy for tissue engineering and regenerative medicine as well as micro-CT (μCT), micro-MRI (μMRI), and nuclear medicine to image regenerating tissues and organs in animal models. Although these imaging technologies can be used to obtain patient-specific information, sample models are currently available for most of tissues and organs on an online repository established by the National Institutes of Health (NIH). The NIH 3D Print Exchange platform provides researchers with scientifically accurate, high-quality 3D models in a ready-to-print format (Coakley et al., 2014).

2.3.1 Magnetic Resonance Imaging

MRI is a sensitive method to monitor structural and functional changes in tissues such as tissue regeneration and death. Such changes are reflected in images via local variations in tissue hydration, its physical state (e.g., freely diffusing or protein bound), and variations in nuclear magnetic resonance times (Xu et al., 2008). It utilizes pulsed radio-frequency electromagnetic waves to excite and generate a detectable radio-frequency signal from hydrogen atoms, which are abundantly present in human body, particularly in water and fat. Changes in the parameters of pulse sequence in radio waves alter nuclear spin energy transition of the protons and hence generate magnetic field gradients, which in turn leads to contrast among the generated images. The generated radio-frequency signals are picked up by a magnetic resonance coil and transferred to computer software for image generation.

MRI has been widely used in scanning of soft tissue components in human body. Since no ionizing radiation is involved, MRI is a preferred imaging method. The highest resolution achieved in 3 Tesla (T) is 250 μm × 250 μm × 0.5 mm with a scan time of 5–40 min (Ballyns and Bonassar, 2009). A higher spatial resolution (5–200 μm) can be achieved with μMRI in very high strength of magnetic fields such as 7–9T (Nam et al., 2014), where the contrast between soft tissues can be further improved by using contrast agents (i.e., magnetic nanoparticles (Terreno et al., 2010)). Anatomical, functional, and cellular information for various soft tissues can be acquired using MRI due to its superior ability to distinguish soft tissue contrast.

Humans cannot withstand higher levels of magnetic fields, which can generate discomfort and sensations of vertigo (Theysohn et al., 2007). In general, the magnetic field that humans are exposed to does not exceed 3T. Longer scan times can improve the resolution of images; however, some patients can still experience anxiety and claustrophobia under longer scans.

2.3.2 Computed Tomography

Computed tomography, also known as computer-axial tomography, is a noninvasive medical scanning technique that has been widely used to image hard tissue components in the human body. It utilizes the principle of two-dimensional (2D) X-ray imaging

(Appel et al., 2011), where an X-ray tube emitting a conic beam of electromagnetic radiation selectively penetrates the body; hard tissue (i.e., bone) attenuates X-rays much more than soft tissue. A detector in the opposite side of the scanner is used to acquire the cross-sectional scans of the tissue, and the resulting data are then processed to generate a cross section of the region of interest in human body. To generate 3D images, a rotational apparatus is used to turn around the scanned body with an angle of increments from 0.25 to 1 degree and covers a scan of 360 degrees producing 360 to 1440 images. The scan images are then stacked using tomographic reconstruction algorithms (Feldkamp et al., 1984).

CT can generate higher resolution images such as 0.24–0.3 mm in relatively short scan times, but the utilized ionized radiation presents a finite risk to patients (Ballyns and Bonassar, 2009). Patients can only be subjected to CT scans at a limited dose at controlled frequencies. CT imaging is not sensitive to metal components so that patients with implants and medical devices with batteries may be safely subjected to the CT-scanning process. Moreover, fewer user manipulations are required in the acquisition of 3D medical images compared to MRI. CT has been utilized in imaging bone and tumor tissue and can differentially display soft tissue along with the boundaries of bone tissue.

In addition to CT, μCT has been used in tissue engineering, particularly to monitor tissue regeneration in small animals such as rodents (Tuan and Hutmacher, 2005). μCT enables high resolution from 1 to 200 μm for a limited volume of samples and is not considered invasive for animals larger than mice (Ballyns and Bonassar, 2009). Contrast agents (i.e., iodine- and nanoparticle-based agents) can be administrated to improve the quality of the image and register the soft tissue components.

2.3.3 Ultrasound Imaging

Ultrasound technology emerged early in the 1960s and is widely used in obstetrics and gynecology (Haller et al., 2004). Ultrasound technology uses sound energy to scan the body via the emission of sound waves at controlled frequencies. As soon as the sound waves hit anatomical interfaces, they are reflected back and detected by a receiver. The frequency, amplitude, and interface profile of the reflected waves is a function of the scanned anatomy, which is further processed and displayed in real time as a computer image.

In contrast to MRI and CT, which require patients to remain in a confined space or exposure to radiation, respectively, ultrasound technology is safe and is easy to administer. Ultrasound has a limited resolution (1 mm × 1.5 mm × 0.2 mm) (Elliot and Thrush, 1996), beyond which abnormal and unclear images with artifacts are generated when compared to MRI and CT scan. One of the major advantages of ultrasound is the scan time, which allows for the capture of real-time images of moving organs and blood flow in vessels. As conventional ultrasound imaging does not support quantitative measurement of tissue mechanical properties, ultrasound elastography can be used to image the mechanical properties of tissues in a quantified and accurate manner (Wells and Liang, 2011).

2.3.4 Other Imaging Modalities

In addition to abovementioned medical imaging modalities, nuclear medicine [i.e., positron emission tomography (PET) and single, photon emission computed tomography (SPECT)] has been used as a powerful tool to visualize functional and molecular data of the imaged target (Dobrucki and Sinusas, 2010). Progenitor and stem cells within engineered tissue constructs have been recently visualized in high resolution to monitor their metabolic and functional activities in regenerating cranium tissue within a critical-size defect model on rabbits (Lin et al., 2012).

Selecting the right imaging modality for design for bioprinting purposes depends on the tissue type to be fabricated as well as other requirements such as image resolution and quality. Recently, researchers have also attempted using multimodal imaging, where multiple modalities can be used in a complementary manner such as MRI/CT, CT/PET, and CT/SPECT (Kim et al., 2009). A detailed comparison of medical image modalities used in tissue engineering is presented in Table 2.2.

2.3.5 Image Segmentation

The acquired noninvasive images [i.e., in the digital imaging and communications in medicine (DICOM) or TIFF format] are processed through image segmentation using image processing software such as open-source ITK-Snap (McCormick et al., 2014) or other commercially available programs such as Materialize Mimics, Amira, and Avizo 3D. Upon loading images onto the software, the region of interest is selected and the approximate threshold value is determined to best capture the tissue anatomy and bioinformatics. Next, all pixel values within the region of interest are merged to a color mask using region growing techniques. Although this approach is the most common segmentation practice used in medical image processing, it does not capture accurate information over a large volume of tissue samples as tissue samples may exhibit heterogeneity. Therefore, a homogenization approach, as demonstrated in (Sun et al., 2004), can be used to better capture the tissue properties over a large volume. In this approach, the region of interest can be divided into a number of subregions, where different threshold values are assigned depending on the tissue properties. The segmentation processes can then be performed independently followed by combination of all subregions for representation as a single 3D object. Therefore, the homogenization approach provides an accurate representation of the native tissues.

2.4 Blueprint Modeling

The generated 3D model as a result of image segmentation is usually represented in stereolithography (STL) format along with other formats such as but not limited to virtual reality modeling language and 3D graphics (Coakley et al., 2014). Here, the STL file format should not be confused with the STL process, a widely used 3D printing

Table 2.2 Comparison of Medical Image Modalities in Tissue Engineering and Regenerative Medicine

Modality	Resolution	Scan Time	Maximum Volume	Preferred Tissue Types	Advantages	Disadvantages
Magnetic resonance imaging	250 μm × 250 μm × 500 μm	5–40 min	Human body	Soft and hard tissue (bone)	• No risk of radiation exposure • Enables imaging of moving components in the body in four dimensional such as heart contractions	• Intolerant of in vivo medical implants and body motions during scanning process • Requires longer scan times for better quality images • Patients may experience anxiety and claustrophobia
Micro-magnetic resonance imaging	5–200 μm	6–24 h	Full body	Soft and hard tissue (bone)	• No risk of radiation exposure • Enables incorporation of contrast agents for molecular imaging • Enables real-time imaging	• High cost • Low portability • Longer scan times
Computed tomography	0.24–0.33 mm	5 min (8–40 s of actual scan time)	Human body	Hard tissue (bone)	• Tolerant of in vivo medical implants (i.e., metallic or with battery) • High-resolution imaging of various tissue types • More tolerant of patient movement during scanning process	• Radiation exposure limits exposure level and frequency; not recommended for pregnant or breast-feeding women • May compromise immune system in children • Iodine contrast material can generate allergic reaction
μCT	1–200 μm	2–4 h	Whole rat	Hard tissue (bone)	• High resolution	• Radiation exposure limits exposure level and frequency
Ultrasound	1 mm × 1.5 mm × 0.2 mm	10–15 min	Neonatal, blood vessels	All tissue types	• Enables real-time images of moving components • Easy to operate and does not involve radiation	• Image quality inferior to other modalities • Cannot detect all abnormalities and melanomas

(Some of data obtained from Ballyns and Bonassar, 2009; Nam et al., 2014; Turnbull and Mori, 2007).

technique discussed in detail in Chapter 6. While STL technique was the first 3D printing process invented in 1980s (Whitaker, 2014), the STL file format emerged as a native file format to the STL CAD software. STL is an exchange file format widely used in various applications, such as 3D printing, 3D scanning, and finite element analysis. Currently, the majority of 3D printers and recent bioprinters accept input files in the STL format. Upon generation of patient-specific tissue or organ models in a digital form, the 3D surface model is further processed to generate an internal architecture to project the anatomy of regenerated tissues. Then, physics-based testing, such as finite element analysis, can be performed to determine the corresponding mechanical and fluid flow properties. This provides a virtual testing tool to rapidly evaluate the properties of the designed tissue construct before bioprinting it, which is a costly and time-consuming endeavor.

As each bioprinting modality supports different process plans and toolpath schemes, the associated compatible software system (specific to the bioprinter) allows the user to follow specific steps for a successful bioprinting mission. For example, working mechanism of the majority of extrusion-based bioprinters is similar to that of fused-deposition modeling (FDM)-based 3D printers (Ozbolat and Hospodiuk, 2016). Other modalities such as droplet-based (i.e., inkjet bioprinting) or laser-based bioprinting modalities have different mechanisms and build platforms which require bioprinter-specific design software. Piezo-inkjet bioprinters (e.g., Jetlab from Microfab Inc.) have software that allows the user to generate a code to define patterns of droplets. Laser-based bioprinters, such as laser-induced forward transfer-based bioprinters, have a similar capability in allowing the operator to define different user-specific patterns. STL and its modifications work with manufacturers' software platforms or simple algorithms to define masks using Microsoft PowerPoint images with white and black patterns defining transparent and opaque sections, respectively. The transparent sections allow ultraviolet light transmission through masks and initiate photopolymerization, which is discussed in Chapter 6.

All these software capabilities enable generation of an internal architecture with a uniform composition with limited design flexibilities to the user, i.e., distance control between printed material and the dimensions of the material footprint. To design tissue constructs with complex internal architecture to recapitulate native tissues and organs with greater fidelity, sophisticated design architectures emerged (Ozbolat et al., 2012), primarily in design of the porous architecture of tissue constructs.

2.4.1 Computer-Aided Design—Based Systems

CAD-based systems have been used in designing tissue constructs for bioadditive manufacturing platforms (Giannitelli et al., 2014). Modeling approaches, such as constructive solid geometry (CSG), boundary representation (B-Rep), and spatial occupancy enumeration (SOE) (Requicha, 1980), can be utilized to develop the design architecture of tissue constructs. CSG modeling relies on solid primitives and Boolean operations to generate different design models, whereas B-rep utilizes boundary elements (i.e., vertices, edges, and faces, etc.) to define closed objects. SOE, on the other hand, combines a number of building blocks, in general, cubic unit elements, to represent larger-scale complex solid objects. Each of these techniques has some limitations and weaknesses with respect to each other. For example, CSG and SOE rely on joining a number of solid primitives, which is computationally expensive and requires a significant amount of data storage; on the other hand, B-Rep uses boundary elements enclosing the entire object. CSG and SOE conveniently model complex shapes compared to B-Rep. Although these approaches are often utilized in the design of tissue constructs using commercial CAD software such as PTC Creo, SOLIDWORKS, and CATIA, current printed samples consist of cylindrical rasters of bioink materials, which are not easily approximated using these modeling approaches. Therefore, researchers used pore-making elements from a design library and subtracted them from the external surface geometry to create porous architecture. With this, an internal architecture with controlled porosity (i.e., pore size, level, and geometry) can be obtained. For example, researchers created algorithms that enabled automatic subtraction of the negative geometry from a CAD model of a femur bone segment obtained from CT images (Cheah et al., 2004). By subtracting the negative geometry (that are assembled in 3D as periodic elements) of the pore-making structure from the surface model of the femur bone segment, 3D porous lattice structures were obtained. The authors also presented different pore-making models such as octahedron, tetrahedron, triangular, and square prisms with tunable geometry as the geometric dimensions are coded as variables in the designed algorithms. Performing Boolean operations, such as combination of pore-making elements or structure-making primitives, Sun et al. (2004) developed a library of unit cells using different CAD-based primitives (see Fig. 2.2A). These unit cells can be further assembled into larger-scale tissue constructs such as femur and spine. In addition, different unit cells can be combined in a composite structure to further improve the heterogeneity of constructs. Despite their great benefit and wide utilization in the generation of porous tissue scaffolds, CAD-based systems are hampered by their poor efficiency and performance in generating biomimetic porous architecture or non-Euclidian solids and have limited control of the biomechanical properties imparted to tissue construct as a whole (Giannitelli et al., 2014).

2.4.2 Image-Based Systems

Current CAD-based modeling systems are highly time-consuming and computationally expensive platforms for design and modeling of tissue constructs. First, medical images are stacked and then segmented to generate the surface model, which is eventually filled by generated unit cells in a repetitive manner. The image-based design approach was first proposed early in 2000s by Hollister et al. (2000), where the defected region of interest in medical images such as CT scans or MRI was identified and filled by a stack of two 3D images made of binary unit cells. In addition to tissue constructs with regular porous architecture, irregular porous scheme can be generated by assigning a random number generator–based approach, where different voxel states are generated randomly throughout the defect. The proposed approach was first implemented for defects in mandibular bone (see Fig. 2.2B1–B4) and orbital floor segments, and sample tissue constructs were 3D printed using a selective-laser sintering process.

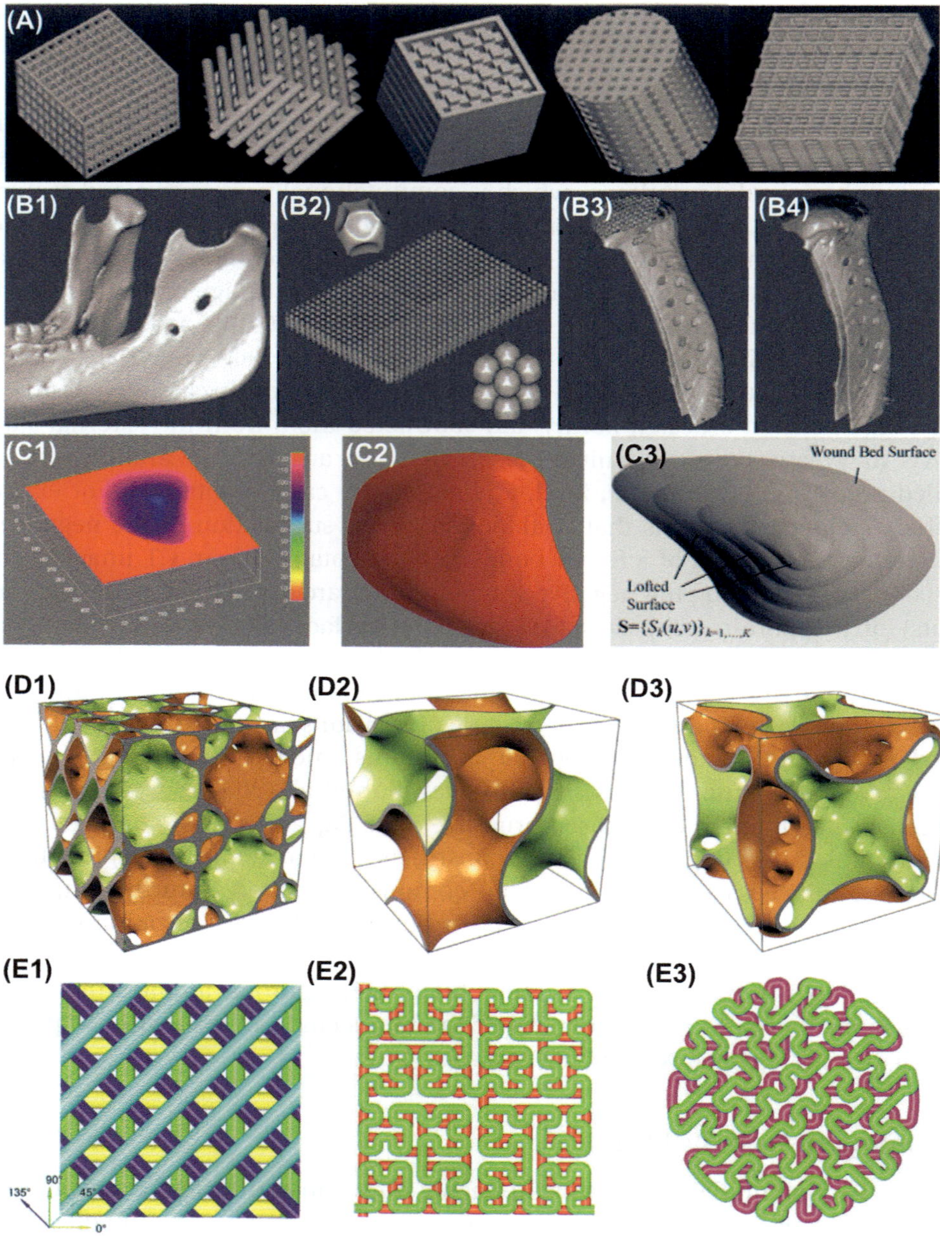

FIGURE 2.2 Blueprint modeling used in design of tissue constructs. (A) A library of unit cells constructed from different primitives using computer-aided design–based systems *(Reproduced and adapted with permission from Sun et al., 2004)*. Image-based design of mandibular condyle scaffolds, where (B1) computed tomography scan of Yucatan minipig condyle was used to generate the external anatomical shape. (B2) A database of porous architecture was used to generate internal architecture, which was then combined with the (B3) external geometry to generate (B4) the complete construct *(Reproduced and adapted with permission from Smith et al., 2007)*. Freeform design of a wound device, where (C1) the wound bed surface was captured using image intensities and (C2) a nonuniform rational B-spline surface was fitted followed by (C3) partitioning the geometric domain using lofting process *(Reproduced and adapted with permission from Ozbolat and Koc, 2012)*. Triply periodic minimal implicit surfaces including cells of (D1) C(D), (D2) Gyroid, and (D3) Manta 35 *(Reproduced and adapted with permission from Kapfer et al., 2011)*. Space-filling curves (E1) using 0/45/90/135 degrees of filament orientation in sequential layers and (E2–E3) Hilbert recursive curves in two consecutive layers. *(Reproduced and adapted with permission from Giannitelli et al., 2014)*.

With direct manipulation of the 3D design architecture using the abovementioned image-based approach instead of generating CAD models, defect models were rapidly generated, which also provided additional freedom to the user in imposing variations in the porosity network by assigning different design architectures to discrete sections within the defect site.

2.4.3 Freeform Systems

CAD- and image-based systems provide porous architectures; however, they mostly generate design architectures with uniform porosity. Freeform-based systems, on the other hand, generate a tissue construct geometry with variations in its architecture since the geometric domain can be partitioned into different regions. These regions can then be populated by different materials and porous architectures. In this regard, wound devices were developed using a surface model obtained from 2D wound images, which were then projected into 3D using image intensity function in Image J software (see Fig. 2.2C1) (Ozbolat and Koc, 2012). Then, the generated surface was approximated into a nonuniform rational B-spline (NURBS) surface followed by lofting process with respect to the center point of the top surface of the wound (see Fig. 2.2C2). This way, a number of regions were defined and each regions was then filled by rasters of different materials; the authors 3D-bioprinted several wound devices with variable biomolecule and sodium alginate concentrations (see Fig. 2.2C3) (Ozbolat and Koc, 2010), which provided synchronous delivery of biomolecules with the wound-healing process (Ozbolat and Koc, 2011). A similar approach was also applied to partition 3D models of vertebrae, femur, and aorta using mesh-based offsetting technique to control the porous architecture (Khoda et al., 2011).

Using the freeform design approach, tissue constructs can be designed and built with spatial control of geometric architecture and material composition as well as spatiotemporal control of release kinetics of biomaterials and biologically active components. These features are not quite feasible using other design techniques.

2.4.4 Design Using Implicit Surfaces

One of the major drawbacks of CAD- and image-based systems is the inability to present highly complex shapes in a short period of time. The geometric complexity of the design is limited by the degree of complexity of the primitives. Thus, implicit functions have been used to illustrate periodic minimal surfaces for complex-shape tissue scaffolds, which can accurately control the spatial porosity distribution within an arbitrarily shaped architecture (Yoo, 2012). Minimal surfaces have several advantages such as possessing lightweight architecture and demonstrating high structural strength (Kapfer et al., 2011). In this regard, triply periodic minimum surfaces (TPMSs) have been established as shown in Fig. 2.2D1–D3. TPMSs are smooth infinite surfaces that split the space into two intertwined labyrinthine domains that are periodic in three distinct lattice directions (Rajagopalan and Robb, 2006). Using TPMSs, Schwarz's Diamond and

Schoen's Gyroid designs were 3D printed for tissue biofabrication (Elomaa et al., 2011; Melchels et al., 2009). Heterogeneous porous scaffold architectures were also demonstrated in a linearly graded way to explore the mechanical responses for stretching and bending dominated deformations for bone tissue engineering (Afshar et al., 2016).

2.4.5 Space-Filling Curves

CAD- or image-based systems utilize solid primitives as building blocks for larger-scale tissue construct models, which are difficult to support with most 3D bioprinting techniques. EBB is the most common bioprinting modality in tissue fabrication, relying on the deposition of straight rasters in each layer using 0/90-degree lay-down pattern. As a result, the abovementioned approaches, except the freeform-design approach, are highly challenging to apply in EBB. Thus, an alternative approach in designing the internal architecture of the tissue construct utilizes space-filling curves as a toolpath. In the literature, design models with different space-filling curves, such as lay-down patterns with various raster deposition angles (i.e., 0/45/90/135 degrees) and Hilbert and Sierpinsky curves, have been demonstrated (Starly and Sun, 2007). The design architecture of the filling curves was changed to generate periodic subpatterns enabling construction of each layer using EBB. For subsequent layers, the orientation of the filling curves was changed to facilitate sufficient mechanical support for structurally integrated constructs. Such examples have been further investigated using Hilbert curves through partitioning the entire design region into unit cells and assigning Hilbert curves at different scales at each region. By combining each Hilbert curve at each region, a continuous toolpath plan could be executed. The use of space-filling curves provides a compatible design platform for EBB and its submodalities (i.e., pneumatic, mechanical, and solenoid microextrusion as detailed in Chapter 4), which is not quite possible using other bioprinting techniques. A similar approach was also performed based on a Lindenmayer system to biomimic vascular networks, where branched structures were printed using LBB (Yasar et al., 2009).

In summary, a number of blueprint modeling approaches have been utilized in design for bioprinting, and each of them possesses different capabilities. Table 2.3 compares different blueprint modeling techniques and presents their strengths and limitations along with their compatibility with different bioprinting modalities.

2.5 Toolpath Planning for Bioprinting

There are currently two different toolpath planning approaches used in bioprinting of tissue and organ constructs. Bioprinting of bulky tissue constructs do not require highly specialized toolpath planning as the goal is to fill a simple primitive geometry such as cubic tissue constructs. Therefore, standard toolpath plans can easily fill the geometry without the need for precision. Such examples are bioprinting of nonporous bulky constructs such as tissue constructs and tissue models for regenerative medicine and pharmaceutics, respectively.

Table 2.3 Comparison of Blueprint Modeling Techniques Used in Tissue Construct Bioprinting

Blueprint Modeling Techniques	Advantages	Disadvantages	Compatible Bioprinting Modalities	References
CAD-based systems	Easy to model; accurately represent simple primitive shapes	Computationally expensive; the complexity is limited to the unit cell resolution; slow processing	DBB and LBB processes based on cell transfer	Wettergreen et al. (2005b); Cheah et al. (2004)
Image-based systems	Directly uses medical images and eliminates their 3D segmentation; facilitates anatomical architecture;	Low accuracy; is not compatible with DBB and LBB	LBB processes based on photopolymerization	Hollister et al. (2000); Smith et al. (2007); Hollister et al. (2002)
Freeform systems	Computationally efficient; facilitates heterogeneous design environment; supports geometric complexity;	Not compatible with majority of CAD software in the market	DBB, LBB, and EBB	Ozbolat and Koc (2010, 2011, 2012)
Implicit surfaces	Computationally efficient; facilitates heterogeneous design environment; support geometric complexity; generates structurally strong design models	Not compatible with majority of CAD software in the market	LBB	Kapfer et al. (2011); Elomaa et al. (2011); Melchels et al. (2009)
Space-filling curves	Computationally efficient; facilitates heterogeneous design environment; supports most of 3D bioprinters and fused-deposition modeling–based 3D printers	Does not support geometrically complex models	EBB	Ozbolat and Khoda (2014); Starly and Sun (2007)

3D, Three-dimensional; *CAD*, Computer-aided design; *DBB*, Droplet-based bioprinting; *EBB*, Extrusion-based bioprinting; *LBB*, Laser-based bioprinting.

In the literature, two different toolpath planning approaches have been proposed including bioprinting rasters in (1) Cartesian and (2) parametric form. As the use of DBB and LBB is greatly less than that of EBB in the bioprinting community and bioprinters associated with these bioprinting modalities utilize manufacturer specific toolpath planning strategies (in Cartesian form), the author here exclude toolpath planning in DBB and LBB modalities.

2.5.1 Toolpath Planning in Cartesian Form

Toolpath planning in Cartesian form has been widely used in all bioprinting modalities including EBB, DBB, and LBB due to its simplicity in creating layers of rasters stacked up in 3D. As EBB has been the most popular among all bioprinting modalities, toolpath planning in EBB has attracted researchers (Ozbolat and Koc, 2012). At each layer during EBB, the deposition direction is reoriented to create a 0/90-degree lay-down pattern. Although different angles can be used (i.e., 0/45 or 0/135 degrees), 0/90 degrees allows for better mechanical and structural integrity than other angles, thus it is commonly used in bioprinting as well as FDM-based 3D printing techniques. For example, Fig. 2.3A1–A2 shows a toolpath designed for continuous deposition and minimal fluid congestion; however, a problem with excess accumulation of bioink at the point of directional change exists with the zigzag pattern. When approaching sharp turns,

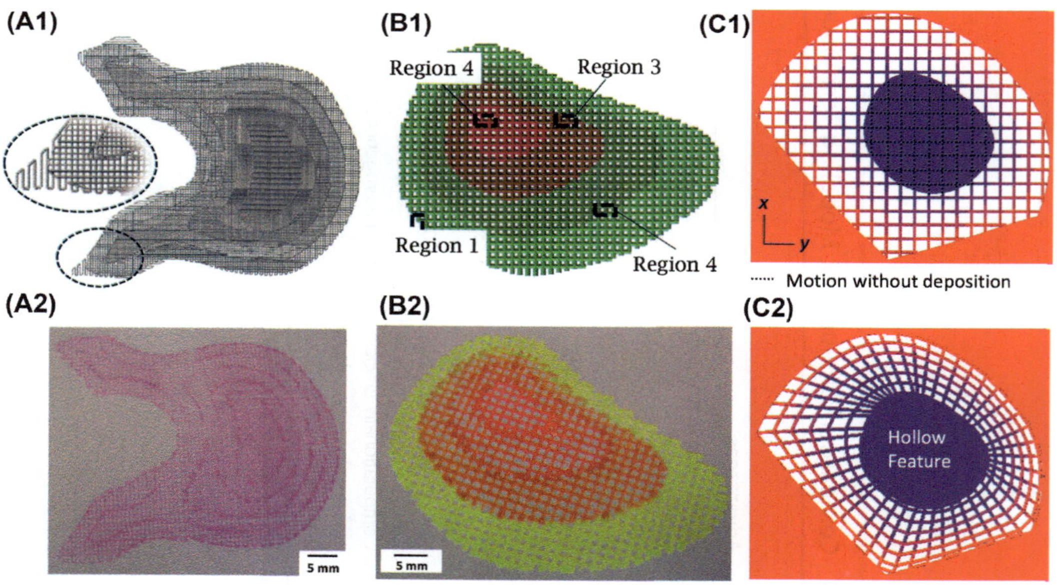

FIGURE 2.3 Toolpath planning in Cartesian coordinates. (A1) Design of a continuous toolpath with variable porosity and (A2) bilayer bioprinted vertebrae; (B1) design of a toolpath for functionally graded wound devices with variable bioink composition and (B2) bilayer bioprinted device; comparison of toolpath planning for functionally graded tissue constructs designed using (C1) Cartesian and (C2) parametric coordinates.

deposition stops, the direction changes, and the feed rate accelerates in the new direction. Although continuous deposition is observable, there is considerable degeneration in the uniformity of deposited filament thickness. This can be alleviated by selecting a higher feed rate while approaching sharp turns; however, it is not completely avoidable. A rational approach to such a problem is to generate a tangential continuity (C^1) along the toolpath.

Toolpath planning in Cartesian form can be also problematic if functionally graded tissue models are desired. For example, a toolpath plan in Cartesian form was used to build multifunctional wound devices (see Fig. 2.3B1–B2) (Ozbolat and Koc, 2012). A 3D blending process was developed to generate functionally graded wound devices with different biomaterial and loaded biomolecule concentrations in different regions. The developed toolpath plan in Cartesian coordinates is, however, no more than an approximation of the actual gradient since the blending direction is independent of toolpath deposition direction. As shown in Fig. 2.3C1, the toolpath follows Cartesian coordinates, but does not follow blending directions between two features. Thus, the toolpath does not capture the geometry; smaller raster size with smaller gaps between adjacent rasters is required for improved accuracy. Moreover, jumps or motion without deposition is substantial due to the nature of the toolpath that is independent of feature geometry.

When any hollow features are introduced into a tissue construct, such as lumen in a blood vessel, toolpath planning in Cartesian coordinates brings further problems. Almost all of the toolpath planning in the literature proposes similar deposition pattern in Cartesian coordinates when any hollow shapes are imposed in object architecture (Ozbolat and Khoda, 2014). Qiu and Langrana (2002) addressed this problem; however, the developed methodology amounted to little more than an improvement in space filling. In that work, they minimized the gap by introducing an adaptive roadwidth toolpath generation method. But the introduction of several hollow shapes resulted in too many starts and stops during deposition. The deposition process again followed Cartesian coordinates independent of hollow feature geometry. Therefore, parametric modeling of the geometric domain that is compatible with the toolpath plan can be a solution to such a problem. An example is provided in Fig. 2.3C2, where the toolpath plan follows the directional gradient in bioink composition.

2.5.2 Toolpath Planning in Parametric Form

To overcome the issues in toolpath planning with Cartesian coordinates, toolpath planning in parametric (u, v) coordinates has been of interest to researchers. In this regard, Ozbolat and his coworkers proposed the idea of using parametric ruling lines in toolpath planning for complex geometric domains, which can dictate the material and porosity composition (Khoda et al., 2013a,b; Ozbolat and Khoda, 2014). First, a medical image-generated CAD file was sliced into several layers, and for each layer, NURBS splines were fitted into the curves. Next, the curves were parameterized and sampled

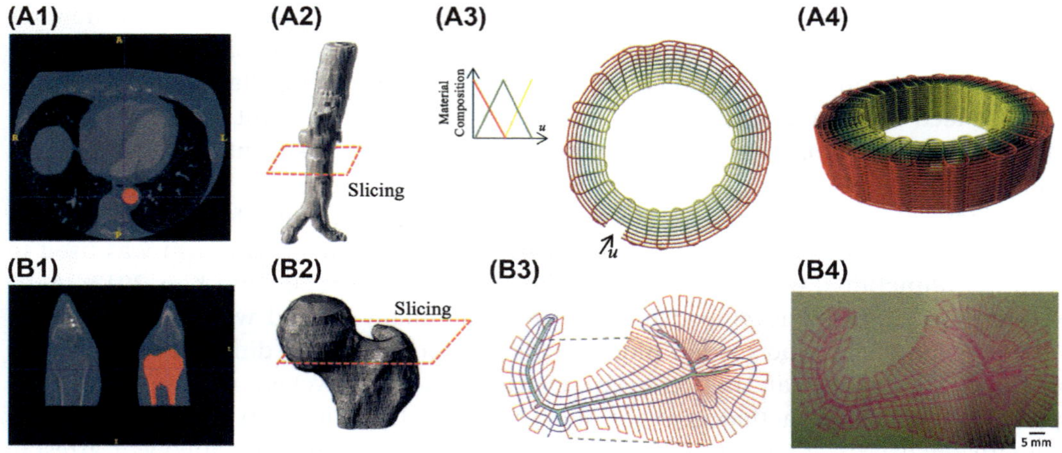

FIGURE 2.4 Toolpath planning in parametric coordinates. (A1) Medical images were processed (A2) to generate a CAD model of aorta, where (A3–A4) a toolpath plan was developed with controlled material composition along the parametric distance *u* (different colors represent different materials) *(Reproduced and adapted with permission from Ozbolat and Khoda, 2014)*. (B1) Using medical image processing, (B2) a femur model was generated and sliced (B3) for toolpath planning with controlled porosity increasing the parametric distance *u*. (B4) A sample double-layer structure was bioprinted using sodium alginate hydrogel. *(Reproduced and adapted with permission from Khoda et al., 2013a,b)*.

into points, and parametric ruling lines were generated between NURBS splines. Then, toolpath generation algorithms were developed to create the toolpath plan in two consecutive layers. The first layer was based on ruling lines and followed a zigzag approach, where arc fitting was introduced at the turns. Arc fitting was used to eliminate two consecutive sharp turns in the zigzag pattern and enabled C^1 tangent continuity with constant feed rate of deposition. This eliminates the aforementioned shortcomings of traditional and recent approaches to hollow object prototyping. To support the zigzag pattern along the ruling lines, a spiral toolpath plan was proposed for the next layer, which was closely perpendicular to ruling lines at the junction point providing better structural support for the next layer. The advantages of the spiral toolpath are that it (1) enables a continuous deposition through a hollow feature compared to the conventional zigzag-based space-filling technique and (2) a smooth transition from one material composition property to another (Fig. 2.4).

2.6 Limitations

Despite the significant progress in designing scaffolds and tissue constructs as generic models, each tissue and organ type has unique requirements and characteristics. Therefore, behavior of different cell types may vary depending on the design architecture of the constructs. For example, the pore size and porous architecture need to be different for specific cell types. For cells that are metabolically highly active such as cardiac or pancreas cells, media transport is crucial; therefore, high porosity for effective transport is of major importance. But for cells such as chondrocytes, the normal cellular environment is hypoxic, thus a less porous architecture would better support formation of cartilage.

A prominent weakness of current bioprinting modalities is the lack of precise control on the cellular microenvironment. Current bioprinting modalities enable a resolution at the submicron level, but smaller features that govern cell attachment, guidance, and spreading cannot be achieved easily. Therefore, researchers devised hybrid fabrication techniques such as bioprinting cells or cell aggregates onto electrospun fibers (Mironov et al., 2009). Nevertheless, little design consideration has been given to multiscale modeling of tissue constructs having both nano- and microscale composition. As multiscale modeling of tissue constructs may be a computationally expensive process, the modeling can be done using computationally efficient approaches such as implicit surfaces in multiple scale.

The majority of research attempts in design and fabrication of tissue constructs have been performed based on uniform composition of design and fabrication elements, for example, bioprinted tissue constructs utilizing uniform microarchitectural and material composition throughout their geometry, but native tissues are anatomically heterogeneous. Therefore, new design approaches should be developed to achieve heterogeneity in tissue constructs with functionally graded or hierarchical properties. Unfortunately, such models with controlled porosity, material composition and biomolecule distribution have rarely been considered in design for bioprinting (Ozbolat et al., 2012).

Significant advances have been made in the design of tissue constructs with intricate geometries in 3D as the design process is quite flexible with minimal limitations. However, manufacturing techniques that incorporate 3D printing processes set stricter limitations as highly intricate shapes can only be manufactured using micro-STL and two-photon polymerization (2PP) processes. Although these techniques facilitate 3D printing of high-definition tissue scaffolds, cells have not yet been bioprinted using these techniques. Particularly, 2PP polymerization enables printing of complex geometries such as porous lattice structures with a resolution of less than a few hundred nanometers (Ovsianikov and Chichkov, 2012). Although this technology may generate structures too small to accommodate high cell densities, it can be used to generate hybrid scaffolds where cells can be bioprinted on the top of prefabricated scaffolds.

Use of soft materials does not support the original design model. The majority of bioprinting work relies on the use of soft materials such as hydrogels and cell aggregates, and these materials do not retain their original shape after bioprinting due to swelling, dehydration, contraction, spreading, and splashing of the bioink materials. Fig. 2.5A1–A2 demonstrates 3D printed heart valve constructs made of poly(ethylene glycol)-diacrylate (PEG-DA) at different scales, where the shape fidelity analysis showed that the deviation from the design model increased when the size of the tissue construct diminished. In DBB and some of LBB processes (see Chapters 5 and 6,

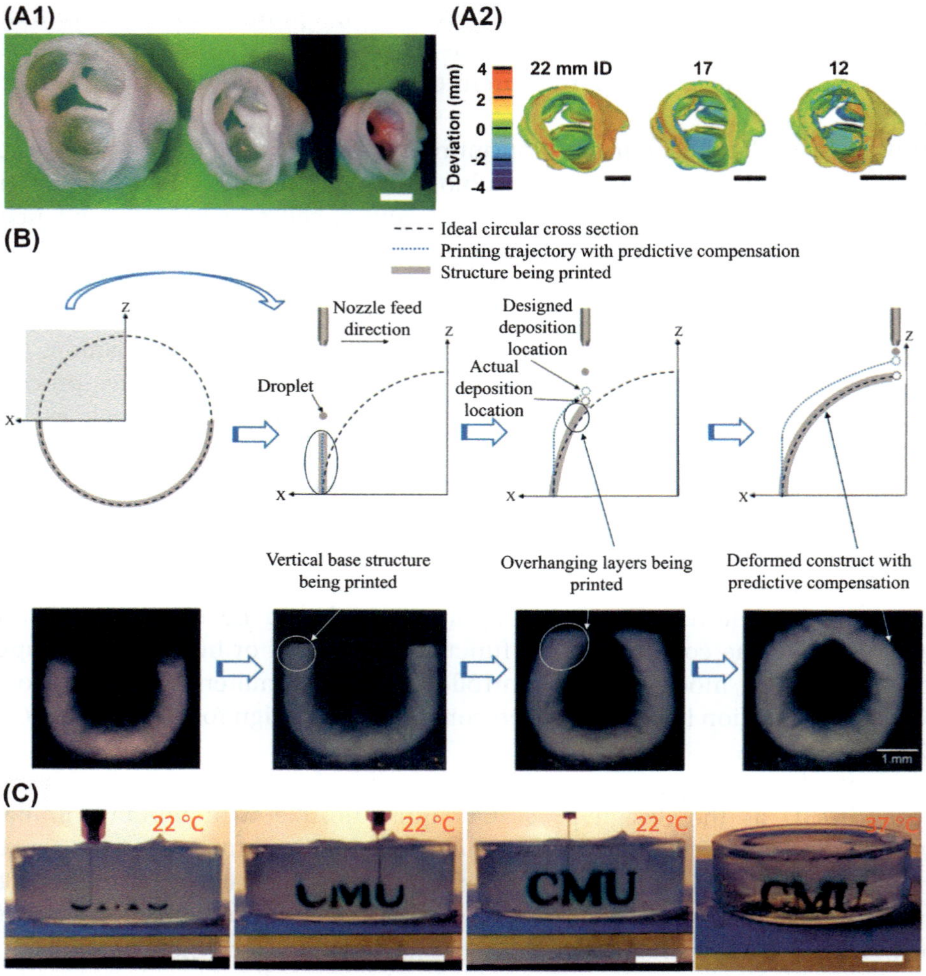

FIGURE 2.5 Recent approaches in bioprinting of high fidelity tissue constructs. (A1) 3D printed heart valve constructs fabricated at different scales using extrusion-based bioprinting with a photo crosslinking apparatus and (A2) their fidelity analysis showing deviations from the original design *(Reproduced and adapted with permission from Hockaday et al., 2012)*. (B) Step-by-step bioprinting trajectory with predictive compensation to inkjet bioprint vascular tubular constructs within an acceptable cylindricity tolerance *(Reproduced and adapted with permission from Xu et al., 2013)*. (C) Step-by-step bioplotting within a hydrogel bath loaded with gelatin microparticles enabling the retention of the original shape of the deposited bioink, where the bioplotted construct was removed when the hydrogel bath was liquefied at 37°C. *(Reproduced and adapted from Hinton et al., 2015)*. Scale bars correspond to 1 cm.

respectively), similar issues can be observed as well even if these processes facilitate bioprinting in higher resolution. Depending on the process parameters, crosslinking, and rheological properties of the bioink solution, the shape accuracy may deviate from the design models. The majority of current toolpath planning approaches do not account for the changes in the shape of soft bioink materials due to reasons discussed previously. As such changes result in variations from the designed toolpath, toolpath compensation approaches can be developed and integrated according to the behavior of different bioink materials. Such toolpath compensation has been widely used in computer numeric control (CNC) machining and other traditional manufacturing techniques. For example, Huang and his coworkers demonstrated piezo-inkjet bioprinting of tubular vascular constructs by depositing sodium alginate into a crosslinker pool by utilizing the buoyancy force to support overhangs (Xu et al., 2013). Due to the substantial weight of the bioink compared to the buoyancy force, bioprinted constructs were deformed and significantly deviated from the original design during construction. Therefore, the group later developed a toolpath strategy with predictive compensation regarding the deflection on bioprinted tubular constructs, which in turn resulted in accurate bioprinting of the design model as can be seen in Fig. 2.5B (Xu et al., 2013). In EBB, similar issues are also observed for the majority of hydrogels used as a bioink material. Although compensation in the lateral plane is important to accurately extrude the bioink in the proper position; compensation in z-axis is also important as majority of the hydrogels contract in z-axis during bioprinting. Additionally, the distance between the nozzle tip and the printing plane is prone to increase over time resulting in imperfections or even failures. Thus, the distance from the nozzle tip to the bioprinting stage should be adjusted automatically during the bioprinting process and should dynamically inform the toolpath plan. To overcome the limitations of bioprinting soft bioink materials, Feinberg's group recently demonstrated a bioplotting process, where the bioink material was extruded and plotted into a hydrogel bath with gelatin microparticles enabling the bath behaving like a Bingham plastic (Hinton et al., 2015). In other words, at 22°C, the bath acts like a liquid facilitating extrusion and plotting of the bioink when the nozzle moves under shear stress and acts like a solid holding the plotted bioink in place when the influence of the nozzle-induced shear stress diminishes. Using this approach, high fidelity constructs were plotted into the hydrogel bath and easily removed at 37°C when the hydrogel bath liquefied (see Fig. 2.5C).

Despite the widespread use of the presented blueprint modeling in design of tissue constructs, a limited number of them are directly relevant and compatible with bioprinting processes. EBB is compatible with space-filling curves as the bioprinter head, and hence, the deposition can directly follow the space-filling curves in a continuous manner. Other blueprint modeling approaches can also be used in bioprinting; however, the accuracy of the design model in general tends to vary greatly from the bioprinted physical models. Conversely, DBB techniques are more compatible with CAD-based models as droplets of spherical shape are deposited as building blocks. Therefore, the sphere can be used as a "primitive" to create the blueprint models for droplet-based bioprinting techniques. For LBB, submodalities determine the choice of the appropriate blueprinting technique. For example, LBB processes involving photopolymerization are compatible with majority of blueprint techniques except the space-filling curves. As such processes have high-resolution capabilities, they are able to capture the blueprint models accurately. Laser-based bioprinting processes based on cell transfer have requirements similar to DBB. As the bioink is deposited on the substrate, it forms a droplet; thus, a CAD-based system with spherical primitives is highly compatible.

Despite the great number of off-the-shelve affordable 3D printers in the market, very few are open-source printers that allow the user to define any toolpath plan on demand using G-code (Trachtenberg et al., 2014). Such a capability would enable the operator to write customized codes according to design needs; however, non open-source 3D printers do not allow such flexibility, and the operator is limited to software-specific automatic toolpath algorithms used for the input CAD model. This feature is particularly useful for researchers who bioprint simple primitive shapes in experimental settings where the added time expenditure of designing a custom toolpath is not required. Rather, the operator can quickly generate the toolpath directly.

2.7 Future Directions

The majority of the design considerations in tissue engineering have been given to scaffold design for cell attachment and growth; however, the current trend in biofabrication is moving toward cell-laden hydrogels, where cells are embedded in hydrated scaffolds and have the ability to migrate in a 3D space. In contrast, cells in traditional polymeric scaffolds are limited to migrate on the scaffold surface only. The porosity within the hydrogel network thus plays a crucial role in stimulating cell growth and proliferation. Although there is a great need for microporous design architecture, such a design has not yet been attempted.

In addition to cell-laden hydrogels, design consideration should also be given to scaffold-free bioprinting. As there is no scaffold to model and design, attention should focus on design of building blocks such as tissue spheroids (Mironov et al., 2009) and tissue strands (Yu et al., 2016) or other form of aggregates. As cell aggregates are subjected to contraction due to cadherin-induced cell—cell integration, the impact of aggregate shape change on the overall tissue fabrication process demands careful consideration (Fleming et al., 2010). There has been a significant amount of theoretical work in modeling fusion dynamics of the 3D constructs, but the majority of these studies do not inform the initial tissue design. Most important, there is no design-driven system that is well integrated with the bioprinting process. For example, a recent work demonstrated toolpath planning for scaffold-free bioprinting of vascular tissue construct (Kucukgul et al., 2015). The authors demonstrated an extensive work on generating the toolpath plan for bioprinting including the path plan for the support material (agarose) and the main material (cell pellet). Upon culturing the samples for sufficient time, the cells were aggregated and the support material was removed. The design toolpath and the fabricated structure differ considerably from each other, and such compensation should be incorporated into the design. Thus, exploring the underlying physics of the process and informing the toolpath decision based on such knowledge will be valuable in optimization of the toolpath plan and fabrication of the tissue constructs, respectively. There is now a current trend in scaffold-free fabrication of tissues, and physics-based model informed design will enable accurate fabrication of tissues.

Physics-based design of cell-laden hydrogels that account for structural and biological changes over time will be highly valuable to the bioprinting research community. Although modeling of degradation and media diffusion has been done in polymeric porous scaffolds (Sengers et al., 2004), degradation of matrix material as well as proliferation of cells in cell-laden hydrogels has not been investigated thoroughly. A thorough understanding of long-term structural stability of hydrogels is of key importance as most of the hydrogels undergo a rapid degradation process. For example, a hydrogel-based environment has been used in the fabrication of microfluidic devices to understand cancer metastasis (Bersini et al., 2014). But, hydrogel materials such as fibrin have quick gelation rates and the device did not retain its integrity for more than two weeks. Researchers have blended different gels such as hyaluronic acid or collagen to improve the degradation and mechanical properties; however, experimentation with combinations of materials at different concentrations is an expensive and time-consuming endeavor. Thus, multiphysics-based design models at multiple scale that can predict the degradation profile of the matrix environment, and the temporal and structural impact of cell proliferation and extracellular matrix (ECM) deposition on the tissue construct will be an invaluable tool in the development of novel biomaterials and bioprinting techniques.

Biologically informed design represents a promising approach in the design and biofabrication of next-generation tissue constructs. Natural tissues possess a heterogeneous architecture with different cell and ECM compositions throughout their structure; this phenomenon should be incorporated into the design environment. Currently, these variations are addressed in a rudimentary fashion rather than devising sophisticated design concepts. Moreover, physics-based modeling of various parameters such as tissue formation and degradation of scaffold-matrix will be highly informative and can contribute significantly toward a complex design environment. Considerations in current design methods for bioprinting of tissue constructs are limited to optimization of porosity for sufficient fluid flow and maximization of mechanical and structural integrity. Although porosity is important in the tissue regeneration process, several other factors affect tissue regeneration such as cell—cell and cell—matrix interactions, scaffold degradation, cell microenvironment in differentiating and proliferating cells, and vascularization; however, majority of these factors have largely been ignored in currently available design approaches and tools. Therefore, more comprehensive design systems need to be developed to integrate other crucial biological factors into the process of building successful tissue constructs.

The majority of the design software currently offered by the bioprinter companies is limited to predefined toolpath planning strategies. For example, the design software enables the user to input a CAD model (that can be obtained from medical images such as CT scan and MRI) and fill contours of each slice generated by the design model similar to FDM-based additive manufacturing processes. But each tissue type or use of different bioink materials and corresponding crosslinking mechanisms necessitates a different path planning strategy. For instance, Pluronic gel has been used as a support material in bioprinting processes as it can quickly retain its shape upon bioprinting. This process can be fine-tuned by using the appropriate concentration of the gel and its temperature profile; however, the other gels utilized in bioprinting do not allow for such a well-defined retention of the gel shape postbioprinting. Therefore, the design models do not actually account for the changes in the printed hydrogel geometry nor compensate for changes in shape caused by swelling and dehydration. Therefore, future design software should take into account bioink solution properties and should enable the user to define distinct path plans for different hydrogels of varying concentrations. Many researchers entering into the bioprinting field invest substantial effort into designing custom toolpath plans for hydrogels. Currently available software does not meet the demands for more sophisticated bioprinting constructs.

2.8 Summary

This chapter elucidates design requirements for bioprinting of tissue and organ constructs and presents the design process for bioprinting starting with acquisition of patient-specific images using medical image modalities (including CT, MRI, and ultrasound), followed by blueprint modeling and a critique of currently available toolpath planning approaches for 3D bioprinting purposes. Contemporary blueprint modeling approaches, used in creating internal architecture of porous tissue constructs, are detailed and discussed along with strengths and limitations. As native tissues and organs are heterogeneous in nature, bioprinting processes should be informed by the appropriate blueprint modeling techniques to recapitulate the native form and function, and bioprinting should complete the process using an appropriate compatible toolpath planning approach.

References

Afshar, M., Anaraki, A.P., Montazerian, H., Kadkhodapour, J., 2016. Additive manufacturing and mechanical characterization of graded porosity scaffolds designed based on triply periodic minimal surface architectures. Journal of the Mechanical Behaviour of Biomedical Materials 62, 481–494.

Appel, A., Anastasio, M.A., Brey, E.M., 2011. Potential for imaging engineered tissues with x-ray phase contrast. Tissue Engineering Part B: Reviews 17 (5), 321–330.

Ballyns, J.J., Bonassar, L.J., 2009. Image-guided tissue engineering. Journal of Cellular and Molecular Medicine 13 (8a), 1428–1436.

Bersini, S., Jeon, J.S., Dubini, G., Arrigoni, C., Chung, S., Charest, J.L., et al., 2014. A microfluidic 3D in vitro model for specificity of breast cancer metastasis to bone. Biomaterials 35 (8), 2454–2461.

Cheah, C.M., Chua, C.K., Leong, K.F., Cheong, C.H., Naing, M.W., 2004. Automatic algorithm for generating complex polyhedral. Tissue Engineering 10 (3–4), 595–610.

Coakley, M.F., et al., 2014. The NIH 3D print exchange: a public resource for bioscientific and biomedical 3D prints. 3D Printing and Additive Manufacturing 1, 137–140.

Dobrucki, L.W., Sinusas, A.J., 2010. PET and SPECT in cardiovascular molecular imaging. Nature Reviews Cardiology 7 (1), 38–47.

Elomaa, L., Teixeira, S., Hakala, R., Korhonen, H., Grijpma, D.W., Seppälä, J.V., 2011. Preparation of poly(ε-caprolactone)-based tissue engineering scaffolds by stereolithography. Acta Biomaterialia 7 (11), 3850–3856.

Elliot, M.R., Thrush, A.J., 1996. Measurement of resolution in intravascular ultrasound images. Physiological Measurement 17 (4), 259–265.

Feldkamp, L.A., Davis, L.C., Kress, J.W., 1984. Practical cone-beam algorithm. Journal of Optical Society of America A 1 (6), 612–619.

Fleming, P.A., Argraves, W.S., Gentile, C., Neagu, A., Forgacs, G., Drake, C.J., 2010. Fusion of uniluminal vascular spheroids: a model for assembly of blood vessels. Developmental Dynamics 239 (2), 398–406.

Giannitelli, S.M., Accoto, D., Trombetta, M., Rainer, A., 2014. Current trends in the design of scaffolds for computer-aided tissue engineering. Acta Biomaterialia 10 (2), 580–594.

Gomez, C., 2007. A Unit Cell Based Multi-scale Modeling & Design Approach for Tissue Engineered Scaffolds. Drexel University.

Gudapati, H., Dey, M., Ozbolat, I., 2016. A comprehensive review on droplet-based bioprinting: past, present and future. Biomaterials 102, 20–42.

Haller, J.O., Slovis, T.L., Babcock, D.S., Teele, R.L., 2004. Early history of pediatric ultrasound (circa 1960-1985). Journal of Ultrasound in Medicine 23, 323–329.

Hinton, T.J., et al., 2015. Three-dimensional printing of complex biological structures by freeform reversible embedding of suspended hydrogels. Science Advances 1 (9), e1500758.

Hockaday, L.A., et al., 2012. Rapid 3D printing of anatomically accurate and mechanically heterogeneous aortic valve hydrogel scaffolds. Biofabrication 4 (3), 035005.

Hollister, S.J., Levy, R.A., Chu, T.M., Halloran, J.W., Feinberg, S.E., 2000. An image-based approach for designing and manufacturing craniofacial scaffolds. International Journal of Oral & Maxillofacial Surgery 29 (1), 67–71.

Hollister, S.J., Lin, C.Y., 2007. Computational design of tissue engineering scaffolds. Computer Methods in Applied Mechanics and Engineering 196 (31–32), 2991–2998.

Hollister, S.J., Maddox, R.D., Taboas, J.M., 2002. Optimal design and fabrication of scaffolds to mimic tissue properties and satisfy biological constraints. Biomaterials 23 (20), 4095–4103.

Kapfer, S.C., Hyde, S.T., Mecke, K., Ams, C.H., Schröder-Turk, G.E., 2011. Minimal surface scaffold designs for tissue engineering. Biomaterials 32 (29), 6875–6882.

Khoda, A.K.M., Ozbolat, I.T., Koc, B., 2013a. Designing heterogeneous porous tissue scaffolds for additive manufacturing processes. Computer Aided Design 45 (12), 1507–1523.

Khoda, A.K.M., Ozbolat, I.T., Koc, B., 2011. Engineered tissue scaffolds with variational porous architecture. Journal of Biomechanical Engineering 133 (1), 011001.

Khoda, A.K.M., Ozbolat, I.T., Koc, B., 2013b. Modeling of variational gradient porous architecture with multi-directional filament deposition in 3D scaffolds. Computer-Aided Design and Applications 10 (3), 445–459.

Kim, J., Piao, Y., Hyeon, T., 2009. Multifunctional nanostructured materials for multimodal imaging, and simultaneous imaging and therapy. Chemical Society Reviews 38, 372–390.

Kucukgul, C., Ozler, S.B., Inci, I., Karakas, E., Irmak, S., Gozuacik, D., et al., 2015. 3D bioprinting of biomimetic aortic vascular constructs with self-supporting cells. Biotechnology and Bioengineering 112 (4), 811–821.

Langer, R., Vacanti, J.P., 1993. Tissue engineering. Science 260 (5110), 920–926.

Lin, C.-Y., et al., 2012. Augmented healing of critical-size calvarial defects by baculovirus-engineered MSCs that persistently express growth factors. Biomaterials 33 (14), 3682–3692.

Lin, C.Y., Kikuchi, N., Hollister, S.J., 2004. A novel method for biomaterial scaffold internal architecture design to match bone elastic properties with desired porosity. Journal of Biomechanics 37 (5), 623–636.

McCormick, M., Liu, X., Jomier, J., Marion, C., Ibanez, L., 2014. ITK: enabling reproducible research and open science. Frontiers in Neuroinformatics 8 (13).

Melchels, F.P., Feijen, J., Grijpma, D.W., 2009. A poly(d,l-lactide) resin for the preparation of tissue engineering scaffolds by stereolithography. Biomaterials 30 (23–24), 3801–3809.

Mironov, V., Visconti, R.P., Kasyanov, V., Forgacs, G., Drake, C.J., Markwald, R.R., 2009. Organ printing: tissue spheroids as building blocks. Biomaterials 30 (12), 2164–2174.

Nam, S.Y., Ricles, L.M., Suggs, L.J., Emelianov, S.Y., 2014. Imaging strategies for tissue engineering applications. Tissue Engineering Part B 21, 1–44.

Ovsianikov, A., Chichkov, B., 2012. Three-dimensional microfabrication by two-photon polymerization technique. In: Liebschner, M. (Ed.), Computer-aided Tissue Engineering. Humana Press, New York, NY, pp. 311–325.

Ozbolat, I.T., Khoda, A.K.M., Marchany, M., Gardella, J., 2012. Hybrid tissue scaffolds for controlled release applications: a study on design and fabrication of hybrid and heterogeneous tissue scaffolds for controlled release applications is presented in this paper. Virtual and Physical Prototyping 7 (1), 37–47.

Ozbolat, I.T., Hospodiuk, M., 2016. Current advances and future perspectives in extrusion-based bioprinting. Biomaterials 76, 321–343.

Ozbolat, I.T., Khoda, A.K.M.B., 2014. Design of a new parametric path plan for additive manufacturing of hollow porous structures with functionally graded materials. Journal of Computing and Information Science in Engineering 14 (4), 041005.

Ozbolat, I.T., Koc, B., 2012. 3D hybrid wound devices for spatiotemporally controlled release kinetics. Computer Methods and Programs in Biomedicine 108 (3), 922–931.

Ozbolat, I.T., Koc, B., 2010. Modeling of spatially controlled biomolecules in three-dimensional porous alginate structures. Journal of Medical Devices 4 (4), 041003.

Ozbolat, I.T., Koc, B., 2011. Multi-function based modeling of 3D heterogeneous wound scaffolds for improved wound healing. Computer-Aided Design and Applications 8 (1), 43–57.

Qiu, D., Langrana, N.A., 2002. Void eliminating toolpath for extrusion-based multi-material layered manufacturing. Rapid Prototyping Journal 8 (1), 38–45.

Rajagopalan, S., Robb, R.A., 2006. Schwarz meets Schwann: design and fabrication of biomorphic and durataxic tissue engineering scaffolds. Medical Image Analysis 10 (5), 693–712.

Requicha, A.G., 1980. Representations for rigid solids: theory, methods, and systems. ACM Computing Surveys 12 (4), 437–464.

Sengers, B.G., Oomens, C.W., Baaijens, F.P., 2004. An integrated finite-element approach to mechanics, transport and biosynthesis in tissue engineering. Journal of Biomechanical Engineering 126 (1), 82–91.

Smith, M.H., Flanagan, C.L., Kemppainen, J.M., Sack, J.A., Chung, H., Das, S., et al., 2007. Computed tomography-based tissue-engineered scaffolds in craniomaxillofacial surgery. The International Journal of Medical Robotics and Computer Assisted Surgery 3 (3), 207–216.

Starly, B., Sun, W., 2007. Internal scaffold architecture designs using Lindenmayer systems. Computer-Aided Design and Applications 4 (1–4), 395–403.

Sun, W., Starly, B., Darling, A., Gomez, C., 2004. Computer-aided tissue engineering: application to biomimetic modelling and design of tissue scaffolds. Biotechnology and Applied Biochemistry 39, 49–58.

Terreno, E., et al., 2010. Challenges for molecular magnetic resonance imaging. Chemical Reviews 110 (5), 3019–3042.

Theysohn, J.M., Maderwald, S., Kraff, O., Moenninghoff, C., Ladd, M.E., Ladd, S.C., 2007. Subjective acceptance of 7 Tesla MRI for human imaging. Magnetic Resonance Materials in Physics, Biology and Medicine 21 (1), 63–72.

Trachtenberg, J.E., Mountziaris, P.M., Miller, J.S., Wettergreen, M., Kasper, F.K., Mikos, A.G., 2014. Open-source three-dimensional printing of biodegradable polymer scaffolds for tissue engineering. Journal of Biomedical Materials Research Part A 102, 4326–4335.

Tuan, H.S., Hutmacher, D.W., 2005. Application of micro CT and computation modeling in bone tissue engineering. Computer Aided Design 37 (11), 1151–1161.

Turnbull, D.H., Mori, S., 2007. MRI in mouse developmental biology. NMR in Biomedicine 20, 265–274.

Wells, P.N.T., Liang, H.-D., 2011. Medical ultrasound: imaging of soft tissue strain and elasticity. Journal of Royal Society of Interface 8, 1521–1549.

Wettergreen, M.A., Bucklen, B.S., Sun, W., Liebschner, M.A., 2005a. Computer-aided tissue engineering of a human vertebral body. Annals of Biomedical Engineering 33 (10), 1333–1343.

Wettergreen, M.A., Bucklen, B.S., Starly, B., Yuksel, E., Sun, W., Liebschner, M.A.K., 2005b. Creation of a unit block library of architectures for use in assembled scaffold engineering. Computer Aided Design 37 (11), 1141–1149.

Whitaker, M., 2014. The history of 3D printing in healthcare. Bulletin of the Royal College of Surgeons of England 96 (7), 228–229.

Xu, C., et al., 2013. Predictive compensation-enabled horizontal inkjet printing of alginate tubular constructs. Manufacturing Letters 1 (1), 28–32.

Xu, H., Othman, S.F., Magin, R.L., 2008. Monitoring tissue engineering using magnetic resonance imaging. Journal of Bioscience and Bioengineering 106 (6), 515–527.

Yasar, O., Lan, S.-F., Starly, B., 2009. A Lindenmayer system-based approach for the design of nutrient delivery networks in tissue constructs. Biofabrication 1, 45004.

Yoo, D., 2012. Heterogeneous minimal surface porous scaffold design using the distance field and radial basis functions. Medical Engineering and Physics 34, 625–639.

Yu, Y., et al., 2016. Three-dimensional bioprinting using self-assembling scalable scaffold-free "tissue strands" as a new bioink. Scientific Reports 6, 28714.

Further Reading

Akkouch, A., Yu, Y., Ozbolat, I.T., 2015. Microfabrication of scaffold-free tissue strands for three-dimensional tissue engineering. Biofabrication 7 (3), 031002.

Koudan, E.V., et al., 2016. Patterning of tissue spheroids biofabricated from human fibroblasts on the surface of electrospun polyurethane matrix using 3D bioprinter. International Journal of Bioprinting 2 (1), 45–52.

3

The Bioink*

CHAPTER OUTLINE

*With contributions by Monika Hospodiuk and Madhuri Dey, The Pennsylvania State University.

3D Bioprinting.

It is the lone worker who makes the first advance in a subject; the details may be worked out by a team, but the prime idea is due to enterprise, thought, and perception of an individual
Alexander Fleming

3.1 Introduction

The need for hierarchical assembly of three-dimensional (3D) heterocellular tissues has been escalating in medicine and biotechnology. It has spurred the development of new technologies with the ultimate goal of creating de novo functional tissues and organs (Ozbolat and Yu, 2013). The principal of bioprinting can be defined as the placement of cells within biomaterials into spatially defined structures using automated 3D bioprinter technologies. This process, first named "cytoscribing," was inspired by classic two-dimensional (2D) paper printers, as the droplets of colored ink are similar in size to biologics (Klebe, 1988). In the last two decades, various bioprinting processes have emerged along with various process-compatible bioink materials. The process of bioprinting requires a delivery medium for cells which can be deposited into designed shapes acquired from computer-aided design (CAD) models. The CAD models can be generated using 3D medical images obtained through magnetic resonance imaging, computed tomography scanning, and other techniques (Lee et al., 2014a; Kucukgul et al., 2015; Pati et al., 2013). Soft biomaterials loaded with living cells are called bioink and are the "raw material" of bioprinting processes.

The development of bioink materials allows scientists to manipulate biological and biochemical environments as well as living cells to create complex biological constructs. The milestones of success are measured by sustained viability of cells during short- and long-term culture, cell spreading and proliferation, cell–cell and cell–extracellular matrix (ECM) interactions, and functionality of the bioprinted constructs. Although a wide array of biomaterials have been developed for tissue engineering and regenerative medicine (Furth et al., 2007), the vast majority are not compatible with existing bioprinting technologies. Some important features of an ideal bioink material are bioprintability, high mechanical integrity and stability, insolubility in cell culture medium, biodegradability at a rate appropriate to the regenerating tissue, nontoxicity and non-immunogenicity, and the ability to promote cell adhesion. In addition, bioink materials should be easily manufactured and processed, affordable, and commercially available. Bioprinted constructs are expected to keep their designed shape and structural strength and integrity, maintain 3D architecture for a defined period of time in vitro, and easily engraft with the host and degrade over time in vivo.

This chapter presents bioink materials used in 3D bioprinting processes including scaffold-based (i.e., hydrogels, microcarriers, and decellularized matrix components), and scaffold-free (i.e., cell aggregates), bioink materials. Limitations and strengths of each bioink material are elucidated, and their characteristics are evaluated based on several criteria including their compatible bioprinting modalities, bioprintability, biomimicry, resolution, affordability, scalability, practicality, mechanical and structural integrity, bioprinting and postbioprinting maturation times, degradability, commercial availability, immunogenicity, and applications. Finally, the chapter provides the reader with limitations and presents future perspectives of bioink materials.

3.2 Bioink Materials

Two major types of bioink materials have been used in bioprinting of 3D tissue and organ constructs (Ozbolat, 2015a). The first and most common one is scaffold-based bioink where cells are loaded in hydrogels or similar exogenous materials and bioprinted into 3D constructs. Cell-laden hydrogels allow cell proliferation and growth and facilitate formation of tissue. In the second type of bioink, cells are bioprinted without the use of an exogenous biomaterial, in a scaffold-free process mimicking embryonic development. Cells are first formed into neotissues that are engineered for bioprinting processes; resulting neotissues are then deposited in specific patterns where they fuse and mature for fabrication of larger scale functional tissues.

3.2.1 Scaffold-Based Bioink Materials

3.2.1.1 Hydrogels

A class of crosslinked polymeric substances capable of absorbing and retaining large quantities of water are generally referred to as hydrogels. Hydrogels in tissue engineering are classified into two groups: naturally derived hydrogels such as gelatin, fibrin, collagen, chitosan, and alginate and synthetically derived hydrogels such as Pluronic® or polyethylene glycol (PEG). They are used in biofabrication and tissue engineering for a wide array of applications such as drug delivery (Yang et al., 2011), contact lenses (White et al., 2011), and wound dressings (Kamoun et al., 2015). Some are able to mimic the native tissue environment as they possess several essential features of the native ECM components (Tibbitt and Anseth, 2009). These ECM-like properties allow cell encapsulation in a highly hydrated, mechanically strong 3D environment; however, both natural and synthetic hydrogels have some limitations. Natural hydrogels generally have weak mechanical properties, while synthetic counterparts lack major components such as bioactive molecules for cell adhesion or migration (Zhu and Marchant, 2011). Biocompatibility of hydrogels is defined by their hydrophilicity. Hydrogels can absorb up to 1000 times their original weight in aqueous medium without dissolving (Ahmed, 2013), making them ideal for cell encapsulation. Because they are highly permeable to oxygen, nutrients, and other water-soluble compounds, hydrogels are attractive materials for fabrication of tissue constructs (Thomas et al., 2009; Zhu and Marchant, 2011). Finally, hydrogels provide 3D niches for embedded cells, which mimic their native tissue environment (Rajan et al., 2006; Drury and Mooney, 2003; Yamamoto et al., 2010;

Benedikt et al., 2000). Distinct features of natural and synthetic hydrogels cannot be clearly stated; however, most of natural hydrogels are cell friendly.

3.2.1.1.1 BIOPRINTABILITY OF HYDROGELS

Over the past few decades, numerous hydrogels have been prepared by altering the chemical backbone of polymers for tissue engineering applications. However, not all hydrogels can be considered "bioprintable." Bioprintability of hydrogels is governed by their rheological properties and the target bioprinting modality. According to their bioprinting mechanisms, bioprinting processes can be classified under three major modalities: extrusion-based bioprinting (EBB), droplet-based bioprinting (DBB), and laser-based bioprinting (LBB) (Gudapati et al., 2016; Ozbolat and Hospodiuk, 2016). Each bioprinting modality has different bioink requirements according to the bioprinting mechanism employed (see Fig. 3.1).

EBB employs pneumatic-, mechanical-, or solenoid-driven microextrusion along with a computer-controlled writing process. Hydrogels used in EBB broadly fall under the category of non-Newtonian fluids, where viscosity is strongly dependent upon shear rate (Jungst et al., 2015). Hydrogels with shear thinning and thixotropic behavior are well suited for EBB processes. In shear thinning hydrogels, shear forces align the random polymer chains in a favorable direction making them extrudable. Thixotropy, a time-dependent shear thinning behavior, enables the bioink to assume a stable form at rest in the barrel, exhibit low viscosity inside the nozzle tip during extrusion, and regain its stability postbioprinting. In addition, the bioink should possess low adhesion and surface tension properties to eliminate its attachment on the surface of the nozzle tip and easily overcome the surface tension–driven droplet formation enabling successful filament extrusion. In addition, the bioink should have rapid gelation characteristics so that it can retain its shape without spreading. Moreover, appropriate substrate (with high surface roughness and low wettability) should be in place so that the bioink can stick to the substrate and retain its shape.

DBB utilizes various energy sources such as electric, sound, and heat to generate droplets of bioink in a high-throughput manner. According to their droplet generation mechanisms, DBB processes can be classified under four groups: inkjet (thermal, piezoelectric, or electrostatic) bioprinting, electrohydrodynamic jetting, acoustic droplet election, and microvalve bioprinting. In general, the bioink used in DBB should have low viscosity and a nonfibrous nature so that it can easily flow through the tubing system and nozzle without clogging problems. In addition, the bioink needs to possess a rheopectic behavior, which is a time-dependent dilatant behavior resulting in increased viscosity as shear is applied triggering droplet formation due to an increase in viscosity following ejection. The bioink should also have appropriate surface tension. It should have sufficient wettability to travel through the cartridge correctly but not leak out, flooding of the print head and wetting the exterior of the nozzle tip. In addition, the droplets should solidify immediately after landing. Droplet–substrate interactions are

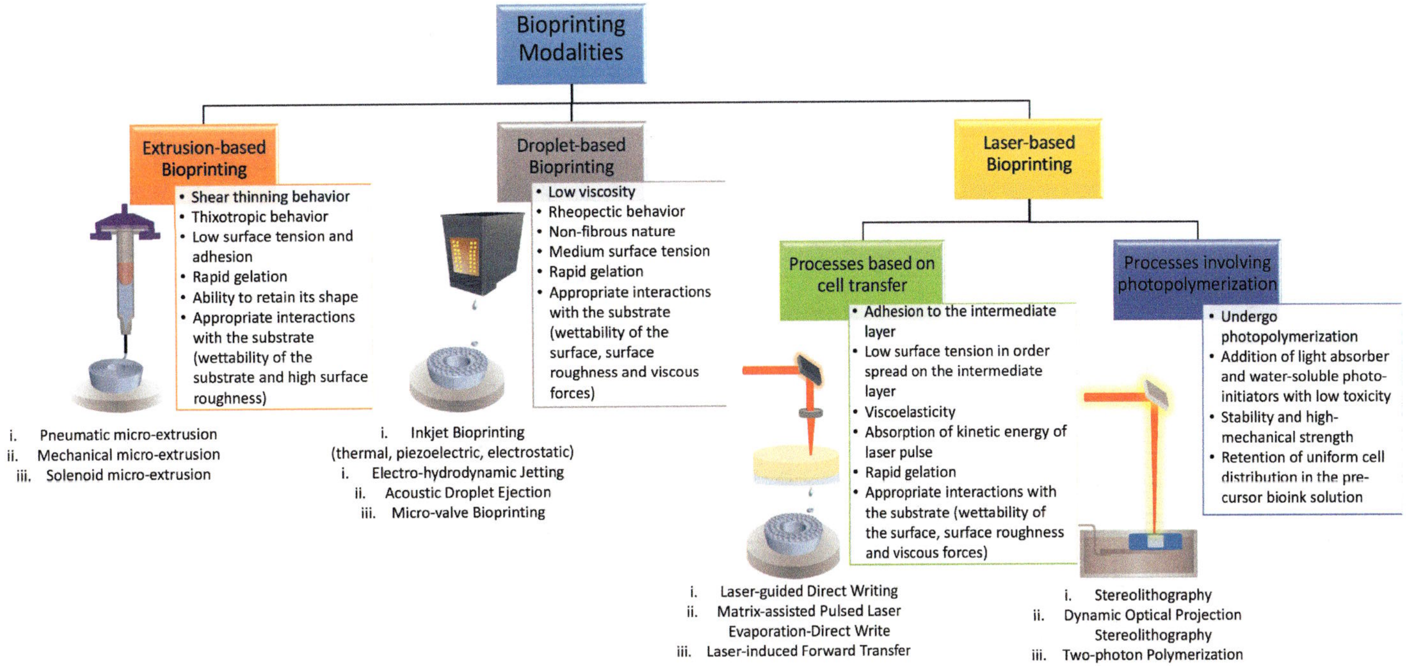

FIGURE 3.1 Modalities of bioprinting processes and their bioink requirements.

also important as appropriate substrate surface properties are needed to prevent spreading, splashing, or rebounding of droplets as extensively discussed in Chapter 5.

LBB utilizes laser energy for fabrication of tissue constructs or high-precision patterning of biologics and can be classified under two groups: processes based on cell transfer [i.e., laser-guided direct writing (Odde and Renn, 1999), matrix-assisted pulsed laser evaporation-direct write (MAPLE-DW) (Riggs et al., 2011), or laser-induced forward transfer (LIFT) (Michael et al., 2013)] and processes involving photopolymerization [i.e., stereolithography (SLA) (Arcaute et al., 2010), dynamic optical projection stereolithography (DOPsL) (Zhang et al., 2012), or two-photon polymerization (2PP) (Ovsianikov et al., 2014)]. In the former approach, the bioink is transferred from a cartridge to a substrate by laser-induced jet formation; however, in the latter approach, the laser beam selectively solidifies a photocurable bioink material (in a vat) through polymerization. The bioink used for cell transfer processes should possess sufficient adhesion and low surface tension characteristics so that it can uniformly spread on the intermediate layer and adhere to it without dripping. The bioink should easily transfer thermal energy into kinetic energy and exhibit high viscoelasticity so that well-defined jets can be formed with rest of the bioink maintained in the cartridge. The bioink needs to have a rapid gelation capability so jets can solidify without spreading. Moreover, jet–substrate interactions are also important (similar to DBB); therefore, an appropriate substrate should be selected to prevent spreading and splashing of the jets. For bioink in processes involving photopolymerization, photopolymerizable hydrogels should be used. The bioink should be further reinforced with nontoxic water-soluble photoinitiators and light absorbers to initiate photopolymerization and enable fabrication of tissue constructs with uniform layer thickness. Stability and high-mechanical strength as well as the ability to retain cells uniformly distributed in the precursor solution are other important requirements of such bioink selection.

In addition, the bioink should possess an appropriate gelation mechanism driven by chemical, physical, or enzymatic crosslinking as outlined in the following section.

3.2.1.1.2 CROSSLINKING MECHANISMS OF HYDROGELS

3.2.1.1.2.1 PHYSICAL CROSSLINKING In the field of tissue engineering, there has been a growing interest in polymers which can be effectively crosslinked without the use of any exogenous agents, thus minimizing the risk of chemical contamination or chemically induced toxicity (Hennink and van Nostrum, 2012). Apart from obvious advantages, such polymeric hydrogels foster a more congenial environment for embedded cells, proteins, and other biologics. Ionic, hydrophobic, and hydrogen bonding interactions, stereocomplexation, self-assembly of amphiphilic peptides or polymers into micellar structures are some of the well-established mechanisms which are known to drive physical crosslinking of hydrogels (Jungst et al., 2015).

Ionic crosslinking involves the association of polymer chains by noncovalent interactions. A crosslinked hydrogel network is formed when molecules containing opposite charges are blended, e.g., polyelectrolyte solution and multivalent ions (Gulrez et al., 2011). The ions of opposite charges electrostatically attract each other giving rise to a crosslinked polymeric network. The network can also be disrupted by using specific chelators to remove the multivalent ions from the polymeric network to reverse the gelation process.

In some hydrogels, hydrophobic interactions or hydrogen bonding interactions play a significant role in crosslinking. These interactions often tend to be temperature dependent and alter the rheology of the hydrogel network with changing temperature. Some hydrogels exhibit a random coil conformation at high temperatures; upon lowering the temperature, the polymer chains adapt a more ordered conformation forming junction points and consequently aggregating as physical gels (Jeong et al., 2002). Others undergo the reverse process. In reverse gelation, polymeric strands mostly contain both hydrophobic and hydrophilic regions (Pradines et al., 2015). At low temperatures, water (solvent) molecules dissolve the hydrophilic parts of the molecule leading to complete dissolution of monomer chains. There is a strong binding affinity between water molecules and monomeric chains, leading to highly ordered water molecules along the monomeric chains. The forces of interaction here are primarily hydrogen bonding forces, where the binding is an enthalpy-driven process; however, when the temperature increases, entropy overcomes enthalpy as water molecules become randomly oriented and hydrophobic interactions between the monomeric chains become predominant. Thus the chains dehydrate as the water molecules break free. With the increase in temperature, the polymeric interactions become more dominant as compared to the hydrogen bonding forces.

The association of disordered molecules into an ordered state by virtue of its nature or by electrostatic or covalent interactions is referred to as "self-assembly," which is a primary mechanism of gelation observed in amphiphilic peptide molecules (Hauser et al., 2015). Synthetic peptides with a cationic polar head group and anionic groups along its backbone undergo rapid self-assembly from a random coil configuration to form ordered α helices and β sheets. With increased concentration, β sheets undergo further self-assembly to form nanofibrous networks that bear close resemblance to the native ECM. Some of the most commonly employed physically crosslinked hydrogels in bioprinting are agarose, alginate, chitosan, collagen, gelatin, Matrigel™, and Pluronic®, which are further discussed in Section 3.2.1.1.3 in detail.

3.2.1.1.2.2 CHEMICAL CROSSLINKING Chemically crosslinked hydrogels, characterized by covalent bonding between polymer chains, often provide better mechanical stability compared to physically crosslinked ones. Chemical crosslinking can involve exogenous crosslinking agents or formation of reactive species by photoirradiation; however, the use of a crosslinker can induce undesirable reactions with the hydrogel surface or result in cytotoxicity (Hennink and van Nostrum, 2012). Some of the widely studied mechanisms for chemical crosslinking of polymers include condensation reactions, crosslinking by Schiff base formation (a compound formed by the nucleophilic addition of an amine and a carbonyl group) (Dragan, 2014), or photo-crosslinking (Wang et al., 2015b).

Schiff base is a compound formed by the nucleophilic addition of an amine to a carbonyl functional group. Amine containing amino acids, natural polysaccharides, or other synthetic polymers can be easily crosslinked under mild reaction conditions in the presence of crosslinkers containing aldehyde functionalities such as glutaraldehyde or other polyaldehydes (Hennink and van Nostrum, 2012). Other complementary functional groups that can also react with aldehydes to form crosslinked hydrogels include alcohol and hydrazides (Hennink and van Nostrum, 2012). The degree of crosslinking depends on the concentration of the crosslinker used. A high degree of crosslinking results in a hydrogel with strong mechanical properties; however, this reduces the degradation time of the hydrogel. Release of drugs, growth factors, or other biologics immobilized in a bioprinted hydrogel matrix might take longer to diffuse into the surrounding tissue region due to stronger encapsulation between the chemically crosslinked polymer chains. Some frequently used crosslinking agents (i.e., glutaraldehyde) are used to induce chemical crosslinking reactions between complementary functional groups. While glutaraldehyde might induce cytotoxicity (Takigawa and Endo, 2006), genipin is a benign naturally derived crosslinker, which has been used to crosslink gelatin (Bigi et al., 2002), collagen (Yan et al., 2010), chitosan (Chen et al., 2004; Moura et al., 2011), and fibrin (Gamboa-Martinez et al., 2015). The amine groups of the amino acids present in fibrin undergo a nucleophilic, ring closure type of reaction to form crosslinked hydrogels with genipin (Gamboa-Martinez et al., 2015).

Photopolymerization is one of the widely used crosslinking mechanisms, where low molecular weight monomers or oligomers undergo a process called curing to form a crosslinked polymeric network, when exposed to radiation[29]. The crosslinking process is initiated in the presence of a photoinitiator that forms excited molecular species on irradiation with light and onsets the polymerization process. Often pure hydrogels do not crosslink by themselves unless an external initiator is added or the molecule is chemically modified with functional groups capable of undergoing free radical polymerization. The physical properties of the hydrogel can be efficiently controlled by proper modulation of the rate and degree of crosslinking by photopolymerization. Some commonly used photoinitiators in bioprinting include Irgacure (2-hydroxy-1-[4-(2-hydroxyethoxy) phenyl]-2-methyl-1-propanone) (Aubin et al., 2010), (Wang et al., 2015b), VA-086 (2, 2′-azobis [2-methyl-N-(2-hydroxyethyl) propionamide]) (Billiet et al., 2014), and Biokey (lithium phenyl-2,4,6-trimethylbenzoylphosphinate) (Fairbanks et al., 2009). While some photoinitiators produce free radicals via unimolecular bond cleavage, others undergo bimolecular reactions by producing excited species which undergo collision with another initiator molecule to generate free radicals. Irgacure is the most widely used photoinitiator in the bioprinting community, but it is only nontoxic below a certain threshold quantity. Even at concentration of 0.5% (w/v), this initiator has proven to be extremely detrimental to cells unless the excess photoinitiator is leached out of fabricated constructs (Arcaute et al., 2006). A few important requirements for photoinitiators are their water solubility, type of radiation, and exposure time required to generate free radicals. Although Irgacure is water soluble, it requires the use of ultraviolet (UV) light which is detrimental to cells with prolonged exposure. Long-term exposure to UV can damage the DNA, can induce undesired crosslinking, or affect cell functionality. In contrast, the use of photoinitiators such as Eosin Y and Biokey is advantageous as crosslinking can occur in visible light within a short span of time (Fairbanks et al., 2009). Using a low concentration (<0.1%) photoinitiator, as recommended by some studies (Fedorovich et al., 2009), can minimize toxicity but diminishes mechanical properties. Low mechanical properties often give rise to increased swelling and enhanced depth of curing, which deteriorates the bioprinted construct quality. Methacrylated gelatin (GelMA) and PEG are two of commonly used polymers capable of undergoing photopolymerization.

3.2.1.1.2.3 ENZYMATIC CROSSLINKING The most popular enzymatically -crosslinked hydrogel in tissue engineering is fibrin (Scheraga, 2004; Benedikt et al., 2000). It is composed of fibrinogen and thrombin, the major precursors involved in blood clotting. Thrombin is a serine protease that converts fibrinogen, a complex glycoprotein, into fibrin. Cytocompatibility and cell adhesive properties make fibrin a widely used bioink in bioprinting (Ehsan et al., 2014; Yu et al., 2015; Lee et al., 2010b). It is possible to manipulate the integrity of other hydrogels, such as gelatin, by using transglutaminase, a bacterial enzyme (Gómez-Guillén et al., 2011). Transglutaminase catalyzes the formation of isopeptide bonds by a transamidation-mediated reaction between the gamma-carbonyl group of a glutamine residue and the epsilon-amino group of a lysine residue (Sakai et al., 2009). Thrombin and transglutaminase are Ca^{2+}-dependent enzymes.

3.2.1.1.3 HYDROGELS USED IN BIOPRINTING

Bioprintability of hydrogels is a key attribute to the success of 3D bioprinting; each hydrogel brings different properties and requirements to the bioprinting process. Hydrogels used in bioprinting technology are herein described in detail with respect to their chemical content, crosslinking behavior, biocompatibility, and bioprintability under EBB, DBB, and LBB.

3.2.1.1.3.1 NATURAL HYDROGELS **Agarose** is a naturally derived polysaccharide molecule which undergoes gradual gelation at low temperatures and liquefies at the temperatures ranging from 20 to 70°C, depending on the hydroxyethylation (Serwer et al., 1983; Tako and Nakamura, 1988). It has been suggested that the gelation mechanism goes through three stages, namely initiation, nucleation, and pseudoequilibrium (Tako and Nakamura, 1988). In solid state, agarose is brittle, but maintains its shape for a long period of time at a broad range of temperatures. Agarose is not as cell friendly as alginate and Pluronic®, as cell proliferation rate and the biosynthesis of cell components is limited (Fedorovich et al., 2008). Low cell adhesion and spreading suggest that agarose is a poor material for cell culture; however, it serves well as a mold material for 3D culture of cell aggregates (Livoti and Morgan, 2010). Its biological properties can, however, be improved by blending with other hydrogels such as collagen (Duarte Campos et al., 2014). Agarose has been used in EBB providing superior stability and construct thickness when compared to collagen/agarose blends. Cell viability was maintained;

however, cells retained a round as opposed to a spread morphology (Duarte Campos et al., 2014). In addition, agarose has been printed for construction of support structures to facilitate aggregation of bioprinted cell aggregates (see Fig. 3.2A). Agarose has a thermally reversible feature and can be used as a sacrificial material in a bulky scaffold of a thermally stable hydrogel. It can be liquefied and drained, leaving a hollow, perfusable structure (Lee et al., 2010a). Agarose has been used in DBB, particularly in microvalve bioprinting of mammalian cells yielding high cell viability (Xu et al., 2005). For microvalve bioprinting, a temperature controller is required to keep agarose in liquid state. In general, its viscous nature does not allow inkjet bioprinting as it can easily clog the nozzle. Agarose is a promising candidate for LBB due to its viscoelastic nature and rapid gelation mechanism. It has been deposited using LIFT technology, successfully maintaining high cell viability (Koch et al., 2010).

Alginate is a popular hydrogel used in bioprinting processes due its biocompatibility, various choices of crosslinking and bioprinting methods, low price, and ease of use in the creation of 3D structures (Ozbolat and Hospodiuk, 2016). It is a polysaccharide made of alternating β-D-mannuronate (M) and its C-5 epimer α-L-guluronate (G) units (Jungst et al., 2015). The G subunits are responsible for forming the gel phase of alginate. As the number of G subunits increase, the degree of gelation increases. Alginate undergoes ionic crosslinking in calcium chloride ($CaCl_2$) or calcium sulfate ($CaSO_4$) solutions. The divalent calcium ions form a bridge, due to the attraction of negatively charged carboxylic acid groups between two neighboring alginate chains (Lai et al., 2016). Alginate has been widely used for cell encapsulation, including neural stem cells (Purcell et al., 2009), skeletal myoblasts (Hill et al., 2006), and articular chondrocytes (Alsberg et al., 2002; Ab-Rahim et al., 2013). Moreover, alginate provides favorable conditions for adipogenic differentiation and does not alter cell morphology (Galateanu et al., 2012). In addition to cell encapsulation, alginate has been successfully used as a 3D matrix for in vitro culture of organoids and embryos, i.e., pancreatic islets (Tomei et al., 2014). However, despite the intrinsic properties of alginate that make it a favorable material for tissue engineering applications, chemical modifications are often required to promote desirable cellular functions, provide a greater range of mechanical properties, and facilitate controlled release of encapsulated factors. It was shown that, due to the highly hydrophilic nature of alginate, proteins are minimally adsorbed thus hampering cell attachment (Rowley et al., 1999). This can be overcome by modifying the alginate surface with peptides, such as RGD, to provide molecule binding sites for cell adhesion. EBB of alginate has been one of the most popular techniques in the bioprinting community (Ahn et al., 2012; Ozbolat and Koc, 2010; Yu et al., 2013). Alginate has several advantages for use in EBB, including the ease of crosslinking and a wide range of concentrations with superior mechanical properties. Alginate can be extruded in one of two forms, precursor and pre–crosslinked, depending on the application. Alginate in 2–4% (w/v) is extrudable, structurally stable and biologically acceptable and, after contacting the crosslinker, solidifies rapidly and maintains its 3D shape (see Fig. 3.2B) (Zhang et al., 2013a,b; Zhang et al. 2015; Ozbolat et al., 2014; Dolati et al., 2014). The concentration of

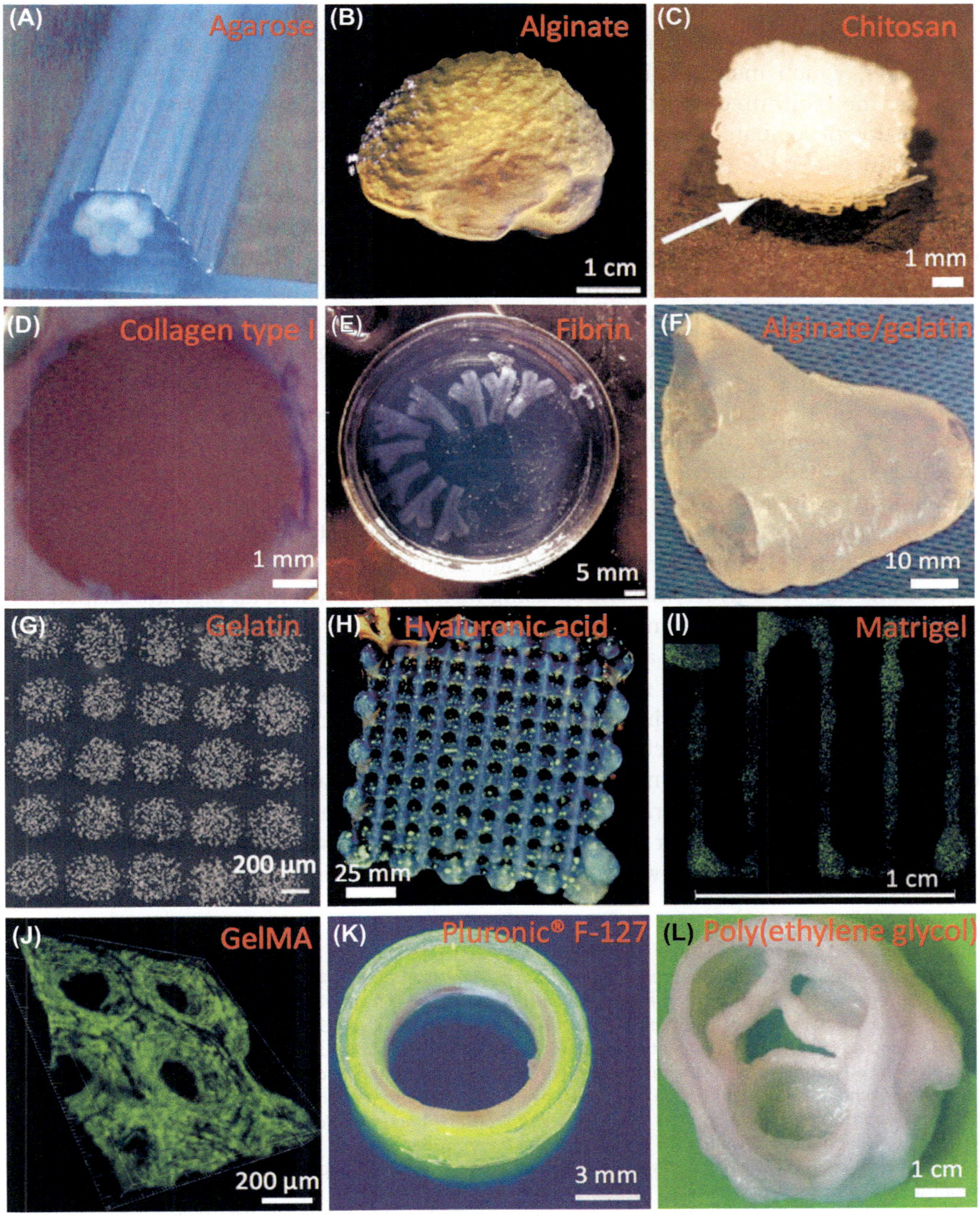

FIGURE 3.2 Bioprinted Hydrogels. (A) Agarose filaments bioprinted to enclose tissue spheroids *(Reproduced/adapted with permission from Norotte et al. (2009))*; (B) three-dimensional (3D) printed alginate in brain shape

alginate determines the viscosity of the solution, porosity and crosslinking time. It is possible to form pre-crosslinked alginate by mixing with low concentrations of the crosslinker, which increases its printability (Cohen et al., 2010b). Depending on the purpose, the bioprinted constructs can be strengthen by further addition of the crosslinker. DBB of alginate is feasible as long as its concentration allows for droplet formation [in general <2% in inkjet bioprinting (Gudapati et al., 2016)]. Exploiting the crosslinking mechanism of alginate with $CaCl_2$, heterogeneous tissue constructs comprised of amniotic fluid–derived stem cells (AFSCs), detrusor smooth muscle cell, and biliary epithelial cells were fabricated (Xu et al., 2013). Mechanical properties of bioprinted constructs can also be improved by combining alginate with other functional materials. For example, bifurcated vascular tissue constructs were fabricated within fluorocarbon employing a blend of 3% (w/v) low melting agarose and 3% (w/v) low viscosity alginate (Blaeser et al., 2013). The buoyant forces of the fluorocarbon solution supported soft tissue constructs. Similarly, zigzag cellular constructs were fabricated by printing 3T3 fibroblast-loaded alginate solution into a $CaCl_2$ crosslinker pool, where the crosslinker provided buoyancy support (Xu et al., 2012). Using an opposite configuration, another work also demonstrated bioprinting of alginate; heartlike tissue constructs were fabricated by bioprinting the crosslinker ($CaCl_2$) solution into an alginate pool using a modified HP inkjet printer (Xu et al., 2009). LBB with alginate of different concentrations has been widely described using MAPLE-DW, where an alginate suspension containing cells was placed on the ribbon then pulsed with a laser (Guillotin et al., 2010; Yan et al., 2013; Gudapati et al., 2014). Successful bioprinting depended upon alginate concentration and viscosity, surface tension, the bioink layer thickness coated onthe intermediate layer, gelation times, wettability, and laser fluence (Gudapati et al., 2014).

Chitosan, a linear polysaccharide molecule obtained from deacetylation of chitin, has a wide range of applications in tissue engineering such as cartilage regeneration, devices for hemostatic and antibacterial activity, formation of sponge scaffolds, and fabrication of wound dressings (Croisier and Jérôme, 2013). The best concentration for optimal biological response is 1.5% (w/w) with a degree of acetylation between 30% and 40%

with recapitulated anatomical features *(Reproduced/adapted from Hinton et al. (2015))*; (C) chitosan scaffold after 4 weeks of culture *(Reproduced/adapted with permission from Ye et al. (2014))*; (D) collagen type I construct for skin tissue regeneration implanted on a wound *(Reproduced/adapted from Michael et al. (2013))*; (E) bioprinted fibrin into 3D tubular scaffolds *(Reproduced/adapted from Hinton et al. (2015))*; (F) 3D bioprinted "half-heart" scaffold using a blend of alginate/gelatin *(Reproduced with permission from Xu et al. (2009))*; (G) gelatin bioprinted by a laser direct-write technique resulted in precise deposition of cells *(Reproduced/adapted with permission from Raof et al. (2011))*; (H) bioprinted hyaluronic acid into a mesh structure *(Reproduced/adapted with permission from Pescosolido et al. (2011))/Copyright (2011) American Chemical Society)*; (I) human mammary epithelial cells bioprinted in Matrigel™ in zigzag shape *(Reproduced/adapted with permission from Snyder et al. (2011))*; (J) a 3D confocal image of cells in a methacrylated gelatin (GelMA) scaffold fabricated by laser-based bioprinting *(Reproduced/adapted with permission from Gauvin et al. (2012))*; (K) a bioprinted Pluronic® F-127 fluorescent tube *(Reproduced/adapted with permission from Müller et al. (2015))*; (L) Polyethylene glycol hydrogel bioprinted into an aortic valve construct *(Reproduced/adapted with permission from Hockaday et al. (2012))*.

(Montembault et al., 2006). Due to its unstable mechanical properties and limited bioprintability (see Fig. 3.2C), chitosan is an appropriate material for cell encapsulation, but not for the formation of large-scale scaffolds (Geng et al., 2005). Chitosan has been used in EBB for bioprinting of perfusable vessel-like microfluidic channels, where chitosan was crosslinked by an ionic crosslinker, sodium hydroxide (NaOH) (Zhang et al., 2013a,b). The polymer and the crosslinker solution were printed simultaneously using a coaxial nozzle unit with the crosslinker solutions in the inner core diffusing out toward the polymer resulting in hollow tubular constructs. Bioprinting of chitosan using DBB and EBB has not yet been attempted.

Collagen type I is a triple helical biocompatible protein obtained from natural sources which has been extensively used in bioprinting (Ferreira et al., 2012). It is one of the major components of connective tissues and occupies about 25% of the entire protein mass in most mammals. Collagen is a highly conserved protein cross-species causing minimal immunological reactions. Collagen matrix facilitates not only cell adhesion but also enhances cell attachment and growth due to abundant integrin-binding domains. Although collagen type I has been used in bioprinting, it has limitations as it remains in a liquid state at low temperatures and forms a fibrous structure with increased temperature or neutral pH. Complete gelation can take up to half an hour at 37°C. This slow gelation rate makes bioprinting of 3D constructs difficult, since deposited collagen remains liquid for more than 10 min. Also, cells deposited in collagen are not homogeneously distributed, as gravity pulls down the cells before gelation takes place. Low mechanical properties and instability along with the abovementioned issues necessitate the use of supportive hydrogels for collagen. EBB has utilized collagen alone as a bioink (Smith et al., 2004); however, mixing it with Pluronic® has generated promising results (Homenick et al., 2011). The cell number increased significantly after 24 h postbioprinting demonstrating that collagen is suitable for cell growth. Fully crosslinked, bioprinted constructs can even be perfused (Lee et al., 2014b). DBB also takes advantage of collagen as a bioink material; however, collagen needs to be deposited before the onset of crosslinking (Deitch et al., 2008). In one study, Boland's group used collagen as a bioink constituent to investigate cell adhesion and proliferation on collagen-coated cell repellant substrates (Roth et al., 2004). Additionally, the same group fabricated a bilayer skin graft that generated neoskins on mice that are near-identical to native skin with microvessels (Yanez et al., 2014). As collagen possesses a fibrous microarchitecture, its use in inkjet bioprinting is highly limited, therefore microvalve bioprinting has been preferred. For example, fibrin-collagen bioink incorporating one of two cell types, AFSCs or mesenchymal stem cells (MSCs), was bioprinted using a valve-based bioprinter into wound sites as a treatment for skin burns (Skardal et al., 2012). Similarly, LBB has been successfully used to coat thin layers of collagen on a laser-absorbing material; due to collagen's sticky nature, it can be easily transferred using a laser source for fabrication of skin tissue constructs (see Fig. 3.2D) (Michael et al., 2013).

Fibrin is a hydrogel formed by the enzymatic reaction between thrombin and fibrinogen, the key proteins involved in blood clotting. It supports extensive cell growth and proliferation (Cui and Boland, 2009), plays a significant role in wound healing, and has been used in fabrication of skin grafts (Skardal et al., 2012; Yanez et al., 2014). Rheology of gelled fibrin has been extensively studied because of its nonlinear elasticity (Janmey et al., 2009). The fibrin network is comprised of filaments forming as soft complex that allows a high degree of deformation without breakage (Janmey et al., 2009). Human umbilical vein endothelial cells (HUVECs) exhibit angiogenic behavior when cocultured with fibroblasts in fibrin. This is an essential factor in the vascularization of large tissue constructs and provides an effective in vitro model for analysis of the fundamentals of the angiogenic process (Nakatsu et al., 2003). The disadvantage of using fibrin for in vivo applications is the possibility of a severe immune reaction or transmission of infectious diseases when heterologous proteins are used. To increase the efficacy and safety of fibrin hydrogels, bacteria and viruses must be inactivated or fibrinogen and thrombin produced as recombinant proteins by mammalian cell lines. In addition, the degradation of fibrin is rapid, which is not conductive to long-term culture. Due to the non–shear-thinning nature of fibrinogen and thrombin, fibrin is rarely extruded (see Fig. 3.2E). However, despite these drawbacks, a few studies have utilized fibrin (Gruene et al., 2011). Weak mechanical properties do not allow manipulation on fibrin after gelation rendering EBB of precrosslinked fibrin a challenge. However, bioprinting of the two components of fibrin is an ideal option for DBB. Bioprinting of thrombin is feasible using inkjet (piezo- or thermal inkjet) bioprinting, but fibrinogen leads to clogging issues with unstable droplet formation due to its fibrous nature. In general, fibrinogen at low concentrations (<2 mg/mL) is usable, but such a concentration range limits the mechanical properties of bioprinted constructs. Therefore, microvalve bioprinting is more convenient for DBB of fibrinogen (Gudapati et al., 2016). For example, thermal-inkjet bioprinting was employed for bioprinting human microvascular endothelial cells (HMVECs), but cell were loaded in culture media and precisely bioprinted on crosslinked fibrin (Cui and Boland, 2009). Cells aligned in fibrin and formed into an extensive capillary network after 21 days of culture. Fibrinogen and thrombin can be bioprinted from separate cartridges and combined on a platform to form a hydrogel; alternating layers of neural cells and fibrin gel were bioprinted generating viable neural constructs with a potential in neural engineering applications (Xu et al., 2006). Because of its prolonged crosslinking time and dependence on thrombin concentration, fibrin is generally difficult to print into a designed shape. Fibrin is not a suitable bioink material for LBB due to its delicate structure; however, it can be mixed with other LBB compatible hydrogels such as hyaluronic acid (HA) (Gruene et al., 2011).

Gelatin, a denatured form of collagen protein, is used in food and pharmaceutical industries (Liang et al., 2004; Gómez-Guillén et al., 2011). It is extracted from bones, skin, and connective tissues of animals (Gómez-Guillén et al., 2002). At low temperatures, gelatin strands self-associate to form helical structures leading to a gel-like form, which reverts back to a random coil conformation as temperature increases (Chiou et al., 2008). Gelatin retains the Arg–Gly–Asp (RGD) sequence from its precursor, is less immunogenic, and promotes cell adhesion, differentiation, migration, and proliferation (Sakai et al., 2009). Gelatin in gel form can be obtained by thermally induced crosslinking, and it can easily liquefy at 37°C. The weight of unmodified gelatin gel decreases by 50% after around 10 h of incubation, and the gel completely dissolves within 24 h (Sakai et al., 2009). To avoid dissolution, a variety of chemical crosslinking methods have been examined; however, such methods are problematic in in situ and in vivo applications as crosslinking agents are toxic to cell-laden constructs (Liang et al., 2004). Popular enzymatic crosslinkers, such as transglutaminase, have been successfully used (Jin and Dijkstra, 2010). Other crosslinkers include horseradish peroxidase (HRP) and hydrogen peroxide (H_2O_2) (Sakai et al., 2009). Gelatin can be successfully gelled in vivo and remained intact for 1 week without inducing necrosis in surrounding tissues (Sakai et al., 2009). Gelatin-encapsulated cells demonstrate long-term viability, but limited cell elongation (Benton et al., 2009; Nichol et al., 2010). Gelatin is rarely bioprinted in its native form due to its poor mechanical properties. To employ gelatin for bioprinting, it has been chemically crosslinked by the addition of agents such as glutaraldehyde (Hellio and Djabourov, 2006). The free amine groups along the gelatin polymer backbone undergo a nucleophilic addition reaction followed by dehydration with the two aldehyde groups of glutaraldehyde that form an imine functional group commonly referred to as a Schiff base (Hennink and van Nostrum, 2012). Often the degree of gelation depends on the pH of the medium. Molecules which are capable of accepting or losing protons with an increase or decrease in pH are sensitive to a change in the local pH environment. Using EBB, hepatocyte-laden gelatin was bioprinted into spatially defined 3D structures. Hepatocytes remained viable and conducted their biological functions for more than 2 months (Wang et al., 2006). Gelatin is, however, not a popular hydrogel for DBB. Some studies have been performed by blending fibrin with gelatin for liver tissue biofabrication (Xu et al., 2007). Boland et al. (2007) presented DBB of gelatin/alginate blend; however, $CaCl_2$ solution was selectively printed onto the blended solution for fabrication of cardiac constructs as can be seen in Fig. 3.2F. Gelatin has been successfully used in LBB due to its viscoelastic properties, stability, and ability to hold cells in precise positions without damaging cells (see Fig. 3.2G) (Raof et al., 2011). Additionally, its thermosensitive properties allow for cell transfer and ease of removal postprinting to reveal an application-specific growth surface.

Hyaluronic acid, a linear nonsulfated glycosaminoglycan, is ubiquitous in almost all connective tissues and a major ECM component of cartilage (Zhang et al., 2009). It behaves similar to collagen type I and has properties that can be beneficial in the treatment of osteoarthritis (Migliore and Granata, 2008). It is comprised of repeating disaccharide units of D-glucuronic acid and N-acetyl-D-glucosamine moieties linked by alternating β-1,4 and β-1,3 glycosidic linkages (Zhong et al., 1994). The three major functional groups, which govern the chemical activity of HA, are the glucuronic carboxylic acid group, the secondary hydroxyl group, and the N-acetyl group. Hyaluronic acid is widely used in tissue engineering due to its excellent biocompatibility and ability to form flexible hydrogels (Luo et al., 2000). Chemical modification of HA is an illustrative example of a bioink molecule polymerized by photo-crosslinking. To use HA as a bioink, chemical modifications of these groups are often carried out to enhance its rheological properties (Burdick and Prestwich, 2011); however, HA has slow gelation rate and poor mechanical properties. Hyaluronic acid is favored due to its role in early embryonic development, cell-friendly nature, and controllable mechanics, architecture, and degradation. Human embryonic stem cells encapsulated in HA, as opposed to 2D culture cells, maintained their phenotype, normal karyotype, and full differentiation capability (Gerecht et al., 2007). Additionally, the high molecular weight of HA adds an essential structural and organizational element into the ECM of native tissues (Kreger and Voytik-Harbin, 2009; Toole, 2004). It is instrumental in cell migration (Baier et al., 2007; Turley et al., 2002), nerve regeneration (Seidlits et al., 2010; Faroni et al., 2015; Ikeda et al., 2003), neuronal (Mészár et al., 2008; Banerjee and Toole, 1991; Margolis et al., 1975; Rauch et al., 2005; Baier et al., 2007) and glial development (Back et al., 2005; Liu et al., 2004), and wound healing (Aya and Stern, 2014). Hyaluronic acid has only minor cross-species variation and excellent biocompatibility (Dana et al., 2004; Leach et al., 2003). Pescosolido et al. (2011) developed a semiinterpenetrating network (semi-IPN) bioink by combining HA with a photopolymerizable dextran derivative (see Fig. 3.2H). In that study, a hydroxyethyl-methacrylate (HEMA) derivative of dextran was prepared by activating the HEMA group with N,N′-carbonyldiimidazole and coupled it to dextran, forming dex-HEMA. Hyaluronic acid/dextran-HEMA solutions were exposed to UV radiations in the presence of a photoinitiator inducing polymerization of the dextran chains. Hyaluronic acid moieties became entangled in the chemically crosslinked dextran network. Hyaluronic acid has been used in EBB but is generally blended with other hydrogels to enhance its bioprintability and solidification ability. For example, Skardal et al., 2010c used hyaluronic hydrogels crosslinked with tetrahedral PEG derivatives for bioprinting vessel-like constructs. To form extrudable ECM hydrogels, the symmetrical tetra-PEG molecules were acrylated to form tetraacrylates (TetraPAcs) then cocrosslinked with thiolated gelatin and HA derivatives. In another study conducted by the same group (Skardal et al., 2010a,b,c), methacrylated derivatives of gelatin and hyaluronic acid were synthesized separately and photo-crosslinked by a two-step process, before and after extrusion, to form more compact firm structures. Dynamic crosslinking of thiol-modified HA by gold nanoparticles was also studied to develop a hydrogel capable of reforming itself during and after bioprinting (Skardal et al., 2010a,b,c). Use of HA in DBB has not been demonstrated so far due to its viscous nature and slow gelation rate; however, it has been employed in LBB when combined with other hydrogels such as fibrin (Gruene et al., 2011) to facilitate faster crosslinking. The bioink consisting of human adipose-derived stem cells or endothelial colony-forming cells combined with hyaluronic acid and fibrinogen was coated on the donor slide and bioprinted using LIFT. The collector slide was blade-coated with HA-fibrinogen as well and subsequently crosslinked by thrombin. Alternating layers of HA-fibrinogen combined with both cell types were bioprinted to study the interaction between the two cell types.

Matrigel™ is a gelatinous ECM protein mixture secreted by Engelbreth-Holm-Swarm mouse sarcoma cells (Kleinman and Martin, 2005). It promotes cellular outgrowth from tissue fragments, vascularization, and differentiation of various cell types (Gaetani et al., 2012; Kleinman and Martin, 2005). One of the major advantages of culturing cells on Matrigel™ is that it promotes complex cellular behavior which is difficult to observe on other surfaces. For example, endothelial cells create capillary sprouts in Matrigel™ (Kleinman and Martin, 2005). Molecules promoting endothelial cell network formation (Paul et al., 2013) are potential candidates for use in tissue regeneration therapies while the molecules that inhibit such formation can be used for anticancer therapies. Matrigel™ has been vital in the development of tumor xenograft models in rodents for discovery of novel cancer treatments (Benton et al., 2011). Matrigel™ is an expensive material; however, it has the ability to create mechanically strong, 3D bioprinted constructs with higher cell survival rates than other popular hydrogels such as agarose and alginate (Melchels et al., 2012). Thermal gelation properties of Matrigel™ and collagen type I are similar; however, gelation of Matrigel™ is thermally reversible. Crosslinking occurs between 24 and 37°C, and gelation takes about half an hour, beginning at temperatures above 4°C. In EBB, Matrigel™ needs to be bioprinted before becoming fully crosslinked; thus, a cooling chamber is essential. To accelerate the crosslinking process after deposition and maintain the printed shape, a heated plate should be employed. In EBB, Matrigel™ has been used in a radioprotection study on human hepatic carcinoma and human mammary epithelial cells (see Fig. 3.2I) (Snyder et al., 2011), and osteo- and endothelial-progenitor cell printing (Fedorovich et al., 2011). For DBB, Matrigel™ has not been used as a bioink material but employed as a substrate to place and pattern cells (Horváth et al., 2015). Its thermal crosslinking property and optimal viscosity make it an attractive bioink for LBB. Matrigel™ has been used for developing cellular constructs with precisely placed cells using MAPLE-DW cell transfer. A study conducted by Schiele et al. (2009) involved encapsulation of many cell types, such as dermal fibroblasts, neural stem, myoblasts, breast cancer cells, and bovine pulmonary artery endothelial in Matrigel™. The donor slide was coated with Matrigel™ containing cells while the receiver was coated only with Matrigel™. In a similar study, 3D cellular constructs were fabricated using multiple layers of human osteosarcoma cells bioprinted onto Matrigel™ substrates, using LIFT technique (Barron et al., 2004).

3.2.1.1.3.2 SYNTHETIC HYDROGELS While natural polymers offer a favorable environment similar to native ECM for tissue engineering applications, synthetic polymers can be adapted according to the requirements of bioprinting processes. Synthetic polymers can be chemically modified not only with crosslinkable functional groups, but also with domains capable of enhancing the structural and mechanical properties of bioprinted constructs. This enables one to carefully engineer the design of the polymer backbone with either cell adhesive domains containing the RGD sequence or with domains responsive to external electric or magnetic stimulus.

Methacrylated gelatin, the denatured form of collagen consisting of methacrylate (MA) groups conjugated to its amine side groups, has been used for tissue engineering due to its favorable biological and adjustable mechanical characteristics (Nichol et al., 2010; Benton et al., 2009). Despite low cell proliferation rates, GelMA has relatively high mechanical strength and low swelling ratio and is amenable to blending with other hydrogels to increase cell survival. In 5% micropatterned GelMA, cells elongated, migrated, and formed interconnected networks with surrounding cells (Nichol et al., 2010). At higher concentrations, 10% or 15%, cells do not migrate; however, individual cells showed limited elongation and some multicellular networks formed. Methacrylated gelatin is frequently used in EBB studies such as bioprinting of chondrocytes (Schuurman et al., 2013), liver cells (Visser et al., 2013; Schuurman et al., 2013; Bertassoni et al., 2014; Billiet et al., 2014), and MSCs (Du et al., 2015). It has low viscosity at room temperature and is easy to extrude, and its crosslinking rate can be manipulated by the length of exposure to UV light. Methacrylated gelatin forms a biomimetic (Nichol et al., 2010) as well as an enzymatically degradable (Hutson et al., 2011) hydrogel that is mechanically strong when photo-crosslinked in the presence of a photoinitiator. For example, Demirci's group bioprinted bone morphogenetic protein-2 (BMP-2) and transforming growth factor (TGF-β1) using DBB on a GelMA substrate to mimic a native fibrocartilage microenvironment. This substrate differentiated bioprinted human MSCs toward osteogenic and chondrogenic lineages in a spatial manner (Gutkan, 2014). Methacrylated gelatin has also been combined with other synthetic polymers such as polyethylene glycol diacrylate (PEGDA) and photo-crosslinked by Eosin Y-based photoinitiator (Wang et al., 2015b). Crosslinking ability with visible light, long-term biocompatibility, bioprintability, and enhanced rheology are some of the advantageous features of this bioink formulation. Scaffolds with a porous architecture based on GelMA have also been bioprinted using LBB, where HUVECs spread over scaffold within 4 days (Gauvin et al., 2012) (see Fig. 3.2J). Recently, Ovsianikov et al. (2014) demonstrated the first bioprinting of cells using 2PP. MG63 cells were encapsulated in GelMA hydrogel loaded with water-soluble photoinitiators. Ying-Yang structures were then bioprinted with solid and hollow parts, where cells exposed to the laser were damaged; however, they were able to proliferate and filled all the available space in 3 weeks of in vitro culture.

Pluronic® F-127 is a trade name for synthetic polymer poloxamer-based polymeric compound. It exhibits a polymeric architecture consisting of two hydrophilic blocks between a hydrophobic block making it an effective surfactant (Mesa et al., 2005). There are 11 types of Pluronic® polymers which differ by molar mass, percentage of composites, functionality, and temperature of crosslinking which can vary from 10 to 40°C (Wang et al., 2015a). Pluronic® undergoes reverse gelation as it starts to crosslink with increasing temperature. Pluronic® copolymer structures erode quickly and cannot hold structural integrity for longer than a few hours; however, Pluronic®, in combination with other hydrogels such as PEG, is useful for drug delivery and controlled release applications (Gong et al., 2009). Increase of mechanical strength was shown also by addition of methacrylated hyaluronic acid (MeHA) and then bioprinted into a fluorescent tube (see Fig. 3.2K) (Müller et al., 2015). The study performed by Vashi et al. (2008) showed that bone marrow–derived MSCs were able to interact with each other in a 3D Pluronic® environment and adipogenic induction started after 4 days of culture. Pluronic®, without any additives, can maintain the viability of cells for up to 5 days with a dramatic decrease thereafter. However, when supplemented with 60 nM hydrocortisone, cell viability was preserved even in higher concentrations of Pluronic® (Khattak et al., 2005). Pluronic® can be cured by UV light for bioink applications; however, the radiation type and duration can impact cell viability, and the concentration of the photoinitiator can affect the metabolic activity of cells. Chemical crosslinking can make the gel more resistant to thermal degradation[33]. Pluronic® can be crosslinked enzymatically whereby two ends of PEO side chains can be formed into self-assembled micelles (Lee et al., 2011). Pluronic® does not lose its thermally reversible properties, but its mechanical strength increases with enzymatic crosslinking. In EBB, acceptable bioprintability of Pluronic® is obtained above 20°C as it becomes more viscous and exhibits shear-thinning behavior. Therefore, Pluronic®, depending on its concentration, requires a heating system around the needle to transition from liquid to gel state; a heated plate to maintain the temperature of the construct after deposition should also be considered. Nonetheless, it is more advantageous to maintain Pluronic® in a semiliquid state to preserve cell viability in homogeneous suspension. In the case of prolonged bioprinting times, a cooling system might be needed to maintain a lower temperature in the bioink reservoir. The reversible properties of Pluronic® can be useful in fabrication of complex constructs. Pluronic® in solid form (at room temperature or higher) can be surrounded by a second type of hydrogel and then placed at 4°C to liquefy the Pluronic®. This procedure creates perfusable channels within bulky cell-laden constructs (Wu et al., 2011). The thermosensitive nature of Pluronic® and its high viscosity is problematic for DBB and so has not been used. LBB has not been attempted as Pluronic® is not viscoelastic, maintains a solid coating on the quartz support, and cannot transfer thermal energy to kinetic energy, which is essential for jet formation.

PEG has been widely used in medical and nonpharmaceutical products (Lin and Anseth, 2009; Pasut et al., 2008; Alexander et al., 2013; Wang et al., 2015a). It is a linear polyether hydrophilic compound which can be conjugated with proteins (Alconcel et al., 2011; Zhang et al., 1998), enzymes (Pasut et al., 2008), liposomes (Ishida et al., 2005), and other biomolecules. It has been employed as a drug delivery agent (Veronese and Pasut, 2005; Lin and Anseth, 2009; Alconcel et al., 2011) and used in biosensing or signaling (Sharma et al., 2004) and pharmaceutical applications (Alconcel et al., 2011). Because PEG is a hydrophilic polymer, it resists protein adsorption and cell adhesion. Hence, some cells, particularly chondrocytes and osteoblasts, encapsulated in PEG survive well even without addition of biological constituents (Benoit et al., 2006). Other cell types may require additional cell adhesion components, such as RGD peptides or fibronectin coating. Fibronectin precoating improves cell adhesion, spreading, and the organization of the actin cytoskeleton (Vladkova et al., 1999). PEGylation inhibits protein adsorption making PEG a very useful synthetic polymer for bioprinting of tissue constructs for regenerative medicine. PEG is water soluble, and its mechanical properties can be manipulated through variation of its chemistry (Gao et al., 2015). Altering the composition of PEG-based hydrogels in tandem with photo-crosslinkage in the presence of a photoinitiator allows alterations to the structural, functional, and mechanical properties of fabricated tissues. One of the major limitations of PEG is its poor mechanical strength; therefore, addition of diacrylate (DA) of MA is highly beneficial. However, additives such as DA and MA require photo-crosslinking by exposure to UV light for a specific length of time to obtain the desired mechanical properties. Excessive exposure to UV light can dramatically reduce cell viability. For example, rat aortic smooth muscle cells have been successfully photoencapsulated in PEG with 20 s of UV exposure (Mann et al., 2001). PEG was also used in creation of microgels that were assembled in seconds using acoustic waves (Xu et al., 2011). PEGDA and polyethylene glycol methacrylate (PEGMA) hydrogels are used in all types of bioprinting modalities: EBB (Hockaday et al., 2012; Wüst et al., 2014; Bertassoni et al., 2014; Skardal et al., 2010c), DBB (Cui et al., 2012a,b), and LBB (Hribar et al., 2014). Photopolymerization of PEG-based hydrogels with tunable mechanical properties has been widely demonstrated using EBB. Hockaday et al. (2012) performed 3D printing of anatomically correct aortic valve scaffolds using PEGDA hydrogels (see Fig. 3.2L). Scaffolds were then seeded with porcine aortic valve interstitial cells, where cells demonstrated adhesion with minimum spreading or proliferation in 21 days. Earlier work, however, demonstrated that the immobilization of cell adhesion sites and growth factors during EBB promoted cell spreading and proliferation (Zhang et al., 1998; Fedorovich et al., 2007). Due to greater mechanical stiffness compared to naturally derived polymers, such as alginate, fibrin, agarose, and collagen type I, PEG has been extensively used in DBB. Using thermal inkjet bioprinting, Cui et al. (2012a,b) bioprinted human articular chondrocytes in PEGDMA into osteochondral plugs in a layer-by-layer fashion with UV exposure following each layer, producing a 3D scaffold with uniform allocation of cells and neocartilage formation. In a similar study, acrylated-PEG was bioprinted with acrylated-RGD peptide, followed by photopolymerization of the bioprinted layer (Gao et al., 2015). Bone marrow–derived human MSCs were suspended in PEGDMA in conjunction with hydroxyapatite (HA) nanoparticles and bioactive glass and bioprinted using a thermal inkjet bioprinter (Gao et al., 2014), which conferred spatial control of the distribution of cells and bioactive ceramic materials in the fabricated bone tissue constructs. PEG-based hydrogels have been widely used in LBB, including SLA and DOPsL. Bioprinting using SLA was first demonstrated with a commercial SLA 3D printer (SLA-250, 3D Systems), where Chinese hamster ovary cells were encapsulated in PEGDMA with over 90% cell viability (Dhariwala et al., 2004). In a similar approach, the same 3D printer equipped with He–Cd laser was used for encapsulation of 3T3 fibroblasts in PEGDMA to fabricate well-defined cylindrical scaffolds with multiple channels (Arcaute et al., 2006). In addition to SLA applications, DOPsL enabled fabrication of vascularized tissue construct using PEGDA hydrogels to study the migration behavior of HeLa cells (Huang et al., 2014). It was demonstrated that HeLa cells migrated significantly when the vasculature diameter was decreased.

Table 3.1 provides sample bioprinting and bioink formulation parameters along with bioprinters used in EBB, DBB, and LBB of all the hydrogels presented in this chapter.

Table 3.1 Detailed Characteristic of Bioprinting Parameters of Hydrogels Using EBB, DBB, and LBB

	Process Type	Crosslinking Properties: Type	Crosslinking Properties: Time	Concen Tration	Bioprinting Parameters	Construct Size	Cell-Related Attributes: Type	Cell-Related Attributes: Density (Million/mL)	Cell-Related Attributes: Viability (%)	Bioprint Ability	Bioprinter Used	References
Agarose	EBB	Thermal	Minutes	0.3%	n/a	2.5 mm	MSCs	0.1	98.8	High	custom-made	(Duarte Campos et al., 2014)
	DBB	Thermal	1–2 h	1.5%	n/a	6 mm × 6.5 mm	CHO: motoneurons	5: 2	90	High	HP Desktop 550C	(Xu et al., 2005)
Alginate	EBB	Ionically: $CaCl_2$	Seconds	2%	200 kPa, 17 mm/s	430 μm diameter	BMSC	0.25	95	High	Bioplotter	(Fedorovich et al., 2008)
		Ionically: $CaSO_4$	10 min	2%	72.3 kPa, 10 mm/s	19 mm × 6 mm	n/a	n/a	n/a	High	Fab@Home	(Cohen et al., 2010a)
		Ionically: $CaCl_2$	Precross linked	3%	n/a	20 mm × 20 mm × 3 mm	gMSCs	10	n/a	High	Bioscaffolder	(Poldervaart et al., 2013)
			n/a	1–2%	50–300 kPa, 1–30 mm/s	20 mm × 20 mm × 2 mm	BMSCs	0.25	95	High	Bioplotter	(Fedorovich et al., 2008)
	DBB	Ionically: $CaCl_2$	n/a	1%	60 Hz, echo and dwell time 45 μs	10 mm × 5 mm	NIH 3T3	5	90.8	High	Platform-assisted 3D inkjet bioprinting system	(Christensen et al., 2015)
	LBB	Ionically: $CaCl_2$	n/a	0.1–1%	4.5–9 μJ, 160-80 cm/s	3 mm × 1.5 mm	HUVECs	40–100	n/a	High	Custom-made	(Guillotin et al., 2010)
			Seconds	1–8%	193 nm, 85% transmit., 1.5 mm/s	100 μm	n/a	n/a	n/a	High	MAPLE-DW	(Yan et al., 2013)
Chitosan	EBB	pH-mediated: CH_3COOH	n/a	3%	89.6 kPa, 15 cm/min	10 mm × 10 mm × 5 mm	Adipose-derived stem cells	0.75	n/a	High	Custom-made	(Ye et al., 2014)
			2 h		200 kPa, 6 mm/s	2 × 2 cm	Porcine bone marrow cells	0.5	n/a	High	Custom-made	(Geng et al., 2005)
Collagen Type I	EBB	pH-mediated	Minutes	0.3%	11.7 kPa, 20 mm/s 10.3 kPa, 15 mm/s	200 μm 800 μm	BAECs	5–20	33 86	Average Low	BioAssembly Tool	(Smith et al., 2004)
		pH: $NaHCO_3$ and cooled under 20°C	1 min	0.223%	0–13.8 kPa, Valve operating time, 600-150 μs	1 mm × 10 mm × 10 mm	Fibroblasts	1	95	High	custom-made	(Lee et al., 2010a)
	DBB	pH-mediated and thermal	1–2 h	0.1%	n/a	6 mm × 6.5 mm	CHO, motoneurons	5;2	90	High	HP Desktop printer HP 550C	(Xu et al., 2005)
		pH-mediated	<2 h	0.025 –0.5%	n/a	23 mm × 3 mm	Rat cardiomyocytes	0.25	n/a	Low	HP DeskJet 500	(Deitch et al., 2008)

Continued

Table 3.1 Detailed Characteristic of Bioprinting Parameters of Hydrogels Using EBB, DBB, and LBB—cont'd

		Crosslinking Properties					Cell-Related Attributes					
	Process Type	Type	Time	Concen Tration	Bioprinting Parameters	Construct Size	Type	Density (Million/ mL)	Viability (%)	Bioprint Ability	Bioprinter Used	References
Fibrin	DBB	Enzymatic fibrinogen [F]–thrombin [T]	Seconds	10 mg/mL [F]; 20 U/ mL [T]	250,000 drops/s	25 mm × 5 mm × 1 mm	NT2 neurons	2	74.27	Low	HP Desktop 550	(Xu et al., 2006)
			6 min	60 mg/mL [F]; 50 U/ mL [T]	Droplets 130 pl; 10 μs pulse	8 mm × 1.8 mm	Human microvascular endothelial cell	1–8	n/a	Low	HP Deskjet 400	(Cui and Boland, 2009)
Gelatin	EBB	Thermal	5 min	20%	5 psi	5 mm × 5 mm × 3 mm	Hepatocytes	1	90 after 45 days	Average	n/a	(Wang et al., 2006)
			n/a	7%	41.4–89.6 kPa, 450 –750 μs valve operating	1 mm × 10 mm × 10 mm	Fibroblasts	1	n/a	High	Custom-made	(Lee et al., 2010a)
	LBB	Thermal	7 min	20%	1.0 J/cm^2	1 mm × 1.5 mm	Fibroblasts	0.6	91	High	MAPLE-DW	(Schiele et al., 2011)
			n/a	n/a	10^7 × g, 122 m/s	n/a	Schwann, astroglial cells	2–6	80–85	Average	AFA-LIFT	(Hopp et al., n.d.)
Gelatin / Alginate	EBB	Ionically: $CaCl_2$	Precross linking	0.06%	5 mm/s	3 × 1 mm	NIH 3T3	10	84.6	High	Fab@Home	(Duan et al., 2013)
	DBB		90% in 5s	2 wt%	96.5–2000 Pa	250 μm × 300 μm × 3.5 mm			n/a	Average	MicroDrop	(Pataky et al., 2012)
Hyaluronic Acid	EBB	Photopoly merization; pH-mediated	3 min	1.5%	n/a	2 mm ring	HepG2, C3A, Int-407, NIH 3T3	25	n/a	Average	Fab@Home	(Skardal et al., 2010a,b,c)
		Photopoly merization	10 min	2–6%	n/a	n/a	Articular cartilage	5	n/a	Average	Bioscaffolder	(Pescosolido et al., 2011)
Matrigels™	EBB	Thermal	n/a	1:1 ratio with cells	11.7 Pa, 1 cm/s	0.75 cm × 1 cm	HepG2 and M10	1	n/a	Low	Roland DXY-1100 plotter	(Snyder et al., 2011)
			n/a	n/a	174 kPa, 30 cm/min	10 mm × 20 mm × 1 mm	gEPCs and MNCs	5	n/a	Low	Bioscaffolder	(Fedorovich et al., 2011)
	DBB		30 min	n/a	24.8 kPa, 20 mm/s, 17.86 Hz	1.12 mm	Alveolar EC, HUVECs	4.5	n/a	Low	BioFactory	(Horváth et al., 2015)
	LBB		n/a	n/a	193 nm, 300 Hz	3 × 3 array	Fibroblast, myoblast, neural stem cells, breast cancer cells	n/a	n/a	Average	MAPLE DW	(Schiele et al., 2009)

GelMA	EBB	Photopoly-merization	Minutes	10–20%	96.5–400 kPa, 30–70 cm/min	150–200 μm	HepG2	1.5	>97	High	Bioplotter pneumatic	(Billiet et al., 2014)
			10–60 s	5–15%	2 mm/s	750 μm	HepG2, NIH3T3	1–6	>75	High	NovoGen MMX Bioprinter	(Bertassoni et al., 2014)
	DBB		10 min	10–20%	300 dpi, 3.6 kHz	4 mm × 2 mm	Articular cartilage	5	63.2	High	HP Deskjet 500	(Cui et al., 2012a,b)
			30 s	5%	6.9 mW/cm^2	8 mm × 8 mm	MSCs, growth factors	1	90	High	custom-made	(Gutkan, 2014)
	LBB		20 s	10–15%	50 mW/cm^2	5 mm × 5 mm × 1 mm	HUVEC	0.02	n/a	High	Custom-made projection stereolithography system	(Gauvin et al., 2012)
Pluronic F-127	EBB	Thermal	Minutes	30%; 27% with cells	250 μm/s	2 mm × 2 mm × 1.5 mm	Human primary fibroblasts	0.8	60	High	BioAssembly Tool	(Smith et al., 2004)
				25%	50–300 kPa, 1–30 mm/s	20 mm × 20 mm × 2 mm	BMSCs	0.25; 0.5	85	High	Bioplotter	(Fedorovich et al., 2008)
			n/a	<10%; 20%	16.5 mW/cm^2, 3–6 mm/s	22 mm × 25 mm, 17 mm × 20 mm, 12 mm × 14 mm	PAVICs	0.5	91.3	High	Fab@Home	(Hockaday et al., 2012)
PEG	EBB	Photopoly-merization	Up to 19 min	10%	300 dpi, 3.6 kHz	4 mm	hMSCs	6	90	High	HP 51626A	(Gao et al., 2015)
	DBB		10 min	10–20%	4–8 mW/cm^2	5 mm	Human articular cartilage	5	89	High	HP Deskjet 500	(Xiaofeng Cui, Breitenkamp, Finn, et al., 2012a)

DBB, Droplet-based bioprinting; *EBB*, extrusion-based bioprinting; *HUVECs*, human umbilical vein endothelial cells; *LBB*, laser-based bioprinting; *LIFT*, laser-induced forward transfer; *GelMA*, methacrylated gelatin; *MAPLE-DW*, matrix-assisted pulsed laser evaporation-direct write; *MSC*, mesenchymal stem cell.

3.2.1.2 Decellularized Matrix Components

Cells secrete specific molecules to create ECM, a localized environment which fosters cell attachment, proliferation, signaling, and tissue development. In an attempt to recapitulate this natural tissue environment, a bioink material based on decellularized extracellular matrix (dECM) has been developed. Preparation of dECM bioink requires removal of cellular material using chemical, physical, and enzymatic processes without damage or loss of ECM (Ott et al., 2008). To determine if the matrix is fully decellularized, samples are evaluated by DNA quantification assays. Successful decellularization methods remove about 98% of the cellular content (Pati et al., 2014). The dECM is then further processed to generate a gel-like substance for use in bioprinting (see Fig. 3.3A1–A2). A recent study showed that bioprinted constructs of dECM and stem cells did not induce cytotoxicity or inflammation after in vivo implantation (Pati et al., 2015). Pati et al. printed a decellularized adipose tissue matrix loaded with human stem cells in tandem with melt extrusion of PCL (see Fig. 3.3B). As the printed dECM could not retain its shape postbioprinting, the printed PCL provided the structural frame necessary to maintain the stability of dECM (see Fig. 3.3C). dECM bioink supported high cell viability over 2 weeks in culture and promoted the expression of adipogenic genes without additional supplementation.

3.2.1.3 Microcarriers

Microcarriers are supportive structures for cell growth and expansion; they are made of synthetic (i.e., dextran, plastic, glass) or natural (cellulose, gelatin, and collagen) materials with specific engineered porosities (Malda and Frondoza, 2006). Typically, they have been used as reinforcement blocks in bioprinting (Turner and Flynn, 2012). The shape of microcarriers, interconnected pores in a spherical architecture, allows cells to attach and grow on the surface (see Fig. 3.4A). They provide an expansive monolayer environment, vastly improving the cell culturing process (Goh et al., 2013). Nutrient and gas transfer between the media and attached cells is more efficient than in 2D culture. Large numbers of cell-laden microcarriers can be suspended in cell media and cultured in environmentally controlled bioreactors. The surface of 1 g of microcarriers is

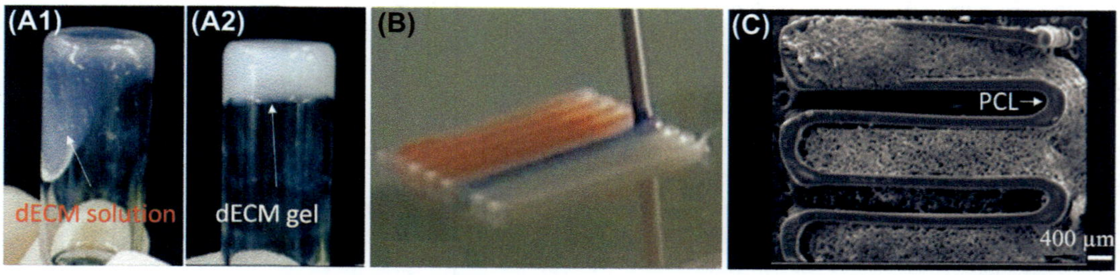

FIGURE 3.3 Bioprinting of Decellularized Extracellular Matrix (dECM). (A1–A2) Sol–gel transition of a dECM-based bioink prepared from porcine cartilage; (B–C) bioprinting of dECM required a PCL structural frame to support gelation of the bioink *(Reproduced/adapted with permission from Pati et al. (2014)).*

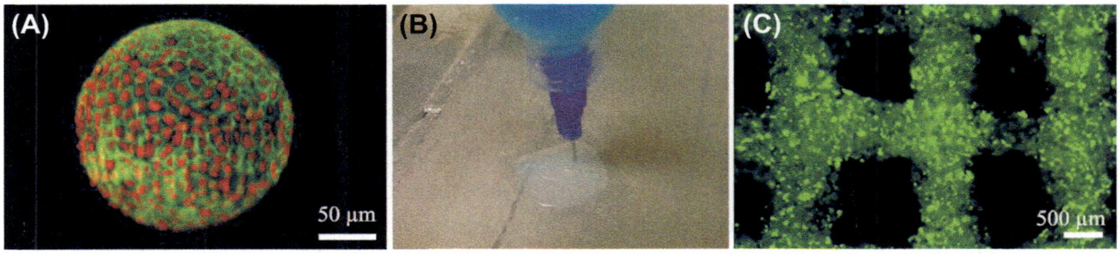

FIGURE 3.4 Bioprinting of Microcarriers. (A) A fluorescence image of a cell-laden microcarrier, where cell surface and nucleus were stained in green and red, respectively *(Reproduced/adapted with permission from Jakob et al. (2016)).* (B) A representative extrusion-based bioprinting process for deposition of microcarrier-laden hydrogels. (C) Bioprinted microcarriers loaded in GelMA hydrogels facilitates better cell–cell interactions *(Reproduced/adapted with permission from Levato et al. (2014)).*

equivalent to the surface of 15 75 cm^2 culture flasks (Malda and Frondoza, 2006). Moreover, they improve the compressive modulus of constructs, support differentiation of stem cells to desired lineages, and preserve phenotypic stability at high cell concentrations (Levato et al., 2014). Using EBB, microcarriers can be loaded and bioprinted in hydrogels, where a representative bioprinting process is illustrated in Fig. 3.4B. The ability to use high cell concentrations without compromising viability makes this a promising approach. Bioprinting MSCs preseeded on polylactic acid (PLA) microcarriers, Levato et al. (2014) showed that cells merely suspended in hydrogels exhibited less interaction, aggregation, and osteogenic differentiation than cell-loaded microcarriers in hydrogels (see Fig. 3.4C).

3.2.2 Scaffold-Free Bioink Materials

Evolution of organ development is based on cellular self-assembly mechanisms (Rivron et al., 2009). The cellular environment of a tissue construct needs to resemble its native counterpart for cells to maintain their phenotype, establish appropriate cell–cell interactions, and express tissue-specific proteins. 3D cell aggregate configurations provide a more hospitable environment for tissue self-assembly to occur than monolayer cell cultures. Tissue morphogenesis is dependent upon the formation of multicellular aggregates bound by cadherin molecules (Heilshorn et al., 2005; Albelda and Buck, 1990). Cadherin facilitates strong intercellular adhesion enabling signal transduction and an increase in integrin expression and binding to RGD motifs in the deposited ECM components (Behrens, 1999).

3.2.2.1 Tissue Spheroids

Tissue spheroids constitute a scaffold-free bioink type, where cells are organized spherically into 200- to 400-μm diameter cell aggregates that can serve as building blocks and tissue models for tissue engineering and pharmaceutics, respectively. Several techniques have been demonstrated for fabrication of tissue spheroids. One of the most popular methods is culturing cells in microwells with rounded ends on a cell adhesion inert mold made of hydrogels such as agarose (Dean et al., 2007; Mehesz et al., 2011; Livoti and Morgan, 2010), MeHA (Wheeldon et al., 2010), and alginate (Yamada et al., 2011). In this approach, thousands to millions of cells are seeded into an array of microwells and cultured for 24–48 h to facilitate cell aggregation (see Fig. 3.5A). Cells fall to the bottom of the microwells and settle in close contact with each other, driving the cells to spontaneously adhere to one another to minimize free energy and develop into a neotissue (Athanasiou et al., 2013). Over time, as tissue spheroids are formed, their size diminishes due to radial contraction; this is attributed to intracellular cytoskeletal reorganization from cadherin-mediated cell–cell binding (Akkouch et al., 2015). Other approaches are also used in tissue spheroid fabrication. One is the hanging drop method (Del Duca et al., 2004), which relies on self-assembly driven by gravity. A cell suspension in a small volume (15–30 μl) is pipetted onto the lid surface of a tissue culture plate. After inverting the lid, the droplets remain attached; however, gravity concentrates the cells at the bottom of droplet facilitating aggregation of cells. Microfluidic-assisted technology is another approach enabling cell aggregation inside cell traps (Jin et al., 2011; Torisawa et al., 2009; Zhang et al., 2014). Usually constructed by polydimethylsiloxane (PDMS) stamping, U-shape traps are created on an angled perfusion channel. During perfusion, cells are entrapped within U-shape and begin aggregation on contact. The device can be set in the vertical position to increase the effect of gravity. The major advantage of this method is the improved oxygen and media flow around the aggregates, which prevents necrosis. The major disadvantage is the difficulty of extraction of intact aggregates from PDMS. Another recent method is acoustic wave–assisted cell assembly (Guo et al., 2015) where cells are deposited onto a membrane, which vibrates in a specific frequency to form defined shapes.

Bioprinting of tissue spheroids has been performed using EBB only (Mironov et al., 2009); as shown in Fig. 3.5B, tissue spheroids within the gel medium can be loaded into a dispensing tip using slight mechanical pressure and extruded one by one to generate a precise spatial conformation (see Fig. 3.5C) for a construct in "T" shape. The speed of this process is driven by a mechanical ram which extrudes the bioink through a pipette

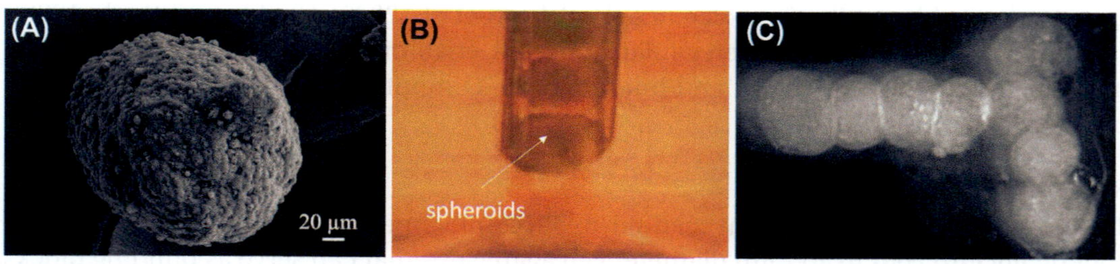

FIGURE 3.5 Bioprinting of Tissue Spheroids. (A) A sample heterocellular tissue spheroid made of beta (β)-TC3 mouse insulinoma and rat heart microvascular endothelial cells. (B) Tissue spheroids can be bioprinted one by one using a piston-driven mechanism in a pipette tip (C) for fabrication of larger scale tissue constructs *(Reproduced/adapted with permission from Mironov et al. (2009)).*

unit. Along with spheroids, an agarose support structure (mold) is also printed to support fusion and maturation of the deposited spheroids. Over time, spheroids fuse to each other creating larger scale tissues that can be easily removed from the mold (Norotte et al., 2009). Instead of using a mold support, a recent work demonstrated the bioprinting of spheroids by picking them from a reservoir and placing and skewering them on a needle array (Itoh et al., 2015).

3.2.2.2 Cell Pellet

The cell pellet technique is based on centrifugal or gravitational forces that concentrate cells at the bottom of conical tube (Khalil et al., 2001). The pellet can then be transferred to a micropipette or other mold where intercellular interactions are further established to improve cohesion (see Fig. 3.6A). The cell pellet technique is a practical method to create aggregates without the need for sophisticated systems; however, medium and oxygen circulation is limited, and cell viability decreases markedly after 24 h. One notable exception is chondrocytes, where a low oxygen level is desirable for enhanced production of ECM, including collagen type II and chondrogenic proteins (Schrobback et al., 2012). Cell pellet–based bioink has been used in EBB where the pellet was extruded into a confined space generated by 3D printing of a supporting agarose mold as demonstrated in Fig. 3.6B (Ozler et al., 2015). As shown in Fig. 3.6C, the agarose support mold facilitated aggregation of cells resulting in tissue constructs [i.e., nerve grafts (Owens et al., 2013) and aortic constructs (Kucukgul et al., 2015)].

3.2.2.3 Tissue Strands

Tissue strands can be defined as cylindrical neotissues that are engineered for bioprinting of scale-up tissues (Yu et al., 2016; Akkouch et al., 2015). The process for tissue strand formation has been recently established (Yu and Ozbolat, 2014). Cells at very high density are injected and packed into hollow alginate tubes. Semipermeable alginate tubes allow the exchange of medium with nutrition and oxygen; the cells grow in given

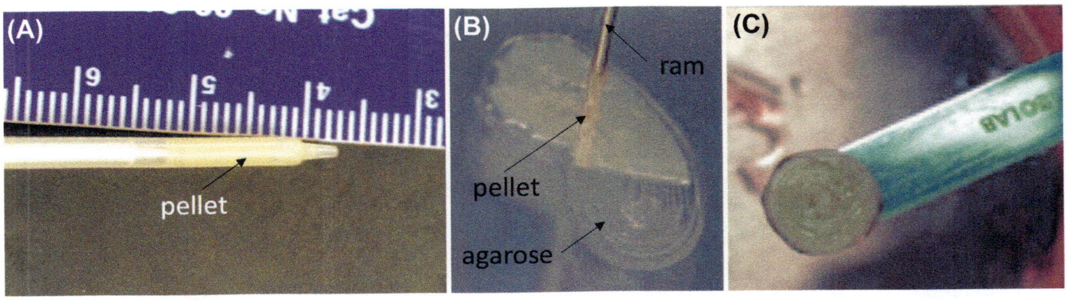

FIGURE 3.6 Bioprinting Cell Pellet. (A) Cell pellet can be injected into in a custom syringe to increase its cohesiveness. (B) Bioprinting of the cell pellet requires three-dimensional printing of an agarose mold structure for facilitation of cell aggregation and tissue maturation, (C) where the bioprinted heterocellular pellet (consisting of mouse aortic smooth muscle cells, 3T3 mouse fibroblasts, and human umbilical vein endothelial cells) aggregated into a tissue construct *(Reproduced/adapted with a permission from Ozler et al. (2015)).*

shape as they do not attach to the alginate luminal surface. When cells aggregate into a neotissue (see Fig. 3.7A), the tube is dissolved using a decrosslinker solution. The formed tissue strand is then placed into a custom-made bioprinter head and extruded mechanically (see Fig. 3.7B). Tissue strands must be optimally matured to ensure appropriate bioprinting conditions. Immature strands that are not fully aggregated may not form the desired shape and can disintegrate during bioprinting. Tissue strands that are overmature may not be malleable enough for deposition. A low level of oxygen in the core of strands may be a drawback for some tissue constructs; however, this method is especially suitable for cartilage formation (see Fig. 3.7C1–C3), as chondrocytes preferentially proliferate in hypoxic conditions (Schrobback et al., 2012).

3.3 Comparative Evaluation of Bioink Materials

In this section, currently available bioink materials are compared and evaluated based on several performance metrics including their (1) compatibility with different bioprinting modalities, (2) bioprintability, (3) biomimicry, (4) resolution, (5) affordability, (6) scalability, (7) practicality, (8) mechanical and structural integrity, (9) bioprinting and postbioprinting maturation times, (10) degradability, (11) commercial availability, (12) immunogenicity, and (13) applications and are summarized in Table 3.2.

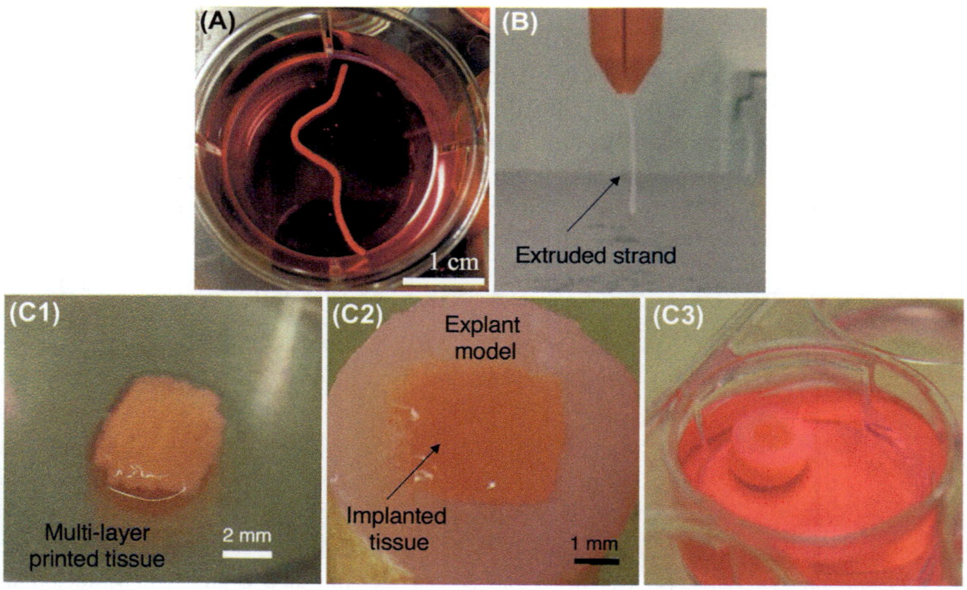

FIGURE 3.7 Bioprinting of Tissue Strands. (A) A tissue strand made of fibroblasts maintains its structural integrity during a prolonged in vitro culture *(Reproduced with permission from Akkouch et al. (2015))*. (B) Cartilage tissues strands were extruded using a custom-made nozzle and (C1) assembled into larger scale tissue patches in 3 weeks (C2–C3) for ex vivo implantation purposes *(Reproduced from Yu et al. (2016))*.

Table 3.2 Comparison of Bioink Types Used in Bioprinting Processes

		Hydrogels	Decellularized Matrix	Microcarriers	Tissue Spheroids	Cell Pellet	Tissue Strands
Process Capabilities	Resolution	High	Medium	Low	Low	Medium	Low
	Accuracy	High	Medium	Low	Low	Medium	Low
	Bioprinting time	Short	Medium–long	Short	Long	Medium–long	Long
	Processing modes	EBB, DBB, LBB	EBB	EBB	EBB	EBB	EBB
	Cell viability	High	Medium–high	High	Medium–high	Medium–high	Medium–high
	Control of single cell printing	High	Low	Low	Low	Low	Low
	Throughput	High	Medium–high	Medium–high	Low	Medium–high	Medium–high
Bioink Capabilities	Bioink mode	Liquid, sol–gel, solid	Liquid	solid	solid	Liquid	solid
	Bioprintability	High	Low–medium	High	Low	Low–medium	Low
	Bioink viscosity	Low–high	Medium–high	n/a	n/a	Medium–high	n/a
	Multicellular feasibility	Yes	Yes	Yes	Yes	Yes	Yes
	Affordability	\$–\$\$\$	\$\$	\$	\$\$\$	\$\$	\$\$\$
	Commercial availability	Yes	No	Yes	Yes	No	No
End Product Capabilities	Cell interactions	Low	Medium	Medium	High	High	High
	Mechanical and structural integrity	Low–high	Low–medium	Very high	Medium–high	Low–medium	High
	Tissue regeneration time	Medium–long	Short–medium	Medium	Short	Short–medium	Short
	Tissue biomimicry	Low–medium	Medium–High	Low	High	Medium–High	High
	Applications	Tissue engineering, transplantation, drug testing, cancer research	Tissue engineering	Tissue engineering, cell proliferation	Tissue engineering, transplantation, drug testing, cancer research	Tissue engineering, drug testing	Tissue engineering, transplantation

Continued

Table 3.2 Comparison of Bioink Types Used in Bioprinting Processes—cont'd

	Hydrogels	Decellularized Matrix	Microcarriers	Tissue Spheroids	Cell Pellet	Tissue Strands
Advantages	Wide range of capabilities, high resolution, easy o bioprint, wide range of bioprinter types	High biomimicry	Great mechanical properties, economical, high cell seeding capacity	High tissue biomimicry and cell–cell interactions	High cell–cell interactions	High tissue biomimicry, and cell–cell interactions, scalable
Disadvantages	Degradation-related issues, limited cell–cell interactions	Expensive and labor intensive, structurally weak, no commercial availability	Low resolution and accuracy, degradation-related issues	Low resolution and accuracy, difficult to bioprint	Need a supporting mold structure, low printing resolution	Difficult to bioprint, low printing resolution, no commercial availability

DBB, Droplet-based bioprinting; *EBB*, extrusion-based bioprinting; *LBB*, laser-based bioprinting.

3.3.1 Compatibility With Bioprinting Modalities

Although there are a wide variety of bioink materials, including hydrogels, dECM, microcarriers, and cell aggregates, not all of the currently available bioprinting modalities are compatible with every bioink material. EBB has the greatest flexibility among existing bioprinting modalities, due to the extrusion mechanism as well as the larger nozzle diameters. EBB can facilitate bioprinting of hydrogels, cell aggregates (in spheroid, strand, and cell pellet form), dECM components, and microcarriers in bulk hydrogels. Other bioprinting modalities including DBB and LBB support bioprinting of hydrogels only. Since the nozzle orifice diameter in DBB is very small [<120 μm (Ozbolat and Hospodiuk, 2016)], bioprinting of cell aggregates and microcarriers is challenging as the nozzle tip can easily clog and does not support formation of droplets as previously discussed (Gudapati et al., 2016). Although not yet attempted, DBB of dECM is technically feasible assuming the dECM viscosity is low and does not generate a fibrous gel. In LBB, bioprinting of cell aggregates, dECM, and microcarriers has not been attempted; however, due to the large mass of microcarriers and cell aggregates, bioprinting with LBB will represent a technical challenge.

3.3.2 Bioprintability

The bioprintability of hydrogels is superior to that of other bioink types. As long as the crosslinking mechanism is incorporated into the layer-by-layer fabrication scheme, bioprinting of hydrogels is relatively straightforward as other bioink types require additional processes and customized systems for the extrusion setup. For example, cell aggregates need to be loaded in a custom-made extrusion head. Tissue spheroids need to be loaded into a pipette unit and delivered in a medium (Tan et al., 2014). The act of loading cell aggregates into the pipette unit can be problematic as tissue spheroids can start to aggregate; this can result in nozzle clogging. In addition, it is difficult to attain the necessary close contact between spheroids postbioprinting, resulting in poor tissue formation. Extrusion of cell pellets, on the other hand, is relatively straightforward; however, an additional support structure (such as agarose mold) should be printed in tandem to support aggregation of cells. Tissue strands, on the other hand, can be bioprinted in solid form without the need for a molding structure or a delivery medium. However, it is crucial that the strands are engineered to be both malleable and mechanically strong to facilitate proper bioprinting (Yu et al., 2016). Bioprinting dECM requires 3D printing of a frame to structurally support the dECM until full gelation is complete. Recent work demonstrated 3D printing of dECM with PCL (Pati et al., 2014), but degradation of the PCL structure is problematic when the printed construct is implanted in vivo. Bioprinting microcarriers is relatively straightforward, but loading them at high densities can cause nozzle clogging issues.

3.3.3 Biomimicry

Cell encapsulation in hydrogels allows patterning of cells; however, subsequent ECM formation, digestion and degradation of the hydrogel matrix, interactions and proliferation of encapsulated cells are all issues that require careful attention. There are intrinsic limitations associated with cell encapsulation in hydrogels such as restricted cell interactions, proliferation, and colonization of immobilized cells within the hydrogel matrix, and the inability of cells to spread, stretch, and migrate to successfully generate the new tissue, particularly at high hydrogel concentrations (Ozbolat, 2015a). Cell aggregate–based bioink materials, however, exhibit better biomimetic characteristics facilitating both homo- and heterocellular interactions due to high cell densities and lack of exogenous matrix immobilization. These tissue constructs closely resemble the native tissue and preserve cell phenotype and functionality for extended periods of times. Microcarriers in hydrogels also allow better interaction between cells due to inherent high cell density. Decellularized matrix components provide a highly biomimetic environment for cell proliferation and differentiation as they are comprised of matrix proteins essential for cellular activities.

3.3.4 Resolution

Resolution of bioprinting processes depends on the bioprinting modality as well as the bioink. When bioprinting cells in hydrogels using LBB, 5.6 ± 2.5 μm resolution can be achieved (Ozbolat and Yu, 2013). In DBB and EBB, the range can increase to approximately 50 and 100 μm, respectively (Ozbolat and Yu, 2013). Incorporating cell aggregates and microcarriers into EBB can further deteriorate the resolution. Particularly, cell aggregates in spheroid and strand forms have a diameter ranging from 250 to 450 μm (Mehta et al., 2012; Yu et al., 2016). Although bioprinting of cell pellet can result in higher resolution compared to bioprinting of tissue spheroids and strands, a reduction in nozzle diameter can have detrimental effect on the cell pellet as cells are directly exposed to the shear stress rather than cushioned within a hydrogel matrix. Although original design structure can be closely fabricated using these bioink materials, most do not retain shape and will spread, shrink, or swell depending on the bioink and culture conditions.

3.3.5 Affordability

Most bioprintable hydrogels are affordable although some naturally derived hydrogels such as Matrigel™, fibrin, and collagen can be expensive. Microcarriers are also quite affordable as they are made of synthetic polymers (Malda and Frondoza, 2006). Cell aggregates, on the other hand, are expensive to produce and can require highly sophisticated approaches to their construction, as discussed previously. Hundreds of millions of cells are needed to prepare them in sufficient quantity, depending on the cell size and the rate of ECM deposition. Expansion of cells in these numbers is labor intensive, costly, and time-consuming. dECM-based bioink can also be expensive as a large amount of native tissue is needed to produce a small volume of bioink.

3.3.6 Scalability

In general, bioprintable hydrogels are scalable; the majority can be obtained in abundant quantities compared to cell aggregates and dECM. Although tissue spheroids are not easy to scale up, cell pellets or tissue strands provide relatively better scalability (Yu et al., 2016). dECM, on the other hand, currently lacks scalability as the original tissue yields a very small amount of dECM. Therefore, dECM can be considered scalable for bioprinting when reinforced with an affordable hydrogel. Microcarriers are smaller in size; however, they are scalable and can be loaded in hydrogels in higher densities as long as they do not clog the nozzle unit during bioprinting.

3.3.7 Practicality

Hydrogel-based bioink materials can be considered the most practical bioink type for bioprinting living tissues; the process can be as simple as loading cells into a hydrogel precursor solution. Different hydrogel types possess varying levels of ease in bioprinting, depending on their crosslinking mechanisms. Other bioink types can be challenging in terms of preparation and processing as well as bioprinting. For example, preparation of cell aggregates is labor intensive and time-consuming. The addition of hydrogels to the process may be necessary for delivery in an extrusion process, support aggregation of cells, or fusion of cell aggregates making the entire process quite complicated. For dECM preparation, well-established protocols are needed to generate the bioink with appropriate biological and biochemical characteristics. Moreover, the bioink needs to be loaded in a compatible hydrogel solution adding complexity to the process. Microcarriers, on the other hand, require the fabrication of porous biodegradable delivery particles for initial seeding of the cells. Upon satisfactory attachment and spreading of cells, microcarriers are then loaded in a hydrogel solution for the bioprinting mission. With the exception of hydrogels (excluding blend hydrogels requiring multiple crosslinking mechanisms), all other bioink types are a multistep approach and, therefore, are not considered practical.

3.3.8 Mechanical and Structural Integrity

Hydrogels and dECM components provide superior structural support for cells in 3D until they are able to secrete their own ECM. Mechanical and structural properties of hydrogels depend on their type and concentration; a lower concentration is more supportive of cell proliferation and growth, but demonstrates inferior mechanical properties. Microcarriers, on the other hand, provide a mechanically strong 3D scaffold as an environment for cells. Cell aggregates have no structural and mechanical support at the beginning of neotissue formation; later, cells support each other through cadherin-mediated cell–cell adhesion followed by ECM deposition (Takeichi, 1988), which lends further integrity to the 3D structure. Depending on the cell type used, mechanical properties alter over time. Parenchymal cells of metabolically highly active organs such as liver, pancreas, and heart do not secrete many ECM components, and the resulting cell aggregates are very weak in their mechanical and structural integrity. Therefore, supporting stromal cells should be cocultured to provide enough strength for bioprinting purposes. Although mechanical properties are important, they can affect the diffusion and permeability of the bioink adversely. In general, permeability of cell aggregates is lower than that of hydrogels, and the diffusion of media and oxygen is limited. Cell aggregates over 400 μm can experience hypoxia at their core, curtailing cell survival (Mehta et al., 2012).

3.3.9 Bioprinting and Postbioprinting Incubation Time

The bioprinting time depends on the size and porosity of the construct as well as the resolution of the bioink. Generally, the bioprinting time of hydrogels and microcarriers loaded in hydrogels is shorter (i.e., few minutes). Bioprinting of dECM takes longer than hydrogels as bioprinting and solidification of the structural PCL support adds extra time. Bioprinting of cell aggregates such as tissue spheroids may take a significant amount of time using a pick-and-place type of robotic dispenser (i.e., minutes to an hour depending on the construct size and complexity) (Itoh et al., 2015). In addition, printing the supporting mold structure also contributes to prolonged fabrication times. Although the bioprinting step takes longer using cell aggregates, postprinting maturation and tissue formation time is significantly shorter than that of hydrogels and microcarrier-loaded hydrogels. Complete tissue fusion and maturation can be obtained successfully in a week, whereas this process is much longer with hydrogels (Yu and Ozbolat, 2014).

3.3.10 Degradability

Degradability of bioink materials depends on the selected hydrogels or their blend, concentrations, temperature, conditions (in vitro or in vivo), and presence of external additives. Hydrogels that are highly sensitive to external conditions are thermosensitive hydrogels, which are easy to dissolve, and thereby lose their shape if environmental conditions are not constant. Also, degradation can be varied by hydrolytic or enzymatic labile components within a hydrogel (Nicodemus and Bryant, 2008). Additionally, the presence of cells within hydrogels limits the choice of chemical formulations while still maintaining mechanical strength. Because of their hard polymer composition, microcarriers degrade slower than hydrogels and may release substance that is toxic to cells. In summary, the degradation rate of 3D constructs must be designed according to the application.

3.3.11 Commercial Availability

Both natural and synthetic hydrogels and microcarriers made of polymers, including PLA, glass, alginate, dextran, and acrylamide in different forms, are commercially available (Jakob et al., 2016; Malda and Frondoza, 2006). As tissue engineering and biofabrication technologies have advanced by leaps and bounds over the past decade, 3D culturing of cells has gained the attention of commercial enterprises and a wide array of spheroid models (such as tumor or other tissue models for drug screening) are now available (Alhasan et al., 2016). Despite substantial progress, there is still a great need for representative spheroid models for several tissue types in the research community. Tissue strands and dECM-based bioink materials are relatively new and are not currently available commercially.

3.3.12 Immunogenicity

The introduction of any biological or nonbiological material has the potential to induce an immune response when implanted into a host. In a recent study, hydrogels obtained from other species such as collagen type I obtained from rat tail generated a low-level of immune response as demonstrated by an in vitro lymphocyte proliferation assay (Murphy et al., 2013). Therefore, the bioink, such as hydrogels and dECM components, obtained from other species can induce an immune response. However, cell aggregates fabricated from autologous cells are not expected to elicit immunogenic issues.

3.3.13 Applications

Bioprinted tissue and organ constructs have been used in various fields including tissue engineering and regenerative medicine, drug screening, cancer research, and high-throughput assays (Ozbolat et al., 2016); however, not all bioink types have been utilized in these application areas yet. Hydrogels have been extensively used in bioprinting for tissue engineering and regenerative medicine as well as drug testing, cancer research, and high-throughput assays. Recently, cell aggregate–based bioink materials have been used in fabrication of tissue models for drug screening (Peng et al., 2016). Although the present bioink types detailed in this chapter have been used in tissue engineering and regenerative medicine research extensively, a clinical trial has yet to be performed.

3.4 Limitations

Despite the recent progress in development of new bioink materials for 3D bioprinting, there are still several challenges in this emerging field. Further advancements are essential in bioink technology including synthesis and processing of new materials for bioprinting. The main objectives are to minimize cell loss and maximize cell–cell interactions, vascularize large-scale tissue constructs, improve mechanical properties, and gain a comprehensive understanding of additional compounds for supporting 3D bioprinted constructs. Although a large number of hydrogels offer great potential for tissue engineering, a limited number has been adopted in bioprinting due to their lack of bioprintability.

Hydrogels are the most favorable material type for cell support; however, there are several weaknesses related to bioprinting. First, hydrogels do not contain specific ECM proteins for particular cell types. Therefore, they are unable to provide a native environment. Second, hydrogels encapsulate and confine cells, limiting their interactions. Also, it is difficult to achieve the same high cell density as in native tissues. The concentration of hydrogels also plays an important role as increased concentration improves mechanical properties, but limits biological activities. Also, more rigid hydrogels require higher pressure levels for extrusion or generation of droplets. A higher concentration of hydrogel lowers the mobility of cells resulting in limited cell proliferation and deposition of ECM proteins. The cellular microenvironment provided in hydrogels may differ significantly from native tissues. Hydrogels degrade much slower in vitro, due to the lack of enzymes, immune response, and blood flow. However, hydrogels must be designed to degrade in vivo in a synchronized manner with respect to the new tissue formation. Another important shortcoming is the toxicity of degradation products that can be harmful to cells or the newly formed tissue. Instability is another important limitation, which may occur at various stages of the bioprinting process. Most hydrogels are extremely soft and can easily spread and lose their structural integrity during the bioprinting process.

Microcarrier technology is an efficient method for cell expansion in a small volume; however, this technology requires bioreactors to provide constant movement of microcarriers and appropriate environmental parameters for cell growth. One of the limitations is the need for a more complex detachment system to harvest cells, depending on the scaffold material. Another limitation is the possibility of nozzle clogging due to inherent adhesive properties of microcarriers, gravitational effects, or high density in hydrogels. In addition, the bioprinting process requires a balance between the media dilution necessary for deposition on the bioprinting stage and close contact between microcarriers in the bioprinted construct. Moreover, degradation products of microcarriers can be toxic to cells if hard polymeric ones are used. Despite its limitations, microcarrier technology has been utilized in other application areas (Malda and Frondoza, 2006) and may be an important and powerful tool for tissue engineering in the near future.

The cell pellet is a dense mass of cells in a suspension with a minimal amount of culture media. Cells quickly form aggregates in the shape that they are cast, i.e., tissue strands or spheroids. It is the most practical scaffold-free bioprinting approach, but the major hurdle is the limited size of constructs to ensure the availability of oxygen in the center of constructs. Also, the need for a temporary molding structure limits the size of tissues to very thin tubular shapes [i.e., blood vessels (Norotte et al., 2009) and nerve conduits (Owens et al., 2013)]. The construct properties ultimately depend on the cell type, the number of cells, and the final construct dimensions.

Despite the variety of tissue spheroid fabrication techniques, there are still limitations with the use of tissue spheroids within the bioprinting domain. Tissue spheroids may experience necrosis in their core, but this can be overcome by vascularization or fabricating lumenized spheroids (Fleming et al., 2010). However, if the culture relies on endothelial cells to create vascularization, the angiogenic process can take more than

48 h. This method is especially important for scale-up fabrication of tissues, where the primary issue is vascularization within the construct (Ozbolat, 2015b). Several difficulties can be encountered during the bioprinting of tissue spheroids. First of all, loading tissue spheroids into a nozzle (i.e., glass pipette) is highly challenging. Spheroids are not a uniform size and can be easily deformed or broken, depending on the cell type and maturity of spheroid. The nozzle must be designed to be large enough to hold the spheroids inside and allow extrusion without clogging. Also, the medium surrounding the tissue spheroids should also have appropriate properties. A characteristic feature of cell aggregates is rapid fusion, which is a desirable attribute postbioprinting, but not during the bioprinting process. On the other hand, if spheroids are too sparse in hydrogels, they will not contact one another upon bioprinting.

Tissue strands are an alternative approach to spheroids, differing in shape and preparation methods. The major drawback is the lack of full automation of the process as loading of tissue strands is performed manually. Also, bioprinting parameters need to be optimized for each tissue-specific strand. Another disadvantage is the requirement for high numbers of cells, depending on the desired length of the strand; additionally, tissue strands shrink substantially during maturation due to contraction. For constructs that require larger diameters for construction of scalable tissues, vascularization of the construct needs to be incorporated.

The most important limitation of dECM-based bioink materials is the need for a live organ source for acquisition of dECM. It can be a complex procedure requiring surgical protocols, donor sources, and involvement of other specialists. Even if a successful extraction is executed, the risk of an immunoreaction by the recipient remains. Moreover, the volume of final product is extremely limited compared to the size of the original organ. Decellularized matrix also loses its mechanical and structural integrity as well as some biochemical properties when homogenized. In addition, toxic residues from the decellularization process can remain. The high cost of the bioink, the need for rigorous protocols, and low yields of product are limitations of dECM-based bioink materials. The major weakness of dECM relative to the bioprinting process is its weak mechanical properties; therefore, 3D printing of a support frame is essential. The cost of dECM depends upon the quantity of ECM in the tissue. If the ECM content is low, the cost of harvesting dECM is high. With some tissue types, the preparation process may result in loss of a large portion of ECM. Other procedures such as chemical treatment can contribute to dECM contamination and toxicity. Finally, cells seeded in dECM can rapidly degrade the bioink due to the production of cellular matrix metalloproteinases (MMPs). Thus, further research is needed to optimize the use of dECM in bioprinting.

While each bioink type has its own advantages over others, hybrid tissue constructs can be envisioned as the combination of two or more complementary bioink types. In hybrid constructs, two types of bioink types can be integrated; in bioprinting a pancreas-on-a-chip model, engineered islets (in tissue spheroid form) can be loaded in hydrogels to create an in vitro vascularized pancreatic tissue model (Peng et al., 2016).

3.5 Future Directions

Despite the great progress in biomaterial development for tissue engineering and regenerative medicine, relatively few research endeavors have been devoted to the development of biomaterials for bioprinting processes; the majority of biomaterial researchers do not consider refinement of their biomaterials for use in the domain of bioprinting. Therefore, further effort should be devoted to engineering new bioprintable materials. A new field of study in the design and development of novel bioink materials is likely to emerge in the near future. To develop such bioink materials, compatible bioprinting processes should be first identified as each bioprinting modality possesses different requirements for the bioink materials.

New bioink development for EBB is crucial as the majority of researchers in the bioprinting domain use EBB due to its practicality and the ability to fabricate larger scale tissue constructs. Bioink materials used in EBB should possess various properties, but the most important characteristics are shear thinning, rapid crosslinking, and solidification capabilities. Hydrogels lacking rapid solidification capabilities tend to spread upon extrusion and cannot retain the originally bioprinted shape. There are currently only a few hydrogel types exhibiting such properties such as Pluronic® and sodium alginate, but these bioink materials do not support cell growth and successful tissue regeneration. Therefore, new bioink materials possessing all these characteristics will be most valuable. In addition, new bioprinting approaches can also be developed to overcome the intrinsic limitations of soft hydrogels. For example, in the recently demonstrated bioplotting approach, hydrogels (such as alginate, fibrin, and collagen) were extruded and bioprinted in a hydrogel bath loaded with gelation microparticles (Hinton et al., 2015). The addition of gelation microparticles at 22°C (when the bath is in solid state) kept the bioprinted gel in place and maintained the shape. In this case, the hydrogel bath acted as a mold support for the bioplotted solution. At the same temperature, when the nozzle moved, the bath near the nozzle acted like a liquid allowing the bioink solution to be extruded and plotted into the hydrogel bath. This behavior of the bath is explained by the Bingham plastic behavior of such materials. Upon increasing the temperature of the hydrogel bath, the bath reverted to a liquid phase and the bioplotted construct could be easily removed.

In DBB, bioink materials are utilized in two different aspects including (1) bioink materials that are ejected for droplet formation and (2) substrate materials for droplet deposition. For bioink materials used in DBB, novel hydrogels should be developed that have lower viscosity, but possess sufficient mechanical and structural properties as well as appropriate gelation properties to allow rapid solidification of droplets. In addition, such bioink materials should not have a fibrous microarchitecture (i.e., collagen and fibrinogen) that can easily clog the nozzle or tubing line within the cartridge head. Bioprinting of larger scale tissue constructs using DBB is limited to a few bioink materials including alginate-agarose blend hydrogels; however, these bioink materials do not favor growth of cells. For substrate biomaterials, where cells are directly patterned on a hydrogel film (substrate), only thin constructs could be obtained and research studies have been limited to 2D patterns. These substrate materials should spread on the printing table uniformly and be easily peeled off by practical means such as thermal alteration of the surface chemistry (i.e., from hydrophobic to hydrophilic), a technique used in cell sheet technology (Yamato and Okano, 2004). For this purpose, a hybrid bioprinting platform can be developed, where the substrate can be applied at a finite thickness followed by bioprinting and patterning of the cell suspension.

For bioink materials used in LBB, two separate considerations are given as the requirements for processes based on cell transfer differ from those involving photopolymerization. For bioink development utilized in cell transfer technologies, new bioink materials should be developed with specific properties such as the ability to spread and create a uniform film on the ribbon, viscoelasticity that facilitates jetting with minimum satellite formation and controlled droplet deposition, quick gelation capabilities to provide sufficient mechanical integrity and hold the entire bioprinted construct in place in 3D. In addition, appropriate substrate biomaterial should be in place, similar to the substrates used in DBB, to provide appropriate landing of the bioink without splashing or spreading. In addition, the bioink should be designed and engineered to easily peel off from the printing stage. For hydrogels used in processes based on photopolymerization, new bioink developments are essential as current photocurable materials are of insufficient strength to generate biologically appealing and mechanically integrated tissue constructs. In processes involving photopolymerization, the photocurable bioink determines the speed of curing and resolution of the process; the bioink should possess certain mechanical, biological, and chemical properties to serve for different tissue fabrication purposes. In this regard, the right combination of photocurable materials, curing agent, solvent, bioreagent, and light absorber should be selected to design the optimal process. Along with photocurable hydrogels, photoinitiators have been used to start the solidification process as well as improve the mechanical stability of the tissue constructs. However, they are not easily applied to bioprinting as photoinitiators are toxic. Low concentration photoinitiators have been used (Fedorovich et al., 2009), but generally result in poor mechanical properties, excessive swelling, and an increased depth of curing. This affects the solidification of other layers and deteriorates the quality of bioprinting. Thus, development of new photocurable materials and water-soluble photoinitiators are essential to the field of bioprinting.

In addition to the bioprintability property, biological properties of hydrogels play a crucial role in successful regeneration of tissues. As synthetically designed hydrogels lack natural proteins with cell adhesion ligands, inclusion of these proteins or RGD peptides can improve cell adhesion. One of the major drawbacks of currently available hydrogel materials is that they do not facilitate differentiation of cells into multiple lineages. As the majority of native tissues and organs have heterocellular niches, where multiple cell types interact in a highly complex microenvironment, only a limited effort has been given to the development of smart bioink materials that can facilitate differentiation of stems cell into different lineages. For example, one of the important problems in regenerative medicine is the development of osteochondral models with smooth transitions between the cellular architecture and the corresponding ECM. Although the use of growth factors or recombinant DNA has been utilized in bioink materials, shortcomings still exist such as limited sustainability and transfection efficiency, respectively. Therefore, bioink materials reinforced with nanomaterials that can induce differentiation of cells with a seamless transition in a chondral bone model would be ideal. In addition, mechanical, chemical, and physical stimuli can be further applied to enhance the differentiation capacity of such bioink materials (Carrow and Gaharwar, 2014).

Scaffold-free approaches should be further investigated to develop physiologically relevant tissue constructs. The majority of available scaffold-free bioink materials and the compatible bioprinting processes utilize a mold support for cell aggregation, tissue fusion, and maturation. This mold support needs to be printed in tandem with the cellular construct limiting the size of the tissues. A recent work demonstrated bioprinting of scaffold-free tissue strands without the use of a mold support; this was attempted for cartilage tissue due to its avascular nature (Yu et al., 2016). Future attempts should include vascularization within scaffold-free aggregates in multiple scales including neovascularization within cell aggregates, capillaries sprouting from the aggregates, and anastomosing capillaries formed within the tissue construct. Alternatively, aggregates can be designed and fabricated in such a way that a porous interconnected network can be integrated within their geometric domain. With integrated pores, cell aggregates should be able to keep their mechanical and structural integrity, while media transport will be enabled throughout the internal architecture. As integration of such porous architecture might be difficult to apply to tissue spheroids due to their small size, tissue strands will be an ideal structure to incorporate such architecture. In addition to efforts in developing scaffold-free bioink materials, compatible bioprinting processes are also required to successfully bioprint cell aggregate–based bioink materials. Mechanical properties of cell aggregates need to be further investigated. The mechanical properties of cell aggregates increase with culture time resulting in more collagen and elastin deposition; however, further maturation limits their fusion capabilities and self-assembly characteristics postbioprinting. Therefore, cells in aggregates should be engineered to overexpress collagen and elastin to increase the cohesiveness in a shorter period of time using maturogens such as TGF-β1, serotonin, and periostin to support collagen accumulation, fibrogenic activity, and collagen fibrilogenesis, respectively (Hajdu et al., 2010). Improvement in cohesion of cell aggregates also eliminates other challenges during bioprinting, such as loading and bioprinting of solid aggregates into custom-made cartridge heads.

Programmable biomaterials based on natural proteins can be one of the future trends in generating superior constructs by altering genetic sequences of biomaterials. With recent advances in CRISPR technology (Doudna and Charpentier, 2014), genetic engineering has become a powerful tool in medicine and such technology can be adopted into design and development of protein or DNA-based biomaterials. Such materials can be programmed to exhibit appropriate properties on demand, such as the ability to facilitate cell attachment, as well as provide a highly porous network for their encapsulation and growth. Having programmable mechanical properties such as the elasticity and tensile/compression strength based on the target tissue type will be extremely valuable. Such biomaterials have been recently used in fabrication of thermoplastics (Jung et al., 2016); however, they can be further refined to generate hydrogel-like environment.

The vast majority of efforts have been devoted to engineering cells; however, engineering ECM produced by cells will have great benefits such as improving mechanical properties of ECM and controlling its microarchitecture (i.e., orientation, thickness and porosity of protein fibers, and composition). For example, successful tissue regeneration for articular cartilage or muscle requires mechanically improved tissue constructs rather than simply implanting freshly bioprinted tissue constructs into lesion sites. For such tissues, the utilized bioink materials can be "trained" to recapitulate the native organization prior to the bioprinting process and the bioprinting process can be used as an assembly platform. As mentioned previously, articular cartilage has a stratified nature with collagen type II fibers orienting horizontally at the superficial layer, where their orientation transitions to random organization in the middle zone and attain a vertical orientation with thicker fibers in the deeper zones. The cell concentration varies throughout the structure as well. New bioink materials can be developed in such a way that the ECM of native tissue can be recapitulated within these bioink materials prior to bioprinting. For example, the density, thickness, and mechanical properties of collagen type II proteins can be enhanced by training the bioink material under cyclic compression and biochemical stimulation. Recent attempts in bioprinting tissue strands demonstrate the ability to control the orientation of collagen fibers along the longitudinal axis of the strands (Yu et al., 2016).

3.6 Summary

This chapter discussed the bioink materials used in 3D bioprinting technology, including hydrogels, microcarriers, dECM, and cell aggregates, and presented a detailed comparative evaluation of these bioink materials under various performance metrics. Future efforts in the evolution of bioink materials need to bring about solutions that will strengthen mechanical properties to stabilize bioprinted constructs, provide biological compounds to allow better cellular interactions, and facilitate an appropriate environment to generate physiologically relevant, functional tissues that are vascularized and can be engrafted with the host tissue after implantation. The abovementioned issues are some of the major reasons that researchers are still far from bioprinting functional organs of the clinically relevant size. However, with newly engineered bioink materials and compatible bioprinting processes on the horizon, 3D bioprinting will be a key technology for the future of tissue engineering, regenerative therapies, and pharmaceutics.

References

Ab-Rahim, S., et al., 2013. Chondrocyte-alginate constructs with or without TGF-β1 produces superior extracellular matrix expression than monolayer cultures. Molecular and Cellular Biochemistry 376 (1–2), 11–20.

Ahmed, E.M., 2013. Hydrogel: preparation, characterization, and applications. Journal of Advanced Research 6 (2), 105–121.

Ahn, S., et al., 2012. Cells (MC3T3–E1)-laden alginate scaffolds fabricated by a modified solid-freeform fabrication process supplemented with an aerosol spraying. Biomacromolecules 13, 2997–3003.

Akkouch, A., Yu, Y., Ozbolat, I.T., 2015. Microfabrication of scaffold-free tissue strands for three-dimensional tissue engineering. Biofabrication 7 (3), 31002.

Albelda, S.M., Buck, C.A., 1990. Integrins and other cell adhesion molecules. FASEB Journal 4 (11), 2868–2880.

Alconcel, S.N.S., Baas, A.S., Maynard, H.D., 2011. FDA-approved poly(ethylene glycol)–protein conjugate drugs. Polymer Chemistry 2 (7), 1442.

Alexander, A., et al., 2013. Poly(ethylene glycol)-poly(lactic-co-glycolic acid) based thermosensitive injectable hydrogels for biomedical applications. Journal of controlled release 172 (3), 715–729.

Alhasan, L., et al., 2016. Rapid enhancement of cellular spheroid assembly by acoustically driven microcentrifugation. ACS Biomaterials Science and Engineering 2 (6), 1013–1022.

Alsberg, E., et al., 2002. Engineering growing tissues. Proceedings of the National Academy of Sciences 99 (19), 12025–12030.

Arcaute, K., Mann, B., Wicker, R., 2010. Stereolithography of spatially controlled multi-material bioactive poly(ethylene glycol) scaffolds. Acta Biomaterialia 6 (3), 1047–1054.

Arcaute, K., Mann, B.K., Wicker, R.B., 2006. Stereolithography of three-dimensional bioactive poly(-ethylene glycol) constructs with encapsulated cells. Annals of Biomedical Engineering 34 (9), 1429–1441.

Athanasiou, K.A., et al., 2013. Self-organization and the self-assembling process in tissue engineering. Annual Review of Biomedical Engineering 15 (1), 115–136.

Aubin, H., et al., 2010. Directed 3D cell alignment and elongation in microengineered hydrogels. Biomaterials 31 (27), 6941–6951.

Aya, K.L., Stern, R., 2014. Hyaluronan in wound healing: rediscovering a major player. Wound Repair and Regeneration 22, 579–593.

Back, S.A., et al., 2005. Hyaluronan accumulates in demyelinated lesions and inhibits oligodendrocyte progenitor maturation. Nature Medicine 11 (9), 966–972.

Baier, C., et al., 2007. Hyaluronan is organized into fiber-like structures along migratory pathways in the developing mouse cerebellum. Matrix Biology 26 (5), 348–358.

Banerjee, S., Toole, B.P., 1991. Monoclonal antibody to chick embryo hyaluronan-binding protein: changes in distribution of binding protein during early brain development. Developmental Biology 197, 186–197.

Barron, J.A., Spargo, B.J., Ringeisen, B.R., 2004. Biological laser printing of three dimensional cellular structures. Applied Physics A 79 (4–6), 1027–1030.

Behrens, J., 1999. Cadherins and catenins: role in signal transduction and tumor progression. Cancer and Metastasis Reviews 18 (1), 15–30.

Benedikt, P., et al., 2000. Fibrin gel as a three dimensional matrix in cardiovascular tissue engineering. European Journal Cardio-Thoracic Surgery 17, 587–591.

Benoit, D.S.W., Durney, A.R., Anseth, K.S., 2006. Manipulations in hydrogel degradation behavior enhance osteoblast function and mineralized tissue formation. Tissue engineering 12 (6), 1663–1673.

Benton, G., et al., 2011. Multiple uses of basement membrane-like matrix (BME/Matrigel) in vitro and in vivo with cancer cells. International Journal of Cancer 128 (8), 1751–1757.

Benton, J.A., et al., 2009. Photocrosslinking of gelatin macromers to synthesize porous hydrogels that promote valvular interstitial cell function. Tissue Engineering: Part A 15 (11), 3221–3230.

Bertassoni, L.E., et al., 2014. Direct-write bioprinting of cell-laden methacrylated gelatin hydrogels. Biofabrication 6 (2), 024105.

Bigi, A., et al., 2002. Stabilization of gelatin films by crosslinking with genipin. Biomaterials 23 (24), 4827–4832.

Billiet, T., et al., 2014. The 3D printing of gelatin methacrylamide cell-laden tissue-engineered constructs with high cell viability. Biomaterials 35 (1), 49–62.

Blaeser, A., et al., 2013. Biofabrication under fluorocarbon: a novel freeform fabrication technique to generate high aspect ratio tissue-engineered constructs. BioResearch Open Access 2 (5), 374–384.

Boland, T., et al., 2007. Drop-on-demand printing of cells and materials for designer tissue constructs. Materials Science and Engineering: C 27 (3), 372–376.

Burdick, J.a, Prestwich, G.D., 2011. Hyaluronic acid hydrogels for biomedical applications. Advanced Materials 23 (12), H41–H56.

Carrow, J.K., Gaharwar, A.K., 2014. Bioinspired polymeric panocomposites for regenerative medicine. Macromolecular Chemistry and Physics 216, 248–264.

Chen, S.-C., et al., 2004. A novel pH-sensitive hydrogel composed of N,O-carboxymethyl chitosan and alginate cross-linked by genipin for protein drug delivery. Journal of Controlled Release 96 (2), 285–300.

Chiou, B.S., et al., 2008. Cold water fish gelatin films: effects of cross-linking on thermal, mechanical, barrier, and biodegradation properties. European Polymer Journal 44 (11), 3748–3753.

Christensen, K., et al., 2015. Freeform inkjet printing of cellular structures with bifurcations. Biotechnology and Bioengineering 112 (5), 1047–1055.

Cohen, D.L., Lipton, J.I., et al., 2010a. Additive manufacturing for in situ repair of osteochondral defects. Biofabrication 2 (3), 035004.

Cohen, D.L., Lo, W., et al., 2010b. Increased mixing improves hydrogel homogeneity and quality of three-dimensional printed constructs. Tissue Engineering: Part C 17 (2), 239–248.

Croisier, F., Jérôme, C., 2013. Chitosan-based biomaterials for tissue engineering. European Polymer Journal 49 (4), 780–792.

Cui, X., Breitenkamp, K., Finn, M.G., et al., 2012a. Direct human cartilage repair using three-dimensional bioprinting technology. Tissue Engineering: Part A 18 (11–12), 1304–1312.

Cui, X., Breitenkamp, K., Lotz, M., et al., 2012b. Synergistic action of fibroblast growth factor-2 and transforming growth factor-beta1 enhances bioprinted human neocartilage formation. Biotechnology and Bioengineering 109 (9), 2357–2368.

Cui, X., Boland, T., 2009. Human microvasculature fabrication using thermal inkjet printing technology. Biomaterials 30 (31), 6221–6227.

Dana, N., et al., 2004. Photocrosslinkable hyaluronan as a scaffold for articular cartilage repair. Annals of biomedical engineering 32 (3), 391–397.

Dean, D.M., et al., 2007. Rods, tori, and honeycombs: the directed self-assembly of microtissues with prescribed microscale geometries. FASEB journal 21, 4005–4012.

Deitch, S., et al., 2008. Collagen matrix alignment using inkjet printer technology. MRS Proceedings 1094.

Dhariwala, B., Hunt, E., Boland, T., 2004. Rapid prototyping of tissue-engineering constructs, using photopolymerizable hydrogels and stereolithography. Tissue Engineering 10 (9–10), 1316–1322.

Dolati, F., et al., 2014. In vitro evaluation of carbon-nanotube-reinforced bioprintable vascular conduits. Nanotechnology 25 (14), 145101.

Doudna, J.A., Charpentier, E., 2014. The new frontier of genome engineering with CRISPR-Cas9. Science 346 (6213).

Dragan, E.S., 2014. Design and applications of interpenetrating polymer network hydrogels. A review. Chemical Engineering Journal 243, 572–590.

Drury, J.L., Mooney, D.J., 2003. Hydrogels for tissue engineering: scaffold design variables and applications. Biomaterials 24, 4337–4351.

Du, M., et al., 2015. 3D bioprinting of BMSC-laden methacrylamide gelatin scaffolds with CBD-BMP2-collagen microfibers. Biofabrication 7 (4), 044104.

Duan, B., et al., 2013. 3D Bioprinting of heterogeneous aortic valve conduits with alginate/gelatin hydrogels. Journal of Biomedical Materials Research: Part A 101A (5), 1255–1264.

Duarte Campos, D.F., et al., 2014. The stiffness and structure of three-dimensional printed hydrogels direct the differentiation of mesenchymal stromal cells toward adipogenic and osteogenic lineages. Tissue Engineering: Part A 21 (3–4), 740–756.

Del Duca, D., Werbowetski, T., Del Maestro, R.F., 2004. Spheroid preparation from hanging drops: characterization of a model of brain tumor invasion. Journal of Neuro-Oncology 67 (3), 295–303.

Ehsan, S.M., et al., 2014. A three-dimensional in vitro model of tumor cell intravasation. Integrative Biology 6 (6), 603–610.

Fairbanks, B.D., et al., 2009. Photoinitiated polymerization of PEG-diacrylate with lithium phenyl-2,4, 6-trimethylbenzoylphosphinate: polymerization rate and cytocompatibility. Biomaterials 30 (35), 6702–6707.

Faroni, A., et al., 2015. Peripheral nerve regeneration: experimental strategies and future perspectives. Advanced Drug Delivery Reviews 82, 160–167.

Fedorovich, N.E., et al., 2011. Distinct tissue formation by heterogeneous printing of osteo- and endothelial progenitor cells. Tissue Engineering: Part A 17, 2113–2121.

Fedorovich, N.E., et al., 2007. Hydrogels as extracellular matrices for skeletal tissue engineering: state-of-the-art and novel application in organ printing. Tissue Engineering 13 (8), 1905–1925.

Fedorovich, N.E., et al., 2009. The effect of photopolymerization on stem cells embedded in hydrogels. Biomaterials 30 (3), 344–353.

Fedorovich, N.E., et al., 2008. Three-dimensional fiber deposition of cell-laden, viable, patterned constructs for bone tissue printing. Tissue Engineering: Part A 14 (1), 127–133.

Ferreira, A.M., et al., 2012. Collagen for bone tissue regeneration. Acta biomaterialia 8 (9), 3191–3200.

Fleming, P.A., et al., 2010. Fusion of uniluminal vascular spheroids: a model for assembly of blood vessels. Developmental Dynamics 239 (2), 398–406.

Furth, M.E., Atala, A., Van Dyke, M.E., 2007. Smart biomaterials design for tissue engineering and regenerative medicine. Biomaterials 28 (34), 5068–5073.

Gaetani, R., et al., 2012. Cardiac tissue engineering using tissue printing technology and human cardiac progenitor cells. Biomaterials 33 (6), 1782–1790.

Galateanu, B., et al., 2012. Layer-shaped alginate hydrogels enhance the biological performance of human adipose-derived stem cells. BMC Biotechnology 12 (1), 35.

Gamboa-Martinez, T.C., et al., 2015. Crosslinked fibrin gels for tissue engineering: two approaches to improve their properties. Journal of Biomedical Materials Research: Part A 103 (2), 614–621.

Gao, G., Yonezawa, T., Hubbell, K., Dai, G., Cui, X., 2015. Inkjet-bioprinted acrylated peptides and PEG hydrogel with human mesenchymal stem cells promote robust bone and cartilage formation with minimal printhead clogging. Biotechnology Journal 10, 1568–1577.

Gao, G., et al., 2014. Bioactive nanoparticles stimulate bone tissue formation in bioprinted three-dimensional scaffold and human mesenchymal stem cells. Biotechnology Journal 9 (10), 1304–1311.

Gauvin, R., et al., 2012. Microfabrication of complex porous tissue engineering scaffolds using 3D projection stereolithography. Biomaterials 33 (15), 3824–3834.

Geng, L., et al., 2005. Direct writing of chitosan scaffolds using a robotic system. Rapid Prototyping Journal 11, 90–97.

Gerecht, S., et al., 2007. Hyaluronic acid hydrogel for controlled self-renewal and differentiation of human embryonic stem cells. Proceedings of the National Academy of Sciences 104 (27), 11298–11303.

Goh, T.K.-P., et al., 2013. Microcarrier culture for efficient expansion and osteogenic differentiation of human fetal mesenchymal stem cells. BioResearch Open Access 2 (2), 84–97.

Gómez-Guillén, M.C., et al., 2011. Functional and bioactive properties of collagen and gelatin from alternative sources: a review. Food Hydrocolloids 25 (8), 1813–1827.

Gómez-Guillén, M.C., et al., 2002. Structural and physical properties of gelatin extracted from different marine species: a comparative study. Food Hydrocolloids 16 (1), 25–34.

Gong, C.Y., et al., 2009. In vitro drug release behavior from a novel thermosensitive composite hydrogel based on Pluronic f127 and poly(ethylene glycol)-poly(epsilon-caprolactone)-poly(ethylene glycol) copolymer. BMC Biotechnology 9, 8.

Gruene, M., et al., 2011. Laser printing of three-dimensional multicellular arrays for studies of cell–cell and cell–environment interactions. Tissue Engineering Part C: Methods 17 (10), 973–982.

Gudapati, H., et al., 2014. Alginate gelation-induced cell death during laser-assisted cell printing. Biofabrication 6 (3), 035022.

Gudapati, H., Dey, M., Ozbolat, I., 2016. A comprehensive review on droplet-based bioprinting: past, present and future. Biomaterials 102, 20–42.

Guillotin, B., et al., 2010. Laser assisted bioprinting of engineered tissue with high cell density and microscale organization. Biomaterials 31 (28), 7250–7256.

Gulrez, S.K., Al-Assaf, S., Phillips, G.O., 2011. Hydrogels: methods of preparation, characterisation and applications. In: Carpi, A. (Ed.), Progress in Molecular and Environmental Bioengineering–from Analysis and Modeling to Technology Applications, InTech.

Guo, F., et al., 2015. Controlling cell-cell interactions using surface acoustic waves. Proceedings of the National Academy of Sciences 112 (1), 43–48.

Gutkan, U., 2014. Engineering anisotropic biomimetic fibrocartilage microenvironment by bioprinting mesenchymal stem cells in nanoliter gel droplets. Molecular Pharmaceutics 7 (11), 2151–2159.

Hajdu, Z., Mironov, V., Mehesz, A.N., Norris, R.A., Markwald, R.R., Visconti, R.P., 2010. Tissue spheroid fusion-based in vitro screening assays for analysis of tissue maturation. Journal of Tissue Engineering and Regenerative Medicine 4, 659–664. http://dx.doi.org/10.1002/term.291.

Hauser, C.A.E., et al., 2015. Peptide bioink: self-assembling nanofibrous scaffolds for 3D organotypic cultures. Nano Letters 15, 6919–6925.

Heilshorn, S.C., Liu, J.C., Tirrell, D.A., 2005. Cell-binding domain context affects cell behavior on engineered proteins. Biomacromolecules 6 (1), 318–323.

Hellio, D., Djabourov, M., 2006. Physically and chemically crosslinked gelatin gels. Macromolecular Symposia 241, 23–27.

Hennink, W.E., van Nostrum, C.F., 2012. Novel crosslinking methods to design hydrogels. Advanced Drug Delivery Reviews 64, 223–236.

Hill, E., Boontheekul, T., Mooney, D.J., 2006. Designing scaffolds to enhance transplanted myoblast survival and migration. Tissue Engineering 12 (5), 1295–1304.

Hinton, T.J., et al., 2015. Three-dimensional printing of complex biological structures by freeform reversible embedding of suspended hydrogels. Science Advances 1 (9), e1500758.

Hockaday, L.A., et al., 2012. Rapid 3D printing of anatomically accurate and mechanically heterogeneous aortic valve hydrogel scaffolds. Biofabrication 4 (3), 035005.

Homenick, C.M., et al., 2011. Pluronics as crosslinking agents for collagen: novel amphiphilic hydrogels. Polymer International 60 (3), 458–465.

Hopp, B., et al. Survival and proliferative ability of various living cell types after laser-induced forward transfer. Tissue Engineering 11(11–12), 1817–1823.

Horváth, L., et al., 2015. Engineering an in vitro air-blood barrier by 3D bioprinting. Scientific Reports 5, 7974.

Hribar, K.C., et al., 2014. Light-assisted direct-write of 3D functional biomaterials. Lab on a Chip 14 (2), 268–275.

Huang, T., et al., 2014. 3D printing of biomimetic microstructures for cancer cell migration. Biomedical Microdevices 16 (1), 127–132.

Hutson, C.B., et al., 2011. Synthesis and characterization of tunable poly(ethylene glycol): gelatin methacrylate composite hydrogels. Tissue engineering: Part A 17 (13–14), 1713–1723.

Ikeda, K., et al., 2003. Hyaluronic acid prevents peripheral nerve adhesion. British Journal of Plastic Surgery 56 (4), 342–347.

Ishida, T., et al., 2005. Accelerated blood clearance of PEGylated liposomes following preceding liposome injection: effects of lipid dose and PEG surface-density and chain length of the first-dose liposomes. Journal of Controlled Release 105 (3), 305–317.

Itoh, M., et al., 2015. Scaffold-free tubular tissues created by a bio-3D printer undergo remodeling and endothelialization when implanted in rat aortae. PLoS One 10 (9), 1–16.

Jakob, P.H., et al., 2016. A 3-D cell culture system to study epithelia functions using microcarriers. Cytotechnology 1–13.

Janmey, P.A., Winer, J.P., Weisel, J.W., 2009. Fibrin gels and their clinical and bioengineering applications. Journal of the Royal Society, Interface 6 (30), 1–10.

Jeong, B., Kim, S.W., Bae, Y.H., 2002. Thermosensitive sol–gel reversible hydrogels. Advanced Drug Delivery Reviews 54 (1), 37–51.

Jin, H.J., et al., 2011. A multicellular spheroid formation and extraction chip using removable cell trapping barriers. Lab on a Chip 11 (1), 115–119.

Jin, R., Dijkstra, P.J., 2010. Hydrogels for tissue engineering applications. Biomedical Applications of Hydrogels Handbook 101 (7), 203–225.

Jung, H., et al., 2016. Molecular tandem repeat strategy for elucidating mechanical properties of high-strength proteins. Proceedings of the National Academy of Sciences 113 (23), 6478–6483.

Jungst, T., et al., 2015. Strategies and molecular design criteria for 3D printable hydrogels. Chemical Reviews 116 (3), 1496–1539.

Kamoun, E.A., et al., 2015. Poly (vinyl alcohol)-alginate physically crosslinked hydrogel membranes for wound dressing applications: characterization and bio-evaluation. Arabian Journal of Chemistry 8 (1), 38–47.

Khalil, M., et al., 2001. Human hepatocyte cell lines proliferating as cohesive spheroid colonies in alginate markedly upregulate both synthetic and detoxificatory liver function. Journal of Hepatology 34 (1), 68–77.

Khattak, S.F., Bhatia, S.R., Roberts, S.C., 2005. Pluronic F127 as a cell encapsulation material: utilization of membrane-stabilizing agents. Tissue Engineering 11 (5–6), 974–983.

Klebe, R.J., 1988. Cytoscribing: a method for micropositioning cells and the construction of two- and three-dimensional synthetic tissues. Experimental Cell Research 179 (2), 362–373.

Kleinman, H.K., Martin, G.R., 2005. Matrigel: basement membrane matrix with biological activity. Seminars in Cancer Biology 15, 378–386.

Koch, L., et al., 2010. Laser printing of skin cells and human stem cells. Tissue Engineering: Part C 16 (5), 847–854.

Kreger, S.T., Voytik-Harbin, S.L., 2009. Hyaluronan concentration within a 3D collagen matrix modulates matrix viscoelasticity, but not fibroblast response. Matrix Biology 28 (6), 336–346.

Kucukgul, C., et al., 2015. 3D bioprinting of biomimetic aortic vascular constructs with self-supporting cells. Biotechnology and Bioengineering 112 (4), 811–821.

Lai, K.K., Renneberg, R., Mak, W.C., 2016. High efficiency single-step biomaterial-based microparticle fabrication via template-directed supramolecular coordination chemistry. Green Chemistry 18, 1715–1723.

Leach, J.B., et al., 2003. Photocrosslinked hyaluronic acid hydrogels: natural, biodegradable tissue engineering scaffolds. Biotechnology and Bioengineering 82 (5), 578–589.

Lee, J.-S., et al., 2014a. 3D printing of composite tissue with complex shape applied to ear regeneration. Biofabrication 6 (2), 024103.

Lee, S.H., et al., 2011. Enzyme-mediated cross-linking of Pluronic copolymer micelles for injectable and in situ forming hydrogels. Acta Biomaterialia 7 (4), 1468–1476.

Lee, V., et al., 2014b. Generation of multi-scale vascular network system within 3D hydrogel using 3D bio-printing technology. Cellular and Molecular Bioengineering 7 (3), 460–472.

Lee, W., et al., 2010a. On-demand three-dimensional freeform fabrication of multi-layered hydrogel scaffold with fluidic channels. Biotechnology and Bioengineering 105 (6), 1178–1186.

Lee, Y.-B., et al., 2010b. Bio-printing of collagen and VEGF-releasing fibrin gel scaffolds for neural stem cell culture. Experimental Neurology 223 (2), 645–652.

Levato, R., et al., 2014. Biofabrication of tissue constructs by 3D bioprinting of cell-laden microcarriers. Biofabrication 6 (3), 35020.

Liang, H.C., et al., 2004. Crosslinking structures of gelatin hydrogels crosslinked with genipin or a water-soluble carbodiimide. Journal of Applied Polymer Science 91, 4017–4026.

Lin, C.-C., Anseth, K.S., 2009. PEG hydrogels for the controlled release of biomolecules in regenerative medicine. Pharmaceutical Research 26 (3), 631–643.

Liu, Y., et al., 2004. CD44 expression identifies astrocyte-restricted precursor cells. Developmental Biology 276 (1), 31–46.

Livoti, C.M., Morgan, J.R., 2010. Self-assembly and tissue fusion of toroid-shaped minimal building units. Tissue Engineering: Part A 16 (6), 2051–2061.

Luo, Y., Kirker, K.R., Prestwich, G.D., 2000. Cross-linked hyaluronic acid hydrogel films: new biomaterials for drug delivery. Journal of Controlled Release 69 (1), 169–184.

Malda, J., Frondoza, C.G., 2006. Microcarriers in the engineering of cartilage and bone. Trends in Biotechnology 24 (7), 299–304.

Mann, B.K., et al., 2001. Smooth muscle cell growth in photopolymerized hydrogels with cell adhesive and proteolytically degradable domains: synthetic ECM analogs for tissue engineering. Biomaterials 22 (22), 3045–3051.

Margolis, R.U., et al., 1975. Glycosaminoglycans of brain during development. Biochemistry 14, 85–88.

Mehesz, A.N., et al., 2011. Scalable robotic biofabrication of tissue spheroids. Biofabrication 3 (2), 25002.

Mehta, G., et al., 2012. Opportunities and challenges for use of tumor spheroids as models to test drug delivery and efficacy. Journal of Controlled Release 164 (2), 192–204.

Melchels, F.P.W., et al., 2012. Additive manufacturing of tissues and organs. Progress in Polymer Science 37 (8), 1079–1104.

Mesa, M., et al., 2005. Morphology and porosity characteristics control of SBA-16 mesoporous silica. Effect of the triblock surfactant Pluronic F127 degradation during the synthesis. Solid State Sciences 7 (8), 990–997.

Mészár, Z., et al., 2008. Hyaluronan accumulates around differentiating neurons in spinal cord of chicken embryos. Brain Research Bulletin 75 (2–4), 414–418.

Michael, S., et al., 2013. Tissue engineered skin substitutes created by laser-assisted bioprinting form skin-like structures in the dorsal skin fold chamber in mice. PloS One 8 (3), e57741.

Migliore, A., Granata, M., 2008. Intra-articular use of hyaluronic acid in the treatment of osteoarthritis. Clinical Interventions in Aging 3 (2), 365–369.

Mironov, V., et al., 2009. Organ printing: tissue spheroids as building blocks. Biomaterials 30 (12), 2164–2174.

Montembault, A., et al., 2006. A material decoy of biological media based on chitosan physical hydrogels: application to cartilage tissue engineering. Biochimie 88 (5), 551–564.

Moura, M.J., et al., 2011. In situ forming chitosan hydrogels prepared via ionic/covalent Co-cross-linking. Biomacromolecules 12, 3275–3284.

Müller, M., et al., 2015. Nanostructured Pluronic hydrogels as bioinks for 3D bioprinting. Biofabrication 7 (3), 035006.

Murphy, S.V., Skardal, A., Atala, A., 2013. Evaluation of hydrogels for bio-printing applications. Journal of Biomedical Materials Research—Part A 101, 272–284.

Nakatsu, M.N., et al., 2003. Angiogenic sprouting and capillary lumen formation modeled by human umbilical vein endothelial cells (HUVEC) in fibrin gels: the role of fibroblasts and Angiopoietin-1. Microvascular Research 66 (2), 102–112.

Nichol, J.W., et al., 2010. Cell-laden microengineered gelatin methacrylate hydrogels. Biomaterials 31 (21), 5536–5544.

Nicodemus, G.D., Bryant, S.J., 2008. Cell encapsulation in biodegradable hydrogels for tissue engineering applications. Tissue Engineering: Part B 14 (2), 149–165.

Norotte, C., et al., 2009. Scaffold-free vascular tissue engineering using bioprinting. Biomaterials 30 (30), 5910–5917.

Odde, D.J., Renn, M.J., 1999. Laser-guided direct writing for applications in biotechnology. Trends in Biotechnology 17 (10), 385–389.

Ott, H., et al., 2008. Perfusion-decellularized matrix: using nature's platform to engineer a bioartificial heart. Nature Medicine 14, 213–221.

Ovsianikov, A., et al., 2014. Laser photofabrication of cell-containing hydrogel constructs. Langmuir 30 (13), 3787–3794.

Owens, C.M., et al., 2013. Biofabrication and testing of a fully cellular nerve graft. Biofabrication 5 (4), 45007.

Ozbolat, I.T., 2015a. Scaffold-based or scaffold-free bioprinting: competing or complementing approaches? Journal of Nanotechnology in Engineering and Medicine 6, 1–6.

Ozbolat, I.T., 2015b. Bioprinting scale-up tissue and organ constructs for transplantation. Trends in Biotechnology 33 (7), 395–400.

Ozbolat, I.T., Chen, H., Yu, Y., 2014. Development of "Multi-arm Bioprinter" for hybrid biofabrication of tissue engineering constructs. Robotics and Computer-Integrated Manufacturing 30 (3), 295–304.

Ozbolat, I.T., Hospodiuk, M., 2016. Current advances and future perspectives in extrusion-based bioprinting. Biomaterials 76, 321–343.

Ozbolat, I.T., Koc, B., 2010. Modeling of spatially controlled biomolecules in three-dimensional porous alginate structures. Journal of Medical Devices 4 (4), 41003.

Ozbolat, I.T., Peng, W., Ozbolat, V., 2016. Application areas of 3D bioprinting. Drug Discovery today 21 (8), 1257–1271.

Ozbolat, I.T., Yu, Y., 2013. Bioprinting toward organ fabrication: challenges and future trends. IEEE Transactions on Biomedical Engineering 60 (3), 691–699.

Ozler, B., Kucukgul, C., Koc, B., 2015. Bioprinting with live cells. In: Turksen, K. (Ed.), Bioprinting in Regenerative Medicine. Springer International Publising, Switzerland, pp. 67–88.

Pasut, G., Sergi, M., Veronese, F.M., 2008. Anti-cancer PEG-enzymes: 30 years old, but still a current approach. Advanced Drug Delivery Reviews 60 (1), 69–78.

Pataky, K., et al., 2012. Microdrop printing of hydrogel bioinks into 3D tissue-like geometries. Advanced Materials 24 (3), 391–396.

Pati, F., et al., 2013. 3D printing of cell-laden constructs for heterogeneous tissue regeneration. Manufacturing Letters 1 (1), 49–53.

Pati, F., et al., 2015. Biomimetic 3D tissue printing for soft tissue regeneration. Biomaterials 62, 164–175.

Pati, F., et al., 2014. Printing three-dimensional tissue analogues with decellularized extracellular matrix bioink. Nature Communication 5, 3935.

Paul, J.D., et al., 2013. SLIT3-ROBO4 activation promotes vascular network formation in human engineered tissue and angiogenesis in vivo. Journal of Molecular and Cellular Cardiology 64, 124–131.

Peng, W., Derya, U., Ozbolat, I.T., 2016. Bioprinting towards physiologically-relevant tissue models for pharmaceutics. Trends in Biotechnology 34 (9), 722–732.

Pescosolido, L., et al., 2011. Hyaluronic acid and dextran-based semi-IPN hydrogels as biomaterials for bioprinting. Biomacromolecules 12 (5), 1831–1838.

Poldervaart, M.T., et al., 2013. Sustained release of BMP-2 in bioprinted alginate for osteogenicity in mice and rats. PloS One 8 (8), e72610.

Pradines, B., et al., 2015. Gelation and micellization behaviors of Pluronic® F127 hydrogel containing poly(isobutylcyanoacrylate) nanoparticles specifically designed for mucosal application. Colloids and Surfaces B: Biointerfaces 135, 669–676.

Purcell, E.K., et al., 2009. Alginate composition effects on a neural stem cell-seeded scaffold. Tissue Engineering: Part C 15 (4), 541–550.

Rajan, N., et al., 2006. Preparation of ready-to-use, storable and reconstituted type I collagen from rat tail tendon for tissue engineering applications. Nature Protocols 1 (6), 2753–2758.

Raof, N.A., et al., 2011. The maintenance of pluripotency following laser direct-write of mouse embryonic stem cells. Biomaterials 32 (7), 1802–1808.

Rauch, U., Zhou, X.H., Roos, G., 2005. Extracellular matrix alterations in brains lacking four of its components. Biochemical and Biophysical Research Communications 328 (2), 608–617.

Riggs, B.C., et al., 2011. Matrix-assisted pulsed laser methods for biofabrication. MRS Bulletin 36 (12), 1043–1050.

Rivron, N.C., et al., 2009. Tissue assembly and organization: developmental mechanisms in microfabricated tissues. Biomaterials 30 (28), 4851–4858.

Roth, E., et al., 2004. Inkjet printing for high-throughput cell patterning. Biomaterials 25 (17), 3707–3715.

Rowley, J.A., Madlambayan, G., Mooney, D.J., 1999. Alginate hydrogels as synthetic extracellular matrix materials. Biomaterials 20 (1), 45–53.

Sakai, S., et al., 2009. An injectable, in situ enzymatically gellable, gelatin derivative for drug delivery and tissue engineering. Biomaterials 30 (20), 3371–3377.

Scheraga, H.A., 2004. The thrombin-fibrinogen interaction. Biophysical Chemistry 112 (2–3), 117–130.

Schiele, N.R., et al., 2009. Laser direct writing of combinatorial libraries of idealized cellular constructs: biomedical applications. Applied Surface Science 255 (10), 5444–5447.

Schiele, N.R., Chrisey, D.B., Corr, D.T., 2011. Gelatin-based laser direct-write technique for the precise spatial patterning of cells. Tissue Engineering: Part C 17 (3), 289–298.

Schrobback, K., et al., 2012. Effects of oxygen and culture system on in vitro propagation and redifferentiation of osteoarthritic human articular chondrocytes. Cell and Tissue Research 347, 649–663.

Schuurman, W., et al., 2013. Gelatin-methacrylamide hydrogels as potential biomaterials for fabrication of tissue-engineered cartilage constructs. Macromolecular Bioscience 13 (5), 551–561.

Seidlits, S.K., et al., 2010. The effects of hyaluronic acid hydrogels with tunable mechanical properties on neural progenitor cell differentiation. Biomaterials 31 (14), 3930–3940.

Serwer, P., Allen, J.L., Hayes, S.J., 1983. Agarose gel electrophoresis of bacteriophages and related particles III. Dependence of gel sieving on the agarose preparation. Electrophoresis 4, 232–236.

Sharma, S., Johnson, R.W., Desai, T.A., 2004. XPS and AFM analysis of antifouling PEG interfaces for microfabricated silicon biosensors. Biosensors and Bioelectronics 20 (2), 227–239.

Skardal, a., et al., 2012. Bioprinted amniotic fluid-derived stem cells accelerate healing of large skin wounds. Stem Cells Translational Medicine 1, 792–802.

Skardal, A., Zhang, J., McCoard, L., Oottamasathien, S., et al., 2010a. Dynamically crosslinked gold nanoparticle–hyaluronan hydrogels. Advanced Materials 22 (42), 4736–4740.

Skardal, A., Zhang, J., McCoard, L., Xu, X., et al., 2010b. Photocrosslinkable hyaluronan-gelatin hydrogels for two-step bioprinting. Tissue Engineering: Part A 16 (8), 2675–2685.

Skardal, A., Zhang, J., Prestwich, G.D., 2010c. Bioprinting vessel-like constructs using hyaluronan hydrogels crosslinked with tetrahedral polyethylene glycol tetracrylates. Biomaterials 31 (24), 6173–6184.

Smith, C.M., et al., 2004. Three-dimensional BioAssembly tool for generating viable tissue-engineered constructs. Tissue Engineering 10 (9), 1566–1576.

Snyder, J.E., et al., 2011. Bioprinting cell-laden matrigel for radioprotection study of liver by pro-drug conversion in a dual-tissue microfluidic chip. Biofabrication 3, 034112.

Takeichi, M., 1988. The cadherins: cell-cell adhesion molecules controlling animal morphogenesis. Development 102 (4), 639–655.

Takigawa, T., Endo, Y., 2006. Effects of glutaraldehyde exposure on human health. Journal of Occupational Health 48 (2), 75–87.

Tako, M., Nakamura, S., 1988. Gelation mechanism of agarose. Carbohydrate Research 180 (2), 277–284.

Tan, Y., et al., 2014. 3D printing facilitated scaffold-free tissue unit fabrication. Biofabrication 6 (2), 024111.

Thomas, B.H., et al., 2009. Hydrophilic-hydrophobic hydrogels for cartilage replacement. Journal of the Mechanical Behavior of Biomedical Materials 2 (6), 588–595.

Tibbitt, M., Anseth, K., 2009. Hydrogels as extracellular matrix mimics for 3D cell culture. Biotechnology and Bioengineering 103 (4), 655–663.

Tomei, A.A., et al., 2014. Device design and materials optimization of conformal coating for islets of Langerhans. Proceedings of the National Academy of Sciences 111 (29), 10514–10519.

Toole, B.P., 2004. Hyaluronan: from extracellular glue to pericellular cue. Nature Reviews Cancer 4 (7), 528–539.

Torisawa, Y., et al., 2009. Microfluidic hydrodynamic cellular patterning for systematic formation of co-culture spheroids. Integrative biology 1 (11), 649–654.

Turley, E.A., Noble, P.W., Bourguignon, L.Y.W., 2002. Signaling properties of hyaluronan receptors. Journal of Biological Chemistry 277 (7), 4589–4592.

Turner, A.E.B., Flynn, L.E., 2012. Design and characterization of tissue-specific extracellular matrix-derived microcarriers. Tissue Engineering: Part C 18 (3), 186–197.

Vashi, A.V., et al., 2008. Adipose differentiation of bone marrow-derived mesenchymal stem cells using Pluronic F-127 hydrogel in vitro. Biomaterials 29 (5), 573–579.

Veronese, F.M., Pasut, G., 2005. PEGylation, successful approach to drug delivery. Drug Discovery Today 10 (21), 1451–1458.

Visser, J., et al., 2013. Biofabrication of multi-material anatomically shaped tissue constructs. Biofabrication 5, 035007.

Vladkova, T., et al., 1999. Preparation of PEG-coated surfaces and a study for their interaction with living cells. Journal of Biomaterials Science: Polymer Edition 10, 609–620.

Wang, S., Lee, J.M., Yeong, W.Y., 2015a. Smart hydrogels for 3D bioprinting. International Journal of Bioprinting 1 (1), 3–14.

Wang, X., et al., 2006. Generation of three-dimensional hepatocyte/gelatin structures with rapid prototyping system. Tissue Engineering 12 (1), 83–90.

Wang, Z., et al., 2015b. A simple and high-resolution stereolithography-based 3D bioprinting system using visible light crosslinkable bioinks. Biofabrication 7 (4), 045009.

Wheeldon, I., Ahari, A.F., Khademhosseini, A., 2010. Microengineering hydrogels for stem cell bioengineering and tissue regeneration. JALA—Journal of the Association for Laboratory Automation 15 (6), 440–448.

White, C.J., et al., 2011. Extended release of high molecular weight hydroxypropyl methylcellulose from molecularly imprinted, extended wear silicone hydrogel contact lenses. Biomaterials 32 (24), 5698–5705.

Wu, W., DeConinck, A., Lewis, J.A., 2011. Omnidirectional printing of 3D microvascular networks. Advanced Materials 23 (24), H178–H183.

Wüst, S., Müller, R., Hofmann, S., 2014. 3D bioprinting of complex channels – effects of material, orientation, geometry and cell embedding. Journal of biomedical materials research—Part A 103 (8), 2558–2570.

Xu, W., et al., 2007. Rapid prototyping three-dimensional cell/gelatin/fibrinogen constructs for medical regeneration. Journal of Bioactive and Compatible Polymers 22 (4), 363–377.

Xu, C., et al., 2012. Scaffold-free inkjet printing of three-dimensional zigzag cellular tubes. Biotechnology and Bioengineering 109 (12), 3152–3160.

Xu, F., et al., 2011. The assembly of cell-encapsulating microscale hydrogels using acoustic waves. Biomaterials 32 (31), 7847–7855.

Xu, T., et al., 2013. Complex heterogeneous tissue constructs containing multiple cell types prepared by inkjet printing technology. Biomaterials 34 (1), 130–139.

Xu, T., et al., 2009. Fabrication and characterization of bio-engineered cardiac pseudo tissues. Biofabrication 1 (3), 035001.

Xu, T., et al., 2005. Inkjet printing of viable mammalian cells. Biomaterials 26 (1), 93–99.

Xu, T., et al., 2006. Viability and electrophysiology of neural cell structures generated by the inkjet printing method. Biomaterials 27 (19), 3580–3588.

Yamada, E., et al., 2011. Replica molding and bonding of microstructured hydrogel plates for tissue engineering applications. In: Conference Proceedings: 15th International Conference on Miniaturized Systems for Chemistry and Life Sciences, pp. 1834–1836.

Yamamoto, M., et al., 2010. Generation of stable co-cultures of vascular cells in a honeycomb alginate scaffold. Tissue Engineering: Part A 16 (1), 299–308.

Yamato, M., Okano, T., 2004. Cell sheet engineering. Materials Today 7 (5), 42–47.

Yan, J., Huang, Y., Chrisey, D.B., 2013. Laser-assisted printing of alginate long tubes and annular constructs. Biofabrication 5, 015002.

Yan, L.P., et al., 2010. Genipin-cross-linked collagen/chitosan biomimetic scaffolds for articular cartilage tissue engineering applications. Journal of Biomedical Materials Research - Part A 95 A (2), 465–475.

Yanez, M., et al., 2014. In Vivo assessment of printed microvasculature in a bilayer skin graft to treat full-thickness wounds. Tissue Engineering: Part A 21 (1–2), 224–233.

Yang, Z., et al., 2011. Thermoreversible Pluronic F127-based hydrogel containing liposomes for the controlled delivery of paclitaxel: in vitro drug release, cell cytotoxicity, and uptake studies. International Journal of Nanomedicine 6, 151–166.

Ye, K., et al., 2014. Chondrogenesis of infrapatellar fat pad derived adipose stem cells in 3D printed chitosan scaffold. PLoS One 9 (6), e99410.

Yu, Y., Ozbolat, I.T., 2014. Tissue strands as "bioink" for scale-up organ printing. In: Conference Proceedings: Annual International Conference of the IEEE Engineering in Medicine and Biology Society. IEEE Engineering in Medicine and Biology Society, pp. 1428–1431.

Yu, Y., et al., 2013. Evaluation of cell viability and functionality in vessel-like bioprintable cell-laden tubular channels. Journal of Biomechanical Engineering. 135 (9), 91011.

Yu, Y., et al., 2015. Use of recombinant human stromal cell-derived factor 1α-loaded fibrin/hyaluronic acid hydrogel networks to achieve functional repair of full-thickness bovine articular cartilage via homing of chondrogenic progenitor cells. Arthritis and Rheumatism 67 (5), 1274–1285.

Yu, Y., et al., 2016. Three-dimensional bioprinting using self-assembling scalable scaffold-free "tissue strands" as a new bioink. Scientific Reports 6, 28714.

Zhang, A.P., et al., 2012. Rapid fabrication of complex 3D extracellular microenvironments by dynamic optical projection stereolithography. Advanced Materials 24 (31), 4266–4270.

Zhang, L., Hu, J., Athanasiou, K.A., 2009. The role of tissue engineering in articular cartilage repair and regeneration. Critical Reviews in Biomed Engineering 37 (1–2), 1–57.

Zhang, L.G., et al., 2014. A microwell pattern for c17.2 cell aggregate formation with concave cylindrical surface induced cell peeling. Biomaterials 35 (35), 9423–9437.

Zhang, M., Desai, T., Ferrari, M., 1998. Proteins and cells on PEG immobilized silicon surfaces. Biomaterials 19, 953–960.

Zhang, Y., et al., 2013a. Characterization of printable cellular micro-fluidic channels for tissue engineering. Biofabrication 5 (2), 24004.

Zhang, Y., et al., 2015. In vitro study of directly bioprinted perfusable vasculature conduits. Biomaterials Science 3 (1), 134–143.

Zhang, Y., Yu, Y., Ozbolat, I.T., 2013b. Direct bioprinting of vessel-like tubular microfluidic channels. Journal of Nanotechnology in Engineering and Medicine 4, 020902.

Zhong, S.P., et al., 1994. Biodegradation of hyaluronic acid derivatives by hyaluronidase. Biomaterials 15 (5), 359–365.

Zhu, J., Marchant, R.E., 2011. Design properties of hydrogel tissue-engineering scaffolds. Expert Review of Medical Devices 8 (5), 607–626.

4

Extrusion-Based Bioprinting*

CHAPTER OUTLINE

To myself I am only a child playing on the beach, while vast oceans of truth lie undiscovered before me
Isaac Newton

4.1 Introduction

Pressure- or extrusion-based method has been used for quite a long time for various processes such as shape forming of metals and plastics (Abeykoon et al., 2012). Later 1990s, with the emergence of fused-deposition modeling (FDM), extrusion-based solid

*With minor contributions by Monika Hospodiuk, The Pennsylvania State University.

3D Bioprinting.

free-form fabrication approach demonstrated three-dimensional (3D) printing of intricate geometries with controlled porous architecture (Lipson and Kurman, 2013). This innovative approach at that time was later introduced into tissue engineering via 3D printing of porous scaffolds (Zein et al., 2002), which are temporary housing for cells to support their attachment, growth, and proliferation. In this regard, several pioneering work has been demonstrated in the literature including development of printable biomaterials and 3D-printing approaches for scaffold fabrication by Hutmacher's group (Ang et al., 2002; Hutmacher et al., 2004; Rai et al., 2005) and efforts in investigating modeling and design aspects for solid free-form fabrication of tissue scaffolds by Hollister's group (Lin et al., 2004; Schek et al., 2006).

With the advent of printing living cells and emergence of first bioprinting technologies via other means such as laser-based bioprinting (LBB) (Odde and Renn, 1999) and droplet-based bioprinting (DBB) (Pardo et al., 2003), extrusion-based bioprinting (EBB) (Mironov et al., 2003) has been started to be investigated for printing living cells including the bioplotting approach, where hydrogel bioink was extruded and bioprinted within a liquid plotting medium resulting in high flexural and mechanical strength, and cell proliferation rate (Pfister et al., 2004). The fledgling technology later received enormous attention and advanced rapidly. Although several groups, including notable contributions of Sun et al. (Khalil Saif, 2007; Khalil et al., 2005), investigated the technology by encapsulating cells in hydrogels solutions, the versatility of the technology allowed other researchers to adopt novel bioink materials into the EBB technology. In 2004, Mironov and Forgacs introduced the concept of printing scaffold-free cell aggregates for bioprinting living tissues and organs (Boland et al., 2003; Jakab et al., 2004). They considered printing cells in clusters in spheroid shape on hydrogel glue called "biopaper" (Mironov et al., 2009) and investigated bioprinting vascular constructs in 3D. After some initial attempts in bioprinting spheroids and assembling them vertically, the technology rapidly evolved into a state generating feasible outcome and resulted in fabrication of blood vessels (Norotte et al., 2009). Further modifications have been applied to the technology, and it currently enables printing tissue constructs that do not require significant vascularization such as thin or hollow (i.e., skin, nerve, and vasculature) and avascular (i.e., cartilage) tissues (Murphy and Atala, 2014).

Due its versatility, affordability, and ability to print porous constructs, EBB is now utilized by numerous researchers worldwide and the technology has already paved the way to bioprint cells (Horváth et al., 2015; Almeida et al., 2014; Bertassoni et al., 2014), tissues (Yu et al., 2016), tissue constructs (Kolesky et al., 2014), organ modules (Marga et al., 2012), and tissue/organ-on-a-chip devices (Kolesky et al., 2014), with a long-term expectations in printing functional scale-up organs (Yu et al., 2014). A wide variety of tissue constructs have been successfully engineered by means of EBB including but not limited to cartilage (Zhang et al., 2014), vasculature (Norotte et al., 2009), bone (Poldervaart et al., 2013), skin (Lee et al., 2009a), liver (Godoy et al., 2013), and cardiac (Gaetani et al., 2012). Currently, EBB technology has been commercialized by several companies and a number of bioprinters are widely available, as detailed in Chapter 7, for new bioprinting researchers entering into the field or researchers using bioprinting as an application to their core fields such as biologists, pharmacists, and medical doctors (Ventola, 2014). The technology has been adopted into various fields including basic research in different areas such as cancer research (Huang et al., 2014; Nöth et al., 2004) and tissue engineering (Liu et al., 2008; Kim and Rajagopalan, 2010; Billiet et al., 2014), pharmaceutics for drug testing (Zhang et al., 2012; Davoodi et al., 2014), and tissue printing for transplantation and clinics (Perkins, 2007).

Several researchers have demonstrated EBB of tissue substitutes in the literature. Different cell types have been loaded and deposited in a wide range of biocompatible hydrogels. Recently, Billiet et al. (2014) used hepatocytes with gelatin-methacrylamide hydrogel to engineer artificial liver tissue constructs. Cell viability after deposition ranged up to 97%. Horváth et al. (2015) demonstrated bioprinting of lung tissue analogs for the first time. The architecture of the air–blood barrier was very precise, comparable to native tissue. Melchels et al. (2014) performed a characterization of a new gelatin-methacrylamide bioink containing gellan gum and mannose. They obtained various 3D structures (pyramid, hemisphere, hollow cylinder) with high cell viability, where hydrogel properties can be tailored by salt concentration. Another group bioprinted human adipose tissue–derived mesenchymal stem cells (hASCs) loaded in decellularized extracellular matrix (dECM) components of adipose tissue (Pati et al., 2015). The bioink was printed in precisely defined and flexible dome-shaped structures, and hASCs in bioprinted structures showed significantly higher-adipogenic differentiation than hASCs cultured in nonprinted decellularized adipose tissue matrix components.

This chapter presents EBB technology including its working principle and physical mechanism behind it, compares EBB with other bioprinting modalities, discusses process configurations, the bioink materials that are applied and the limitations of EBB, and describes future prospects to the reader.

4.2 Extrusion-Based Bioprinting

4.2.1 Working Principle

EBB technique is a combination of a fluid dispensing and an automated robotic system for extrusion and bioprinting, respectively (Mironov et al., 2003). During bioprinting, bioink is dispensed by a deposition system, under the control of a computer, resulting in precise deposition of cells encapsulated in cylindrical filaments of desired 3D custom–shaped structures. This rapid fabrication technique provides relatively better structural integrity due to continuous deposition of filaments. Moreover, this method easily can incorporate computer software such as computer-aided design (CAD) software, which enables users to load a CAD file to automatically print the structure (He et al., 2003). The CAD file can be obtained from medical images or a free-form design per demand (Giannitelli et al., 2014) as detailed in Chapter 2. Therefore it is considered as the most convenient technique in producing 3D porous cell-laden structures. Fluid dispensing system can be driven by (1) pneumatic-, (2) mechanical- (piston or screw driven), or (3) solenoid-based system, as shown in Fig. 4.1.

Pneumatic-based system utilizes pressurized air using valve-free (Fig. 4.1A1) or valve-based (Fig. 4.1A2) configuration. Although valve-free configuration has been widely used due to its simplicity, valve-based configuration can be preferable with controlled pressure and pulse frequency for high-precision applications. Valve-free configuration works sufficiently for hydrogels with shear-thinning property; however, bioink materials with highly low viscosity can easily flow through the nozzle even if there is no pressure applied. Therefore valve-based configuration is highly recommended for low-viscosity bioink materials or crosslinker solutions. Pneumatic-driven EBB systems require sterilization of the used air from the air dispenser compressor. Thus using a filter on the airway would be ideal to minimize contamination of the bioprinted constructs. Pneumatic-driven systems do not generate smooth extrusion of the semisolid or solid bioink (i.e., cell aggregates) and requires another liquid or gel medium to deliver the bioink through the nozzle tip. Otherwise, the bioink can easily attach on the nozzle wall. No issues are foreseeable for hydrogel-based bioinks due to its liquid- or sol-gel nature, where bioink in liquid- or sol-gel state can easily transmit forces equally in all directions without any entrapment inside the nozzle.

Mechanical microextrusion systems utilize piston- (Fig. 4.1B1) or screw-driven (Fig. 4.1B2) configurations. Piston-driven configuration generally provides more direct control over the flow of bioink through the nozzle. Screw-driven configuration may give more spatial control and is beneficial for dispensing of bioinks with higher viscosities. However, screw-driven configuration can generate larger-pressure drops along the nozzle, which can potentially harm the loaded cells. Thus the design of rotating screw gear needs to be carefully performed to use it in EBB. In addition, mechanical-driven systems are highly affordable, easy to program, and portable, and do not need air compressor unit and necessary accessories. Mechanical-driven systems provide better printing abililty for semisolid or solid bioink materials such as cell aggregates.

Solenoid microextrusion (Fig. 4.1C) utilizes electrical pulses to open a valve by canceling magnetic pull force generated between a floating ferromagnetic plunger and a ferromagnetic ring magnet. A similar configuration can be developed using piezoelectric-actuated system; however, it is not convenient for EBB while the process mode is droplet. Solenoid-based microextrusion enables dispensing of sub-μL range volume of bioink (Bammesberger et al., 2013) and is convenient for bioprinting of low-viscosity bioink materials with ionically or ultraviolet (UV) irradiation–based cross-linking mechanism. Although high accuracy can be obtained, there are a number of factors affecting the accuracy and reproducibility of solenoid-based microextrusion systems including the time-lapse between actuation time (where the coil is energized) and the time when the valve opens, soft nature of the sealing between the plunger and the valve seat resulting in compression of the sealing and time delays, and the need for high-actuating pressure to dispense highly viscous bioink.

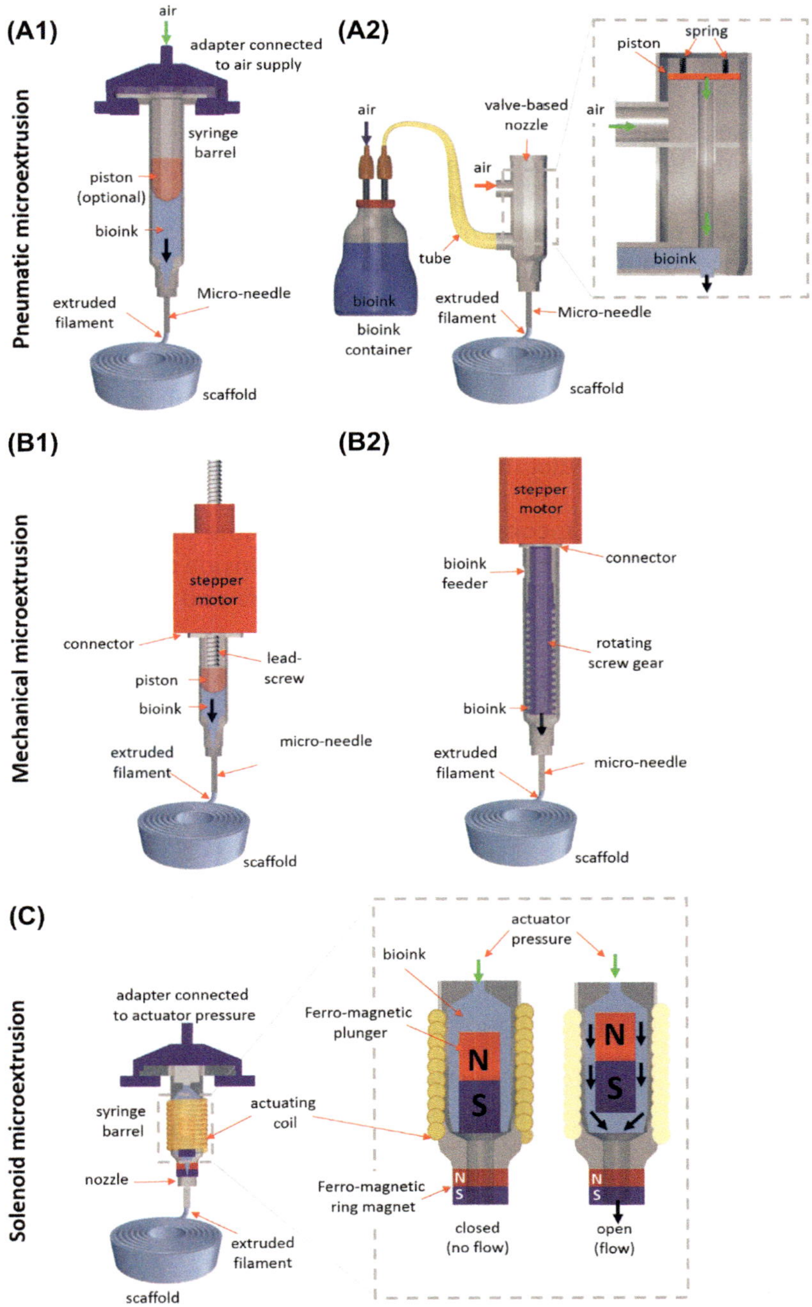

FIGURE 4.1 Extrusion-based bioprinting systems: (A) pneumatic microextrusion including (A1) valve-free and (A2) valve based, (B) mechanical microextrusion including (B1) piston- or (B2) screw-driven, and (C) solenoid microextrusion.

4.2.2 Physical Explanation of Extrusion-Based Bioprinting Process

Majority of EBB bioprinting processes utilize a simple setup (see Fig. 4.2A), where hydrogel-based bioink materials are loaded into a syringe barrel and extruded through a micronozzle tip, and printed onto a stage layer by layer. As the pressure applied to the syringe, the polymer oozes out through the nozzle tip. If the space between the nozzle tip and the stage is too sparse, then the bioink solution accumulates and solidifies at the tip without successful deposition. On the other hand, if the nozzle tip is highly close to the printing stage, then the bioink solution breaks out and fine lines are traced on the stage. Therefore adjusting the space between the tip and the stage is highly important for bioprintability and it is recommended that a space with a distance roughly equal to the diameter of the tip should be used. In addition, other bioprinting parameters such as extrusion and printing speed as well as printed filament diameter are also important during EBB process. In this section, the physical formulation is presented to the reader, which is highly essential to predict the bioprinting parameters to successfully print well-defined tissue constructs.

In a steady state laminar incompressible flow for time-independent bioinks, the linear momentum balance on a cylindrical fluid element inside the nozzle (see Fig. 4.2B) with radius r and length L can be formulated as (Chhabra and Richardson, 2008):

$$P(\pi r^2) = (P + \Delta P)(\pi r^2) + 2\pi \mathrm{r} L \tau_{\mathrm{rz}} \tag{4.1}$$

where P is the pressure applied from the source of flow, ΔP is the pressure drop, and τ_{rz} is the shear stress on the cylindrical fluid element. In Eq. (4.1), gravitational force is

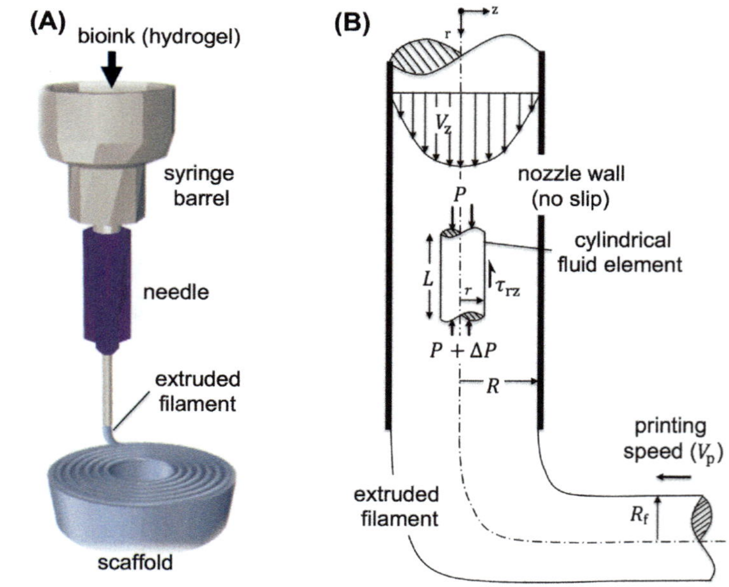

FIGURE 4.2 Extrusion-based bioprinting: (A) a general setup for extruding bioink solution through a micronozzle tip and (B) the schematic representation of extrusion process at the end of the nozzle tip for formulation of bioprinting parameters.

neglected. By rearranging Eq. (4.1), the shear stress on the fluid element can be written as:

$$\tau_{rz} = \left(\frac{r}{2}\right)\left(\frac{-\Delta P}{L}\right) \tag{4.2}$$

The shear stress can also be represented as a function of shear rate using a power-law fluid relationship (Richardson et al., 1991) as presented in Eq. (4.3), where K is the flow consistency index, μ_{eff} is the apparent viscosity, V_z is the velocity in the axial direction at radius r, and n is the dimensionless flow behavior index. According to literature (Faghri and Zhang, 2006), $n < 1$ for pseudoplastic or shear-thinning fluids, $n = 1$ for Newtonian fluids, and $n > 1$ for dilatant or shear-thickening fluids.

$$\tau_{rz} = K\left(\frac{\mathrm{d}V_z}{\mathrm{d}r}\right)^n = \mu\frac{\mathrm{d}V_z}{\mathrm{d}r} \tag{4.3}$$

By combining Eqs. (4.2) and (4.3) (assuming no-slip condition at the nozzle wall) and integrating it with respect to r, the following expression can be derived for the velocity distribution:

$$V_z = \left(\frac{n}{n+1}\right)\left(\frac{-\Delta P}{KL}\frac{R}{2}\right)^{1/n} R\left[1 - \left(\frac{r}{R}\right)^{\frac{n+1}{n}}\right] \tag{4.4}$$

As can be derived from the expression of the velocity distribution, the velocity of the bioink flow is maximum in the core and equal to 0 when the radius is equal to R (at the nozzle wall) (see Fig. 4.2B). The average velocity profile, on the other hand, can be formulated as the volumetric flow rate (Q) per cross-sectional area of the nozzle. The volumetric flow rate can be represented as integration of V_z with respect to r:

$$V = \frac{Q}{\pi R^2} = \frac{1}{\pi R^2}\int_0^R 2\pi r V_z \mathrm{d}r \tag{4.5}$$

Then the integration yields as presented in Eq. (4.6):

$$V = \left(\frac{n}{3n+1}\right)\left(\frac{-\Delta P}{2KL}\right)^{1/n} R^{n+1/n} \tag{4.6}$$

Using the preservation of volumetric flow rate before and after the fluid ejection from the nozzle tip, where V_p is the printing speed (robot speed) and R_f is the radius of the printed filament,

$$V\pi R^2 \cong V_p \pi R_f^2 \tag{4.7}$$

the equation can be further arranged by combining Eqs. (4.6). and (4.7) as follows:

$$R_f \cong V_p^{-1/2}\left(\frac{n}{3n+1}\right)^{1/2}\left(\frac{-\Delta P}{2KL}\right)^{-1/2n} R^{3n+1/2n} \tag{4.8}$$

By using the previously mentioned equations, bioprinting parameters for EBB can be easily obtained for different bioink solutions of power-law fluids with various rheological properties. The presented formulations on the other hand cannot be used for solid-based bioink materials such as cell aggregates.

4.3 Process Configurations

EBB is highly versatile in depositing a wide array of bioink types including hydrogels (Khalil and Sun, 2009; Murphy et al., 2013), tissue spheroids (Boland et al., 2003; Mironov et al., 2009; Jakab et al., 2010; Mehesz et al., 2011), cell pellets (Owens et al., 2013), microcarriers (Levato et al., 2014), decellularized matrix components (Pati et al., 2015), and tissue strands (Yu and Ozbolat, 2014) as shown in Fig. 4.3. This versatility originates due to larger nozzle diameter ranges applied, ability to deposit small building blocks in fugitive liquid delivery medium, flexibility in nozzle tip design, and the ability to extrude bioink in near solid-state.

A wide variety of process configurations have been demonstrated in the literature of EBB due to a number of solidification or crosslinking mechanism experimented for hydrogels using EBB including physical [temperature (Norotte et al., 2009), and light (Billiet et al., 2014)] and chemical [pH (Smith et al., 2004), ionic compound (Cohen et al.,

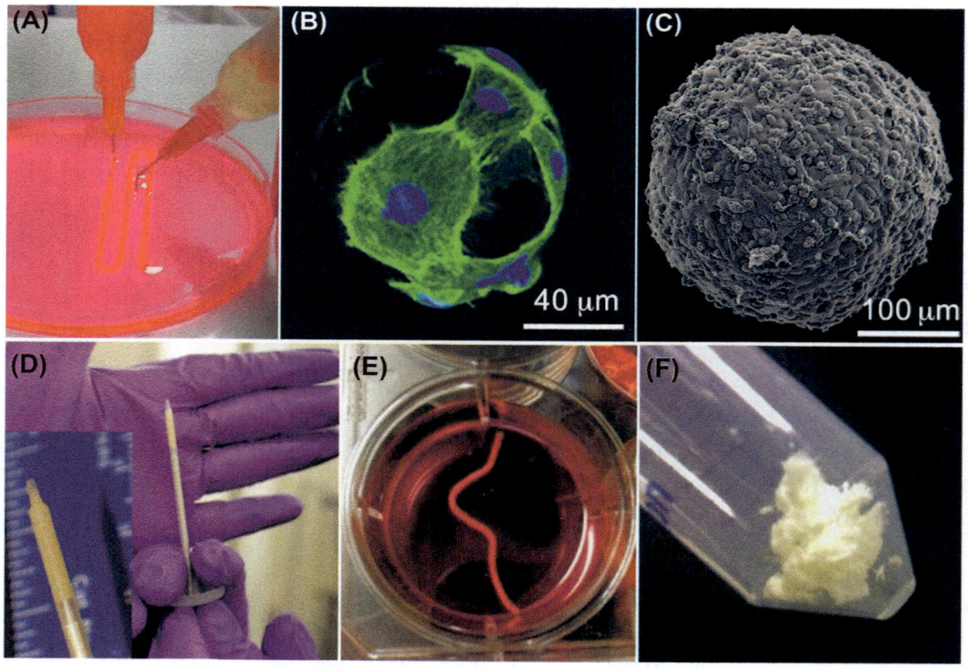

FIGURE 4.3 Bioink types used in EBB: (A) cells loaded in hydrogels, (B) polymer microcarriers preloaded with cells *(Reproduced/adapted with permission from Levato et al. (2014))*, (C) tissue spheroids made of cells and extracellular matrix (ECM) (Reproduced/adapted with permission from Norotte et al. (2009)), (D) cell pellet in nozzle tip, (E) tissue strands *(Reproduced/adapted with permission from Akkouch et al. (2015))* and (F) dECM before loading cells *(Reproduced/adapted with permission from Pati et al. (2015))*.

2010)] crosslinking. Processing configurations in EBB can be therefore classified based on the bioink types used as process configuration for (1) ionically crosslinking hydrogels, (2) UV-crosslinking hydrogels, (3) thermally crosslinking hydrogels, (4) enzymatically crosslinking hydrogels, (5) microcarriers, (6) cell aggregates, and (7) decellularized matrix components.

4.3.1 Nozzle Configuration for Ionically Crosslinking Hydrogels

Different EBB systems have been experimented due to instant gelation properties of hydrogels in ionic solutions (such as alginate and chitosan). These mechanisms are (1) bioplotting (Pfister et al., 2004), (2) bioprinting hydrogel with a secondary nozzle (Duan et al., 2013) using crosslinker deposition or spraying system (Sato et al., 2010), (3) or coaxial nozzle system (Ozbolat et al., 2014), (4) bioprinting precrosslinked hydrogel and further crosslinking it thereafter (Chung et al., 2013), and (5) bioprinting with an aerosol crosslinking process (Tan et al., 2014). Although some researchers use the term "bioplotting" and "bioprinting" interchangeably, there is a misconception about the "bioplotting" term. In bioplotting approach (see Fig. 4.4A), cells in a hydrogel solution are extruded into a plotting medium (crosslinker pool), where the extrusion process takes place within the pool and the bioprinted construct stays inside the pool until the process is completed. Therefore extrusion of hydrogels without a crosslinker plotting medium shall not be classified under "bioplotting" approach. In bioplotting, the density of the extruded bioink needs to be greater than that of the plotting medium for successful

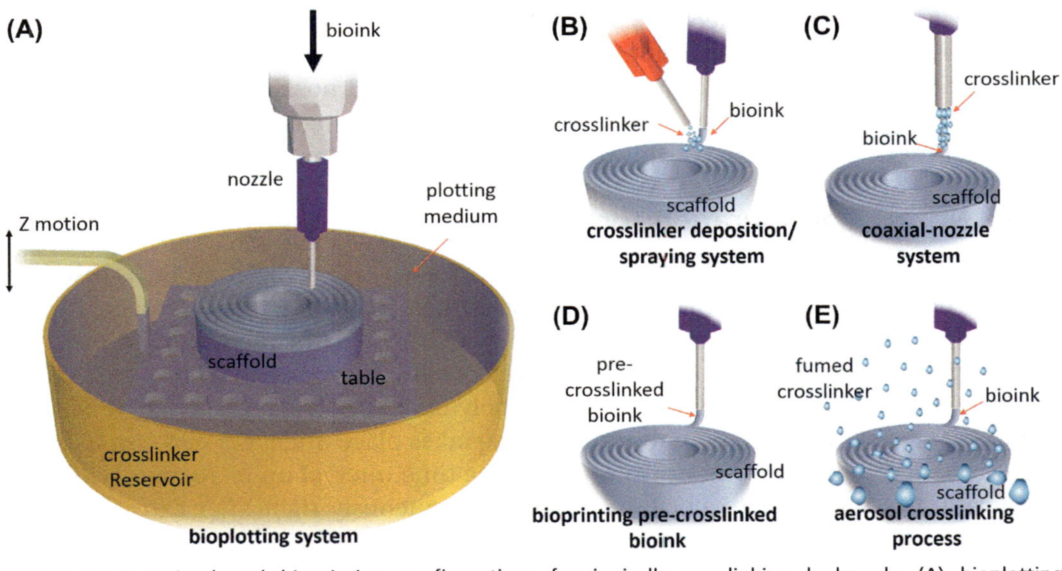

FIGURE 4.4 Extrusion-based bioprinting configurations for ionically crosslinking hydrogels: (A) bioplotting, (B) crosslinker deposition or spraying system, (C) coaxial nozzle system, (D) bioprinting precrosslinked bioink, and (E) aerosol crosslinking system.

deposition. By altering the temperature and the viscosity of the plotting medium, extrusion and deposition process can be controlled easily. In the second technique as show in Fig. 4.4B, the crosslinker solution is deposited or sprayed onto the bioprinted hydrogel using a secondary nozzle, where the nozzle position can change using a motorized system. In the third technique (see Fig. 4.4C), hydrogel bioink is bioprinted using a coaxial nozzle apparatus, where the hydrogel is bioprinted through the core and the crosslinker solution is ejected through the sheath section of the outer nozzle that is slightly shorter than the core nozzle providing better control on the extrudability of the bioink.

In the fourth technique (see Fig. 4.4D), precrosslinked hydrogel (with low crosslinker concentration) is bioprinted providing sufficient deposition quality of the bioink and structural integrity of the scaffold followed by enhancing crosslinking by exposing the bioprinted scaffold to a high concentration of crosslinker solution. In this approach, mechanical properties of printed constructs are better, but pressure level for extrusion process is higher relative to the density of precrosslinked hydrogel. In addition, the bioink is not even, which brings discontinuities and nonuniformities during extrusion. In the fifth approach using an aerosol crosslinking system (see Fig. 4.4E), the hydrogel bioink is printed onto a table, where the entire system is enclosed in a moisture intensive environment with evaporated crosslinker solution (generated by an ultrasonic humidifier) fumed over the entire bioprinting space. The difference between the fifth and the spraying approach is that fuming process generates highly small particles of the crosslinker solution in near-vapor state that can be uniformly distributed over the entire structure as oppose to the spraying approach. This enables simultaneous crosslinking between layers, generating mechanically and structurally integrated constructs. All these approaches have pros and cons with respect to each other but it has been demonstrated that bioprinting precrosslinked hydrogel or using a coaxial nozzle–assisted crosslinker deposition system shows promising results in terms of printing accuracy and the ability to 3D bioprint tissue constructs with well-integrated interlayers (Fedorovich et al., 2008).

4.3.2 Nozzle Configuration for Ultraviolet-Crosslinking Hydrogels

In nozzle configuration for UV-crosslinking hydrogels, a UV light guide is used to crosslink the deposited hydrogel. The process configuration for this approach is presented in Fig. 4.5. Upon bioprinting hydrogels such as gelatin methacrylate (GelMA) (Bertassoni et al., 2014; Billiet et al., 2014), hyaluronan methacrylate (Dana et al., 2004; Skardal et al., 2010b; Skardal and Atala, 2014), poly(ethylene glycol) diacrylate (PEG-DA) (Hockaday et al., 2012), where photo-crosslinking takes place under 6.9 mW/cm UV light with wavelength ranging from 360 to 480 nm for a time interval up to 10 min. While the solidification of the gel does not take place instantaneously right after extrusion, bioprinting of UV-crosslinked hydrogels does not generate structurally and mechanically integrated tissue constructs. As the period for UV exposure prolongs, mechanical strength of the hydrogel increases, but bioprinting in 3D becomes not efficient while a

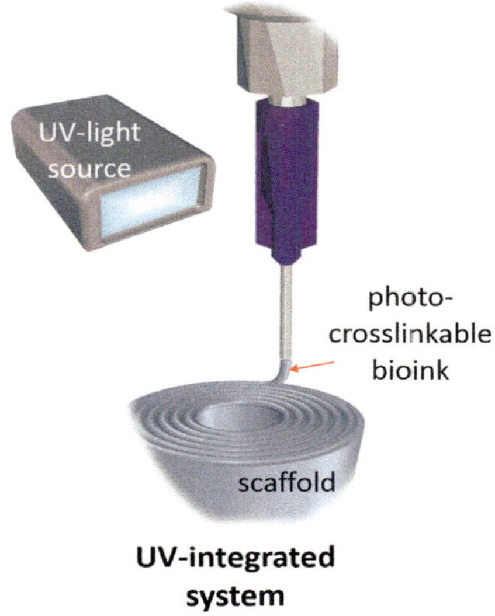

FIGURE 4.5 Extrusion-based bioprinting configurations for UV-crosslinking hydrogels.

substantial idle time is acquired between two layers. During this time, a new calibration might be needed ascribed to layer thickness change due to hydrogel contraction, dehydration, or swelling. Therefore this configuration is not convenient for bioprinting porous tissue constructs but works for bioprinting bulk hydrogel tissue constructs. In addition, exposing cells to UV for prolonged times can also be detrimental for cells.

4.3.3 Nozzle Configuration for Thermally Crosslinking Hydrogels

In addition to ionically crosslinking and photocurable hydrogels, there has been a plethora of work done in bioprinting of thermally crosslinking hydrogels (Wu et al., 2011; Chang et al., 2011). There are two different configurations for thermally crosslinking hydrogels ascribed to the crosslinking mechanism including hydrogels that solidify under either heating or cooling.

An EBB configuration, presented in Fig. 4.6A, can be used to bioprint thermally crosslinking hydrogels such as agarose that have low melting temperature, where extruded agarose in liquid state rapidly solidifies when bioprinted onto a freezing stage. Using EBB system, researchers extruded agarose as supporting gel for cell aggregation (Norotte et al., 2009). This configuration can also be used for another temperature-sensitive hydrogel, gelatin, where gelatin has been used as a sacrificial material to fabricate 3D-printed scaffolds with open fluidic channels (Lee et al., 2010). Upon printing, gelatin can be liquefied after incubating the scaffold at 37°C, leaving empty and perfusable channels. In the second approach, thermally reversible hydrogels crosslinking at higher temperatures can be used in a configuration presented in Fig. 4.6B. For example, 20% Pluronic® F-127 solution is sol at room temperature and gels above 20°C, where the sol-gel transition can be modified by changing the solution concentration (Skardal and Atala, 2014). Pluronic® F-127 has a great potential in EBB process (Wu et al., 2011;

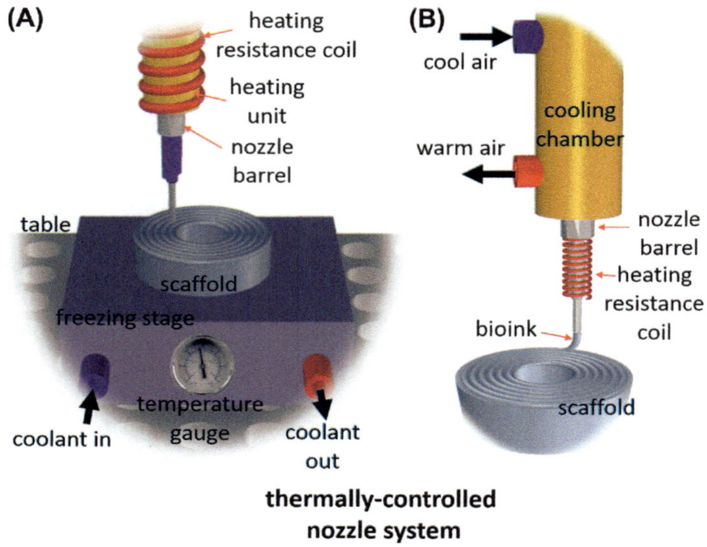

FIGURE 4.6 Extrusion-based bioprinting configurations for thermally crosslinking hydrogels: (A) a heating unit–assisted barrel with cooling unit–assisted bioprinting stage and (B) a cooling unit–assisted barrel with a heating unit–assisted nozzle tip.

Chang et al., 2011), but requires special bioprinting apparatus. Thus the configuration presented in Fig. 4.6B is used to solidify the bioink as extrusion takes place. When the bioink is loaded into the barrel in liquid state, it is kept at low temperature using a cooling chamber if the melting temperature is below room temperature. A heating unit around the dispensing tip enables precise control of the temperature while the bioink is extruded. In this way, the bioink can be extruded in solid filament form. Optionally, a heating plate can be used to prevent melting of hydrogel and lose of the structure and shape. Using Pluronic®, spatially well-defined constructs can be printed accurately (Smith et al., 2004). Similarly, Matrigel™, which is a thermosensitive material, but not reversible can be used in the process configurations. Once it crosslinks at 24–37°C, it does not decrosslink when cooled. Gelation time takes about 30 min and starts above 4°C in the barrel. To extrude Matrigel™, it is necessary to possess temperature-controlled bioprinting system to retain the hydrogel at 4°C (Snyder et al., 2011). Otherwise, dispensing needle clogs and makes bioprinting highly challenging. In addition, collagen type I can also be used in a similar configuration, where the bioink is kept in low temperature ranges and heated up to physically relevant temperature ranges, full crosslinking of collagen can be achieved in half an hour time period in incubation.

4.3.4 Nozzle Configuration for Enzymatically Crosslinking Hydrogels

Enzymatically crosslinking hydrogels such as fibrin can be extruded and bioprinted using different combinations. For example, fibrinogen and thrombin can be mixed on ice preventing gelation and then extruded using a configuration presented in Fig. 4.6B.

Alternatively, a multichamber single-nozzle apparatus can be used to blend both fibrinogen and thrombin into one solution at the very end of the extrusion process (Gregor and Hošek, 2011) as shown in Fig. 4.7.

In addition to bioprinting single type of bioink, the multichamber single-nozzle configuration shown in Fig. 4.7 has been used to blend and print multiple bioinks with different material properties or loaded biomolecule concentrations to generate heterogeneous filaments with varying properties of biomaterials along the longitudinal direction of filaments (Ozbolat and Koc, 2011a). Using such a nozzle assembly, biofabrication of hybrid tissue-engineered porous scaffolds, where multiple functional properties can be obtained by changing biomaterial type and concentration spatially (Ozbolat and Koc, 2011b). Material flow and concentration through the mixture chamber can be controlled by regulating positive nozzle pressures connected to an air pressure control unit. A similar approach has been extended to triple chambers by (Mogas-Soldevila et al., 2014), where scaffolds were fabricated by bending materials, chitosan, sodium alginate, and chitin powder using a static mixer nozzle mounted on a 6-axis robotic printer (Mogas-Soldevila et al., 2014).

A detailed list of hydrogels used in EBB are presented in Table 4.1 with their crosslinking mechanism, solidification reversibility, extrusion configuration along with advantages and disadvantages.

4.3.5 Nozzle Configuration for Microcarriers

Bioprinting of microcarriers (see Chapter 3 for details about microcarriers) can be performed using EBB systems only while microcarriers can easily block the orifice of DBB and laser energy in LBB is not sufficient enough to repel microcarriers. Upon culturing cells on microcarriers, they allow cells to quickly proliferate. Matured microcarriers

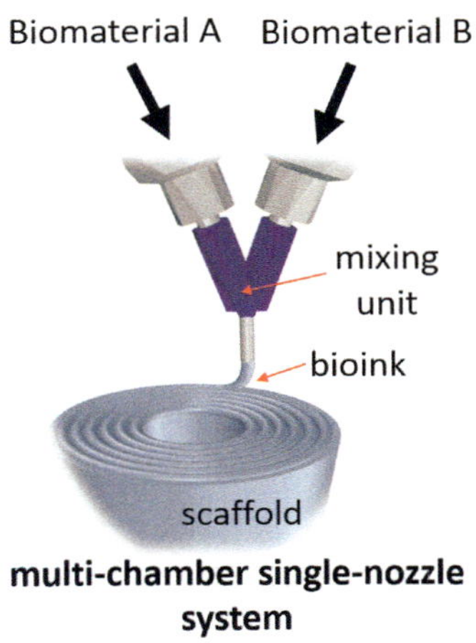

FIGURE 4.7 Extrusion-based bioprinting configuration for enzymatically crosslinking hydrogels.

Table 4.1 Hydrogels Used in EBB

Hydrogel Type	Bioink	Crosslinking Mechanism	Solidification Reversibility	EBB System	Advantages	Disadvantages	Sample Tissue Construct	References
Alginate	Aggregates, proteins, encapsulated cells [skeletal myoblasts, bone marrow stem cells (BMSCs), smooth muscle cells (SMCs), mesenchymal stem cells (MSCs), adipose stem cells (ASCs), cartilage progenitor cells (CPCs), chondrocytes, cardiomyocytes]	Ionic	–	Pneumatic microextrusion and bioplotting	Biocompatibility, good extrudability and bioprintability, fast gelation, good stability and integrality of printed construct, medium elasticity, low cost, nonimmunogenic	Low cell adhesion and spreading without modification of hydrogel	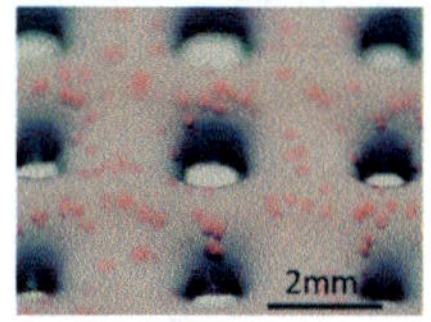 Reproduced/adapted with permission from Poldervaart et al. (2013).[a]	Tan et al. (2014); Fedorovich et al. (2008); Poldervaart et al. (2013); Duan et al. (2013); Fedorovich et al. (2012); Gaetani et al. (2012); Lee et al. (2014a,b,c); Zhang et al. (2013)
Collagen type I	Encapsulated cells [bovine aortic endothelial cells, keratinocytes, fibroblasts, rat neural cells, MSC, amniotic fluid –derived stem cells (AFSs)]	pH-mediated or thermal	–	Pneumatic microextrusion	Cell-adherent, promote proliferation, signal transducer, good extrusion and bioprinting abilities, nonimmunogenic	Poor mechanical properties, slow gelation, unstable	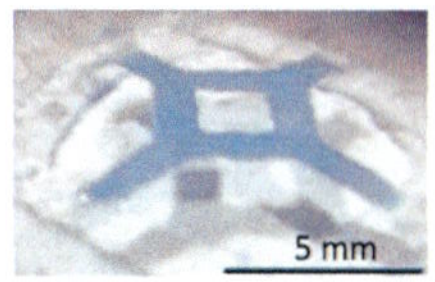 Reproduced/adapted with permission from Lee et al. (2010).[a]	Smith et al. (2004); Rücker et al. (2006); Lee et al. (2010); Lee et al. (2014b,c); Lee et al. (2009b); (2009a); Skardal et al. (2012)
Gelatin	Encapsulated cells (HepG2, hepatocytes, fibroblasts, SMC)	Thermal	+	Mechanical and pneumatic microextrusion	cell-adherent, biocompatible, nonimmunogenic	Unstable, fragile, weak mechanical properties at physiological temperature and low abilities to extrude and print without modification	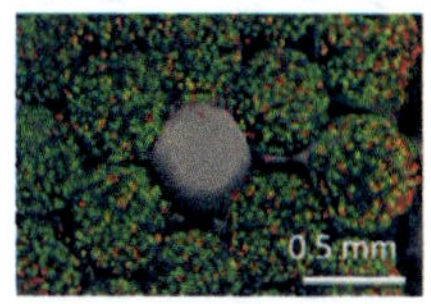 Reproduced/adapted with permission from Bertassoni et al. (2014).[a]	Billiet et al. (2014); Lee et al. (2010); Duan et al. (2013); Tocchio et al. (2015); Bertassoni et al. (2014); Wang et al. (2006)

Poly ethylene glycol	Encapsulated cells (BMSCs or porcine aortic valve interstitial cells)	Ionic, physical, or covalent agents	–	Pneumatic microextrusion	Support cell viability, biocompatible, nonimmunogenic, widely used in tissue engineering when modified	Low proliferation rate, low cell adhesion, weak mechanical properties and stability without modification	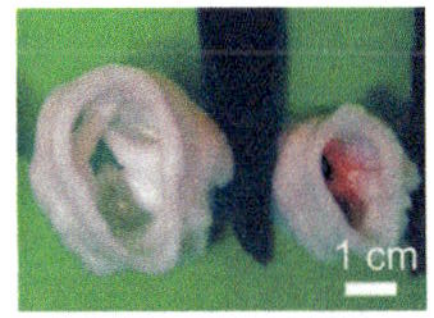 Reproduced/adapted with permission from Hockaday et al. (2012).[a]	Fedorovich et al. (2008); Hockaday et al. (2012)
Fibrin	Acellular scaffolds or encapsulated cells [AFS, human umbilical vascular endothelial cells (HUVECs)]	Enzymatic	–	Pneumatic microextrusion	Promote angiogenesis (causes inflammatory response), fast gelation, good integrality, medium elasticity	Difficult to control geometry, low mechanical properties, limited EBB printability	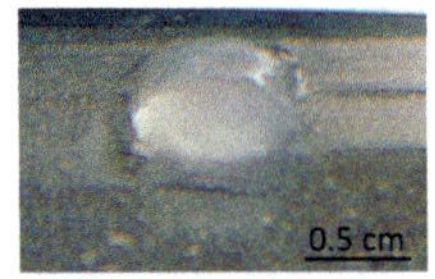 Image courtesy of Prof. Hosek from Czech Technical University in Praque.[b]	Gregor and Hošek (2011); Wei et al. (2007); Skardal et al. (2012); Lee et al. (2014b,c)
Matrigel	Encapsulated cells [HepG2, BMSCs, MSC, endothelial progenitor cells (EPC)]	Thermal	–	Pneumatic microextrusion	Promote cell differentiation and vascularization of construct, support cell viability, good bioprintability, highly suitable particularly for cardiac tissue engineering	Slow gelation, which affects mechanical stability, requires cooling system for EBB, expensive	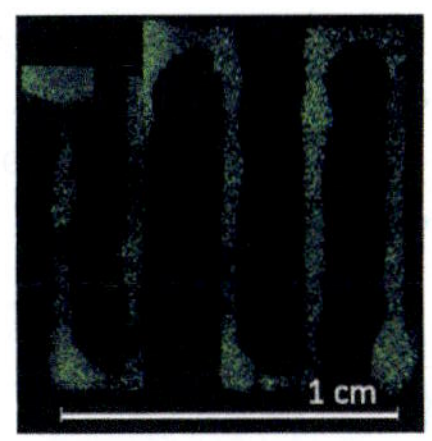 Reproduced/adapted with permission from Snyder et al. (2011).[a]	Fedorovich et al. (2008); Fedorovich et al. (2011); Snyder et al. (2011)

Continued

Table 4.1 Hydrogels Used in EBB—cont'd

Hydrogel Type	Bioink	Crosslinking Mechanism	Solidification Reversibility	EBB System	Advantages	Disadvantages	Sample Tissue Construct	References
Agarose	Acellular supporting gels	Thermal	+	Pneumatic and mechanical microextrusion	Stable mechanical properties, stable, resistant for protein adsorption, low cost, good integrality, nonimmunogenic	Low cell adhesion, fragile, require heating system for EBB	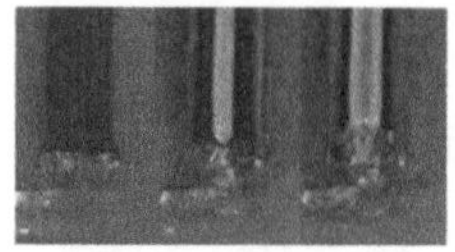 Reproduced/adapted with permission from Norotte et al. (2009).[a]	Norotte et al. (2009); Bertassoni et al. (2014)
Chitosan	Acellular scaffolds, encapsulated cells (MSCs, CPC)	Ionic or covalent agents	–	Pneumatic microextrusion	Antibacterial and antifungal, medium printability, nonimmunogenic	Weak mechanical and stability properties without modification, slow gelation rate	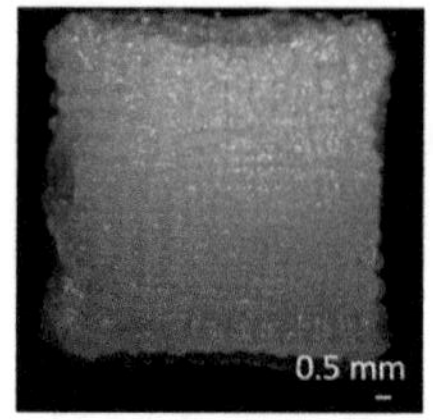 Reproduced/adapted with permission from Ye et al. (2014).[a]	Ye et al. (2014); Rinaudo (2006); Zhang et al. (2013)
Pluronic® F-127	Encapsulated cells (human primary fibroblasts, BMSCs, HepG2)	Thermal	+	Pneumatic and mechanical microextrusion	High printability, good bioprintability, nonimmunogenic	Poor mechanical and structural properties, slow gelation, rapid degradation, require heating system for EBB	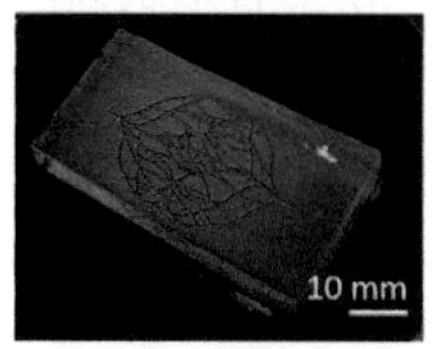 Reproduced/adapted with permission from Wu et al. (2011).[a]	Smith et al. (2004); Wu et al. (2011); Fedorovich et al. (2008); Khattak et al. (2005)

Hyaluronic acid	Encapsulated cells (chondrocytes, HepG2, C3A, fibroblasts)	Ionic, covalent agents	−	Pneumatic and mechanical microextrusion	Promote proliferation and angiogenesis, fast gelation, good bioprintability, nonimmunogenic	Rapid degradation, poor mechanical properties, and low stability without modification	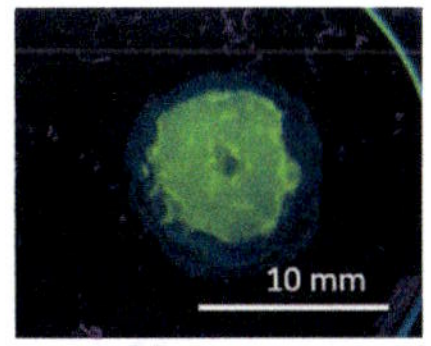 Reproduced/adapted with permission from Skardal et al. (2010a,b).[a]	Dana et al. (2004); Skardal et al. (2010a,b)
Methylcellulose	Encapsulated chondrocytes	Thermal, pH-mediated	+	Mechanical microextrusion	High printability, nonimmunogenic	Low bioprintability, sensitive on common cell culture media, unstable	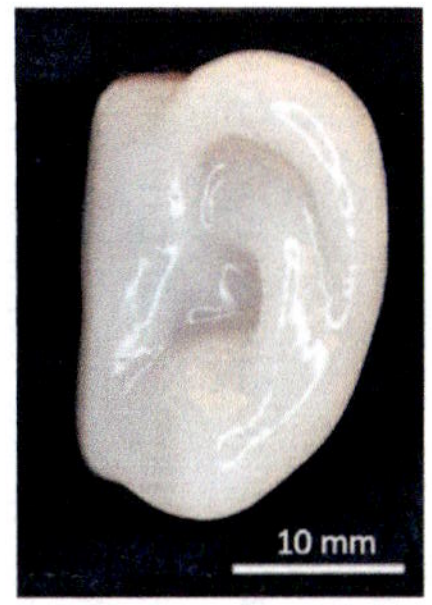 Reprinted (adapted) with permission from Markstedt et al. (2015).[a] Copyright (2015) American Chemical Society	Markstedt et al. (2015)

[a]*All sample figures are reprinted with permission from the respective publishers as indicated in the reference source.*
[b]*Image courtesy of the author.*

can be bioprinted in a delivery medium such as hydrogels as shown in Fig. 4.8. One of the previously described hydrogel crosslinking mechanisms can be used during bioprinting of microcarriers and EBB bioprinting works efficiently as it offers larger nozzle selections for extrusion of large microparticles.

4.3.6 Nozzle Configuration for Cell Aggregates

For bioprinting cell aggregates (see Chapter 3 for details about cell aggregates), different process configurations have been demonstrated based on the bioink applied including tissue spheroids, cell pellets, and tissue strands. Prefabricated tissue spheroids are loaded in pipettes and dispensed using a mechanical ram–driven EBB system in a carrier hydrogel that is inert to cell adhesion (see Fig. 4.9A). In the meantime, a mold structure is 3D printed, where the bioprinted spheroids are cast inside the mold, which allows them fusing and maturating into tissue followed by removal of the mold material. Instead of delivering cells in high density in aggregated mature spheroid form, delivering them directly in pellet form works more efficiently (Owens et al., 2013). In that case, bioprinting cells into printed micromolds is essential to confine cells inside the molds and trigger them to aggregate in the shape of the molds (see Fig. 4.9B). Thus two materials need to be deposited into the construct, where cell pellet can be printed inside hydrogels that are inert to cell adhesion such as agarose or alginate. There is a controversy among some scientists about when the applied molding approach should be considered a scaffold. Although the mold itself supports the tissue to grow and maturate, cells do not use mold matrix to proliferate through; thus the applied mold can be considered as a support structure, which is very common in traditional additive manufacturing technologies used for supporting overhangs. The major hurdle with this

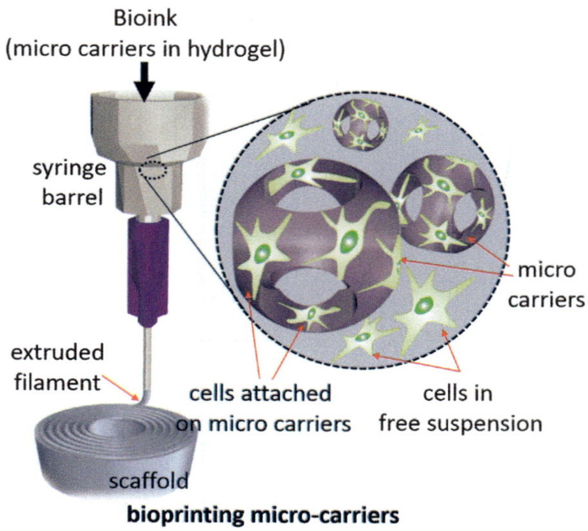

FIGURE 4.8 Extrusion-based bioprinting configuration for bioprinting microcarriers.

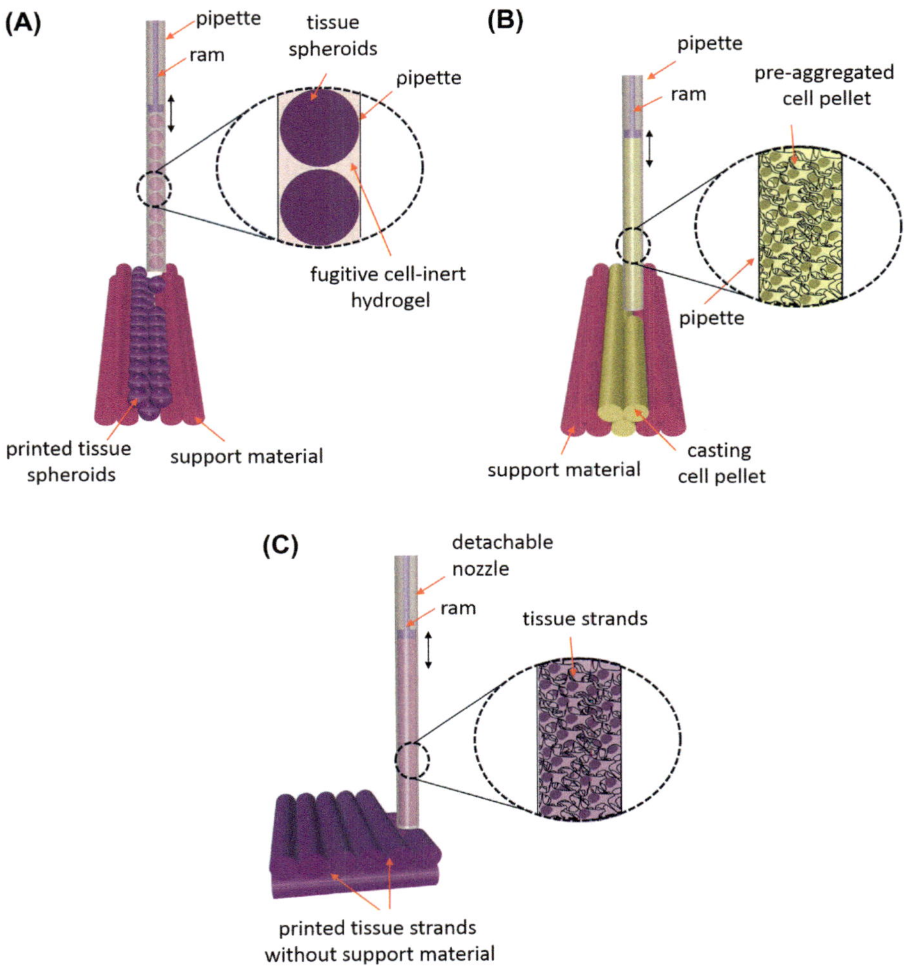

FIGURE 4.9 Extrusion-based bioprinting configuration for bioprinting cell aggregates: (A) a mechanically driven pipette unit bioprinting tissue spheroids in a hydrogel, (B) a mechanically driven pipette unit for bioprinting cell pellet into a cell adhesion inert mold, and (C) a mechanically driven detachable nozzle unit for bioprinting of tissue strands.

approach is the difficulty of making large-scale tissues without using a temporary molding material. Thus tissue strands can be considered as an alternative approach to tissue printing, where long strands of tissues can be fabricated and printed using a custom-made nozzle apparatus Fig. 4.9C (Yu et al., 2016). In this case, the laborious nature of spheroid preparation and loading can be eliminated, and the need for printing an enclosure mold is eliminated for cell pellets. Although this approach provides the unique advantage of printing tissue strands in tandem with vasculature, increasing the size of the tissue strands or the need for neovascularization within them can be considered as milestones on the way to generate larger-scale tissues and organs in the future (Ozbolat, 2015).

4.3.7 Nozzle Configuration for Decellularized Matrix Components

Bioprinting of dECM components have been recently used in bioprinting of living tissue and organ constructs. In their recent study, Dong-Woo et al. (Pati et al., 2015) decellularized natural tissues and chopped them into smaller fragments, which were then loaded with cells and printed with PCL frame to support the tissue analogs. A represent figure of the process is illustrated in Fig. 4.10. Human adipose–derived stem cells (hASCs) were tested using the proposed technology that demonstrated natural differentiation of cells when they were loaded in their native dECM. The approach seems to have a great benefit toward biomimetic tissue and organ printing when the dECM bioink compounds can be tuned in a way that they can be printed with enhanced mechanical properties without need of a polymer frame for future studies.

4.3.8 Other Nozzle Configurations

Extrusion process has been used for extruding plastics and metals, and several nozzle designs have been considered to extrude different geometries (McGuinness et al., 2005). One example can be aluminum extrusions, which are commonly used in construction of frames of 3D printers, with very complex geometric configurations (Ozbolat et al., 2014).

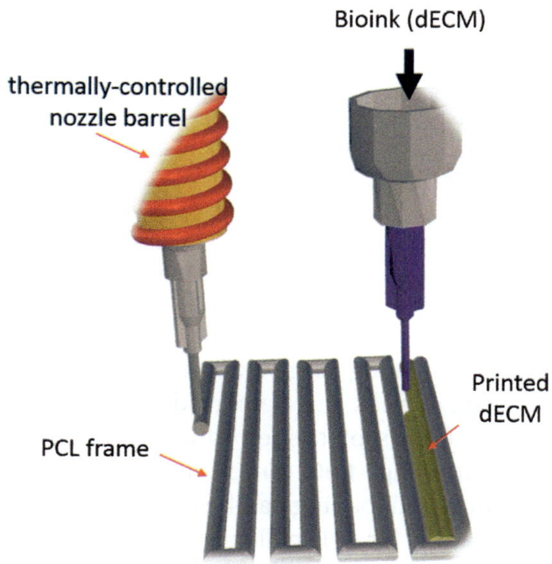

FIGURE 4.10 EBB configuration for bioprinting dECM components where a frame is 3D printed to support integrity of the bioprinted dECM until solidification is achieved.

The most common nozzle configuration used in bioprinting is the circular cross-section while most of the polymers are soft and cylindrical strands are easy to preserve its original shape. In general, the higher the viscosity of the polymer, the easier for the polymer to overcome surface tension–driven droplet formation so that the polymer can be drawn in the form of a filament; however, higher viscosity decreases when the polymer is extruded through nozzle tip due to shear-thinning behavior of non-Newtonian bioink materials. Although square or rectangular cross-section can be used for 3D printing of hard polymers such as hydroxyapatite or PCL, no study has reported that due to the common sense among the scientific community. In addition to nozzles with circular cross-section, coaxial nozzle has been used in several applications such as creating multimaterial fibers for controlled drug delivery (Zhang et al., 2012; Davoodi et al., 2014), bioprinting blood vessels (Yu et al., 2013), or microfluidic channels for tissue engineering applications (Zhang et al., 2013), encapsulating cell pellet to grow cell aggregates in strand shape (Akkouch et al., 2015). Similar configuration was further integrated to high-voltage source in electrospinning process to create nanofibers with multiple materials (Yoshimoto et al., 2003; Li et al., 2004, 2006). For composite biomaterials, both materials flow together creating an integrated filament with core and sheath made of different components. For single material to create tubular shapes, the crosslinker solution flows through the core and the biomaterial flows through the sheath section and crosslinking occurs when two contact immediately. By controlling coaxial nozzle configurations such as inner diameter of the outer nozzle, the outer diameter of the inner nozzle, and the bioprinting flow rheology including the viscosity and flow speed of the bioink, one can control the anatomy of the tubular conduits.

In addition to commercially available conventional nozzles in different dimensions and configurations made of different materials by companies such as Nordson EFD, Spraying Systems Co., and The Lee Company, researchers continue investigating new nozzle designs for advanced bioprinting technologies. Depending on the bioink, its flow rheology, solidification needs, and desired final shape, different nozzle architecture can be considered. Nozzle design is also determined by final tissue construct and the applied crosslinking mechanism. Printing nonporous constructs is relative straightforward while one can solidify the printed construct using other means such as culturing the construct for some period until full crosslinking is achieved such as fibrin and collagen or using UV irradiation to crosslink the construct if the bioink is photocurable such as GelMA, PEG-DA, and carboxymethylcellulose. In addition, past work demonstrated vaporization- (Soler-Illia et al., 2002) and diffusion-based crosslinking (Cheng and Landry, 2007; Hatch et al., 2004) showing possibility of creating strong bonding between the layers. In general, fusion of chemically crosslinked hydrogels is highly challenging and the previously mentioned approaches can lessen the issues arisen between the two layers of hydrogels when they are chemically crosslinked at different times.

4.4 Comparison of Extrusion-Based Bioprinting With Other Bioprinting Techniques

EBB technique has several advantages and disadvantages with respect to other bioprinting techniques including DBB [inkjet-based (Xu et al., 2013), electrohydrodynamic jetting (Gasperini et al., 2015; Eagles et al., 2006), and acoustic droplet ejection (Demirci and Montesano, 2007)] or LBB [stereolithography and its modifications (Lin et al., 2013), laser-guidance direct writing (Odde and Renn, 2000), and laser-induced forward transfer (Mézel et al., 2010)]. It has greater deposition and printing speed than others that can facilitate scalability in relatively short period of time. In addition, the hardware is affordable and a wide array of bioprinting technologies are commercially available by companies including nScrypt, EnvisionTec, Fab@Home, MicroFab, etc. (see Chapter 7). Besides, EBB enables bioprinting a wide array of bioink materials including cell aggregates (Boland et al., 2003; Mironov et al., 2009; Jakab et al., 2010; Mehesz et al., 2011), cell-laden hydrogels (Chung et al., 2013; Khalil and Sun, 2009), microcarriers (Levato et al., 2014), and decellularized matrix components (Pati et al., 2015), where other techniques can only facilitate printing cell-laden hydrogels. Bioprinting high cell density is currently feasible with EBB technologies only. The process is highly biocompatible with reasonably small process–induced cell damage and injury. Moreover, the technology is easy to implement and use by operators that have limited exposure to the technology. The last but the most important, EBB enables bioprinting anatomically correct porous constructs (Gou et al., 2014), which is highly challenging using other means except modifications of stereolithography.

Despite its versatility and great benefits, EBB has some disadvantages with respect to other technologies. First of all, the resolution of the technology is highly limited in a sense that the minimum feature size is over 100 μm in general (Duan et al., 2013), which is considerably lower than the resolution in other bioprinting techniques (Chang et al., 2011). Therefore cells cannot be precisely patterned and organized due to limited resolution. In addition, the bioink, in liquid- or solgel state, should possess shear-thinning ability to overcome surface tension–driven droplet formation to be extruded in the form of cylindrical filaments. Gelation and solidification requirements during extrusion process limits the hydrogels used in EBB. Besides, shear stress on nozzle tip wall induces significant drop in the number of living cells when the cell density is high. The time for bioprinting larger constructs also affects cell viability. Printing large tissue construct into cell culture media is not practical and current attempts do not allow incorporating cell media during bioprinting of scale-up tissue constructs, except bioplotting approach where tissue construct is bioprinted in a plotting medium (Hinton et al., 2015); therefore cells are exposed to lack of nutrients and dehydration.

4.5 Limitations

EBB systems provide relatively better structural integrity due to the continuous deposition of cylindrical struts, which makes it the most convenient technique for rapidly fabricating 3D porous cellular structures (Yeong et al., 2004). Although this technology lays the foundation for cell patterning for scale-up tissue and organ fabrication technologies, it has several limitations, including low resolution, shear stress–induced cell deformation, and limited material selection due to the need for rapid encapsulation of cells via gelation. Shear stress on the nozzle tip wall induces a significant drop in the number of living cells when the cell density or the bioink concentration is high. The author's past work demonstrated that the bioprinting process could induce quantifiable cell death due to changes in dispensing pressure, nozzle geometry, and bioink concentration (Yu et al., 2013). As the nozzle diameter decreases, or the viscosity of bioink increases, or the extrusion pressure increases, the viability of cells decreases. Therefore using optimum process parameters such as bioink concentration, nozzle pressure (ideally minimum), nozzle diameter, and loaded cell density, one can overcome these limitations and challenges to some extent.

Restricted bioink selection and low resolution and accuracy limit applicability of EBB systems (Dababneh and Ozbolat, 2014). Although certain errors can be induced due to other system components such as errors associated with the motion system, the extrusion process itself has an enormous contribution to the low resolution. Despite very small nozzle tips that can be considered possible in EBB, decreasing the nozzle size results in a considerable increase in the shear stress and corresponding cell damage and death. In addition, sufficiently high viscosity is essential for the bioink suspension to overcome surface tension–driven droplet formation and be drawn in the form of straight filaments. High viscosity, on the other hand, triggers clogging inside the nozzle tip and should be optimized considering the diameter of the nozzle tip. In addition, nozzle clogging is one of the most common problems faced in EBB, and the bioink solidifies inside the nozzle tip for several reasons, such as imprecise adjustment of the temperature on the heating chamber (for thermally crosslinked bioink), splashing/diffusion of the crosslinker solution into the nozzle (for ionically crosslinked bioink), early fusion of spheroids before extrusion (for tissue spheroid–based bioink), coagulation of the bioparticles loaded in the bioink in relatively small inner-nozzle diameter (for microcarriers), discontinuity in the pressure overholding the bioink inside the nozzle tip, and nonuniform bioink solutions with large fragments stacking the nozzle opening. Thus EBB systems should be modified to alleviate this issue. In addition, lowering the size further increases issues such as nozzle clogging and the need for elevated dispensing pressure levels.

Bioprinting porous cell-laden constructs on the other hand requires solidification to be realized immediately after or during extrusion process due to structural stability and integrity requirements of the constructs. Therefore more sophisticated nozzle designs should be developed. For thermally reversible hydrogels, the crosslinking mechanism determines the nozzle and the bioprinter head design. For example, hydrogels such as gelatin and agarose crosslinks at room temperature, thus loading them in a hot reservoir allows them to be extruded in liquid state and solidify rapidly as they come out from the nozzle tip. In contrast, hydrogels such as Pluronic® F-127, Matrigel™, and methylcellulose solidify in room temperature and stay in liquid state in lower temperatures. Thus a heating-assisted nozzle design is required to solidify the bioink as extrusion takes place.

In addition to the previously mentioned limitations, EBB faces hardware-related challenges. Pneumatically driven EBB systems require sterilization of the used air from the air dispenser compressor. Thus using a filter on the airway would be ideal to minimize contamination of the printed structures. Sterilization of a mechanically driven system is more trivial while the mechanical dispenser head can be easily autoclaved. Mechanically driven systems are affordable, easy to program, portable, and do not need an air compressor unit and accessories. Pneumatically driven systems are very precise and accurate; a microdroplet size of 0.5 nL (Nordson Coorporation, 2015) can be generated using a valve-based system. However, the cost of the system increases as the precision of the deposition volume increases. A mechanically driven system necessitates a tighter tolerance selection on the ram and the nozzle unit. An incorrect selection during bioprinter head development results in an unnecessary power requirement on the motor, additional friction forces and leakage of bioink, or failure of the nozzle assembly due to overloading. Mechanically driven systems provide a better printing ability for semisolid or solid bioink such as cell aggregates. Pneumatically driven systems do not generate smooth extrusion of the semisolid or solid bioink and require another liquid or gel medium to deliver the bioink through the nozzle tip. One of the most important aspects of nozzle selection is the friction coefficient on the wall of the nozzle tip because the friction coefficient mediates the shear stress, which might be detrimental for cells. Thus a surface with a small friction coefficient and one that is easy to sterilize would be ideal for printing cells, e.g., glass pipettes (Bruzewicz et al., 2012). Solenoid-based microextrusion enables dispensing of a sub-μL range volume of bioink (Bammesberger et al., 2013) and is convenient for bioprinting of low-viscosity bioink materials with an ionic- or UV-irradiation–based crosslinking mechanism. Although high accuracy can be obtained, a number of factors affect the accuracy and reproducibility of solenoid-based microextrusion systems, including the time lapse between actuation time (where the coil is energized) and the time when the valve opens; the soft nature of the seal between the plunger and the valve seat, resulting in compression of the sealing and time delays; and the need for high-actuating pressure to dispense highly viscous bioink. In addition, temperature, and hence viscosity, variations considerably affect the valve-opening time when the bioink has to be displaced for moving the plunger. Therefore solenoid-based microextrusion systems may not be convenient for thermally controlled nozzle configurations. In addition, fabrication of tolerances on the nozzle is important. For each different dispensing tip mounted, calibration of the valve may be needed, especially for very long-dispensing tips.

4.6 Future Directions

EBB stands as a promising technique among all bioprinting modalities due to its versatility in printing various bioink types, its capability in printing porous tissue analogs for enhanced media diffusion and perfusion capabilities, its ability to print fully biological large tissue constructs rapidly, and in reasonable acceptable mechanical and biological properties, which cannot be achieved using other bioprinting techniques including DBB and LBB. Despite the great progress and remarkable achievements in the last decade, there is much more still to be investigated to generate robust and viable end products for various applications such as pharmaceutics, transplantation, and clinics. The below directions can be considered under future perspectives in EBB technology.

Extrusion-based deposition system stands as a promising technique in organ printing technologies while scaffold-free bioink can be easily delivered to the printing stage in solid form, which is highly critical for structural integrity and handling of the printed tissue constructs. Other bioprinting techniques including DBB and LBB currently do not allow scaffold-free bioprinting of fully biological tissue constructs. Currently, scaffold-free tissue models can be bioprinted for drug screening; however, further advancement in EBB will have a great potential in generating scaffold-free scale-up tissues and organs that are at the clinically relevant volumes. This will definitely necessitate integration of tissue bioprinting process with vasculature bioprinting as larger tissue models require incubation under perfusion culture.

Bioprinting living tissue constructs or cell-laden scaffolds in vitro has been well studied in the literature, where successful results have been achieved with growing tissues in laboratory settings such as thin tissues or tissues that do not need vascularization including skin (Koch et al., 2010) and cartilage (Zhang et al., 2014). In situ bioprinting, on the other, can enable grow of thick tissues in critical defects with the help of vascularization driven by the nature in the body. Therefore in situ bioprinting stands as a promising direction for bioprinting porous tissue analogs that can engraft with the endogenous tissue and generate the new tissue along with vascularization through recruitment of endothelial cells into the tissue construct and sprouting of capillaries from the endogenous tissue. Very few attempts have been made in situ bioprinting where only DBB and LBB have been considered in limited capacity (Ozbolat, 2015). EBB, on the other hand, has the flexibility and capability in bioprinting tissue analogs with controlled porous architecture. To take the EBB into robust state in clinical settings, bioprinting ex vivo on explants can be considered as a transitional stage, where explants can be harvested from the animal model and the tissue construct can be built and engineered inside the defect. EBB has thus a great potential for printing porous tissue construct directly into defects, which will one day translate into operating rooms for repair and regeneration of organs.

One of the future prospects for EBB is to increase its bioprinting resolution for construction of tissues with precise control on cell positions. Although a low electric field can be applied to reduce the size of the printed filaments as widely used in electrohydrodynamic printing (Gasperini et al., 2015), cells should be kept away from the electric field to safely deliver them. A previous work in the application of electrohydrodynamic jetting in inkjet-based bioprinting demonstrates the safe usage of the system with cells; this approach has the potential to be used in EBB (Eagles et al., 2006). The other potential of increasing the resolution is to use a cone-shaped nozzle (i.e., Taylor cone or regular cone) that has a relatively alleviated shear stress, which reaches its maximum at the end of the nozzle tip, affecting cells at a minimum duration (Franco et al., 2011). In addition to these approaches, a highly innovative approach might be using a nozzle-free extrusion system that enables the bioink to overcome surface tension–induced droplet formation.

Although great progress has been made with novel biomaterials and biomaterial processing techniques, the development of bioink materials that suit well with EBB and allow one to bioprint biomechanically and biologically enhanced tissue constructs is still a great need. Particularly, new biomaterials with very quick gelation or solidification capabilities providing mild environment for cells would be highly desirable. Despite the great success in developing new hydrogels for tissue engineering; unfortunately, not all of them have been adopted to bioprinting. Particularly, new materials with very quick gelation or solidification capabilities providing mild environment for cells would be highly desirable. Thus a new field of study such as "extrudable biomaterials" potentially under biomaterials and biofabrication fields can be a great leap to promote research in this direction.

4.7 Summary

This chapter discusses EBB technique and its fundamentals for tissue biofabrication. The physics behind the process is formulated for extrusion and bioprinting of incompressible time-independent liquid bioink materials. Despite the great benefits and flexibility in printing a wide range of bioink types including tissue spheroids, tissue strands, cell pellets, and cells in hydrogels as well as dECM components, the technology currently faces with several limitations. Although the technology currently enables bioprinting of living cells, tissues, tissue constructs, organ modulus, and organ-on-chip devices for tissue engineering, regenerative medicine and pharmaceutics, it vitally needs further advancement in process, bioink, and hardware-related capabilities. In addition, the chapter instructs the reader with the limitations and the near-future trends in technology that will enable viable solutions for wide span of applications ranging from tissue engineering and pharmacy to clinics.

References

Abeykoon, C., et al., 2012. A review and evaluation of melt temperature sensors for polymer extrusion. Sensors and Actuators, A: Physical 182, 16–27.

Akkouch, A., Yu, Y., Ozbolat, I.T., 2015. Microfabrication of scaffold-free tissue strands for three-dimensional tissue engineering. Biofabrication 7 (3), 031002.

Almeida, C., et al., 2014. Impact of 3-D printed PLA- and chitosan-based scaffolds on human monocyte/macrophage responses: unraveling the effect of 3-D structures on inflammation. Acta Biomaterialia 10 (2), 613–622.

Ang, T.H., et al., 2002. Fabrication of 3D chitosan–hydroxyapatite scaffolds using a robotic dispensing system. Materials Science and Engineering: C 20 (1–2), 35–42.

Bammesberger, S.B., et al., 2013. A low-cost, normally closed, solenoid valve for non-contact dispensing in the sub-μl range. Micromachines 4, 9–21.

Bertassoni, L.E., et al., 2014. Direct-write bioprinting of cell-laden methacrylated gelatin hydrogels. Biofabrication 6 (2), 024105.

Billiet, T., et al., 2014. The 3D printing of gelatin methacrylamide cell-laden tissue-engineered constructs with high cell viability. Biomaterials 35 (1), 49–62.

Boland, T., et al., 2003. Cell and organ printing 2: fusion of cell aggregates in three-dimensional gels. The Anatomical Record Part A: Discoveries in Molecular, Cellular, and Evolutionary Biology 272A (2), 497–502.

Bruzewicz, D.A., Reches, M., Whitesides, G.M., 2012. Low-cost printing of PDMS barriers to define microchannels in paper. Changes 29 (9), 997–1003.

Chang, C.C., et al., 2011. Direct-write bioprinting three-dimensional biohybrid systems for future regenerative therapies. Journal of Biomedical Materials Research. Part B, Applied Biomaterials 98 (1), 160–170.

Cheng, K., Landry, C.C., 2007. Diffusion-based deprotection in mesoporous materials: a strategy for differential functionalization of porous silica particles. Journal of the American Chemical Society 129 (20), 9674–9685.

Chhabra, R.P., Richardson, J.F., 2008. Non-newtonian Flow and Applied Rheology, second ed. Elsevier, Oxford, UK.

Chung, J.H.Y., et al., 2013. Bio-ink properties and printability for extrusion printing living cells. Biomaterials Science 1 (7), 763.

Cohen, D.L., et al., 2010. Additive manufacturing for in situ repair of osteochondral defects. Biofabrication 2 (3), 035004.

Dababneh, A.B., Ozbolat, I.T., 2014. Bioprinting technology: a current state-of-the-art review. Journal of Manufacturing Science and Engineering 136 (6), 061016.

Dana, N., et al., 2004. Photocrosslinkable hyaluronan as a scaffold for articular cartilage repair, 32 (3), 391–397.

Davoodi, P., et al., 2014. Coaxial electrohydrodynamic atomization: microparticles for drug delivery applications. Journal of Controlled Release 205, 70–82.

Demirci, U., Montesano, G., 2007. Single cell epitaxy by acoustic picolitre droplets. Lab on a Chip 7 (9), 1139–1145.

Duan, B., et al., 2013. 3D Bioprinting of heterogeneous aortic valve conduits with alginate/gelatin hydrogels. Journal of Biomedical Materials Research - Part A 101 A, 1255–1264.

Eagles, P.A., Qureshi, A.N., Jayasinghe, S.N., 2006. Electrohydrodynamic jetting of mouse neuronal cells. The Biochemical Journal 394, 375–378.

Faghri, A., Zhang, Y., 2006. Transport Phenomena in Multiphase Systems, first ed. Academic Press, USA.

Fedorovich, N.E., et al., 2012. Biofabrication of osteochondral tissue equivalents by printing topologically defined, cell-laden hydrogel scaffolds. Tissue Engineering. Part C, Methods 18 (1), 33–44.

Fedorovich, N.E., et al., 2011. Distinct tissue formation by heterogeneous printing of osteo- and endothelial progenitor cells. Tissue Engineering. Part A 17, 2113–2121.

Fedorovich, N.E., et al., 2008. Three-dimensional fiber deposition of cell-laden, viable, patterned constructs for bone tissue printing. Tissue Engineering. Part A 14 (1), 127–133.

Franco, J., et al., 2011. Direct-Write assembly of calcium phosphate scaffolds using a water-based hydrogel. Acta Biomaterials 6 (1), 218–228.

Gaetani, R., et al., 2012. Cardiac tissue engineering using tissue printing technology and human cardiac progenitor cells. Biomaterials 33 (6), 1782–1790.

Gasperini, L., et al., 2015. An electrohydrodynamic bioprinter for alginate hydrogels containing living cells. Tissue Engineering-Part C, Methods 21 (2), 123–132.

Giannitelli, S.M., et al., 2014. Current trends in the design of scaffolds for computer-aided tissue engineering. Acta Biomaterialia 10 (2), 580–594.

Godoy, P., et al., 2013. Recent advances in 2D and 3D in vitro systems using primary hepatocytes, alternative hepatocyte sources and non-parenchymal liver cells and their use in investigating mechanisms of hepatotoxicity, cell signaling and ADME. Archives of Toxicology 87 (8), 1315–1530.

Gou, M., et al., 2014. Bio-inspired detoxification using 3D-printed hydrogel nanocomposites. Nature Communications 5, 3774.

Gregor, A., Hošek, J., 2011. 3D printing methods of biological scaffolds used in tissue engineering. Romanian Review Precision Mechanics, Optics and Mechatronics 3, 143–148.

Hatch, A., Garcia, E., Yager, P., 2004. Diffusion-based analysis of molecular interactions in microfluidic devices. Proceedings of the IEEE 92 (1), 126–139.

He, Y., Xue, G., Fu, J., 2003. Fabrication of low cost tissue prostheses with the desktop 3D printer. Scientific Reports 4, 6973.

Hinton, T.J., et al., 2015. Three-dimensional printing of complex biological structures by freeform reversible embedding of suspended hydrogels. Science Advances 1 (9), e1500758.

Hockaday, L., et al., 2012. Rapid 3D printing of anatomically accurate and mechanically heterogeneous aortic valve hydrogel scaffolds. Biofabrication 4, 035005.

Horváth, L., et al., 2015. Engineering an in vitro air-blood barrier by 3D bioprinting. Scientific Reports 5, 7974.

Huang, T.Q., et al., 2014. 3D printing of biomimetic microstructures for cancer cell migration. Biomedical Microdevices 16, 127–132.

Hutmacher, D.W., Sittinger, M., Risbud, M., 2004. Scaffold-based tissue engineering: rationale for computer-aided design and solid free-form fabrication systems. Trends in Biotechnology 22 (7), 354–362.

Jakab, K., et al., 2004. Engineering biological structures of prescribed shape using self-assembling multicellular systems. Proceedings of the National Academy of Sciences of the United States of America 101 (9), 2864–2869.

Jakab, K., et al., 2010. Tissue engineering by self-assembly and bio-printing of living cells. Biofabrication 2 (2), 22001.

Khalil, S., Sun, W., 2009. Bioprinting endothelial cells with alginate for 3D tissue constructs. Journal of Biomechanical Engineering 131, 111002.

Khalil, S., Nam, J., Sun, W., 2005. Multi-nozzle deposition for construction of 3-D biopolymer tissue scaffolds. Rapid Prototyping Journal 11, 9–17.

Khalil Saif, S.W., 2007. Biopolymer deposition for freeform fabrication of hydrogel tissue constructs. Material Science and Engineering: C 27 (3), 469–478.

Khattak, S.F., Bhatia, S.R., Roberts, S.C., 2005. Pluronic F127 as a cell encapsulation material: utilization of membrane-stabilizing agents. Tissue Engineering 11 (5–6), 974–983.

Kim, Y., Rajagopalan, P., 2010. 3D hepatic cultures simultaneously maintain primary hepatocyte and liver sinusoidal endothelial cell phenotypes. PLoS One 5 (11), e15456.

Koch, L., et al., 2010. Laser printing of skin cells and human stem cells. Tissue engineering. Part C, Methods 16 (5), 847–854.

Kolesky, D., et al., 2014. Bioprinting: 3D bioprinting of vascularized, heterogeneous cell-laden tissue constructs (Adv. Mater. 19/2014). Advanced Materials 26 (19), 2966.

Lee, J.-S., et al., 2014a. 3D printing of composite tissue with complex shape applied to ear regeneration. Biofabrication 6 (2), 024103.

Lee, V., et al., 2014b. Design and fabrication of human skin by three-dimensional bioprinting. Tissue Engineering. Part C, Methods 20 (6), 473–484.

Lee, V., et al., 2014c. Generation of multi-scale vascular network system within 3D hydrogel using 3D bio-printing technology. Cellular and Molecular Bioengineering 1–13.

Lee, W., et al., 2009a. Multi-layered culture of human skin fibroblasts and keratinocytes through three-dimensional freeform fabrication. Biomaterials 30 (8), 1587–1595.

Lee, W., et al., 2010. On-demand three-dimensional freeform fabrication of multi-layered hydrogel scaffold with fluidic channels. Biotechnology and Bioengineering 105 (6), 1178–1186.

Lee, W., Pinckney, J., et al., 2009b. Three-dimensional bioprinting of rat embryonic neural cells. Neuroreport 20, 798–803.

Levato, R., et al., 2014. Biofabrication of tissue constructs by 3D bioprinting of cell-laden microcarriers. biofabrication 6 (3), 35020.

Li, D., et al., 2004. Electrospinning nanofibers as uniaxially aligned arrays and layer-by-layer stacked films. Advanced Materials 16 (4), 361–366.

Li, M., et al., 2006. Electrospinning polyaniline-contained gelatin nanofibers for tissue engineering applications. Biomaterials 27, 2705–2715.

Lin, C.Y., Kikuchi, N., Hollister, S.J., 2004. A novel method for biomaterial scaffold internal architecture design to match bone elastic properties with desired porosity. Journal of Biomechanics 37, 623–636.

Lin, H., et al., 2013. Application of visible light-based projection stereolithography for live cell-scaffold fabrication with designed architecture. Biomaterials 34 (2), 331–339.

Lipson, H., Kurman, M., 2013. Fabricated: The New World of 3D Printing. Wiley.

Liu, C.Z., et al., 2008. Novel 3D collagen scaffolds fabricated by indirect printing technique for tissue engineering. Journal of Biomedical Materials Research. Part B, Applied Biomaterials 85 (2), 519–528.

Marga, F., et al., 2012. Toward engineering functional organ modules by additive manufacturing. Biofabrication 4 (2), 22001.

Markstedt, K., et al., 2015. 3D bioprinting human chondrocytes with nanocellulose-alginate bioink for cartilage tissue engineering applications. Biomacromolecules, 150325142328001.

McGuinness, P., Drenckhan, W., Weaire, D., 2005. The optimal tap: three-dimensional nozzle design. Journal of Physics D: Applied Physics 38, 3382–3386.

Mehesz, A.N., et al., 2011. Scalable robotic biofabrication of tissue spheroids. Biofabrication 3 (2), 25002.

Melchels, F.P.W., et al., 2014. Development and characterisation of a new bioink for additive tissue manufacturing. Journal of Materials Chemistry B 2, 2282.

Mézel, C., et al., 2010. Bioprinting by laser-induced forward transfer for tissue engineering applications: jet formation modeling. Biofabrication 2 (1), 014103.

Mironov, V., et al., 2003. Organ printing: computer-aided jet-based 3D tissue engineering. Trends in Biotechnology 21 (4), 157–161.

Mironov, V., et al., 2009. Organ printing: tissue spheroids as building blocks. Biomaterials 30 (12), 2164–2174.

Mogas-Soldevila, L., Duro-Royo, J., Oxman, N., 2014. Water-based robotic fabrication: large-scale additive manufacturing of functionally graded hydrogel composites via multichamber extrusion. 3D Printing and Additive Manufacturing 1 (3), 141–151.

Murphy, S.V., Atala, A., 2014. 3D bioprinting of tissues and organs. Nature Biotechnology 32 (8), 773–785.

Murphy, S.V., Skardal, A., Atala, A., 2013. Evaluation of hydrogels for bio-printing applications. Journal of Biomedical Materials Research Part A 101A (1), 272–284.

Nordson Coorporation, November 5 , 2015. Available from: http://www.nordson.com.

Norotte, C., et al., 2009. Scaffold-free vascular tissue engineering using bioprinting. Biomaterials 30 (30), 5910–5917.

Nöth, U., et al., 2004. In vivo determination of tumor oxygenation during growth and in response to carbogen breathing using 15C5-loaded alginate capsules as fluorine-19 magnetic resonance imaging oxygen sensors. International Journal of Radiation Oncology, Biology, Physics 60 (3), 909–919.

Odde, D.J., Renn, M.J., 1999. Laser-guided direct writing for applications in biotechnology. Trends in Biotechnology 17 (10), 385–389.

Odde, D.J., Renn, M.J., 2000. Laser-guided direct writing of living cells. Biotechnology and Bioengineering 67 (3), 312.

Owens, C.M., et al., 2013. Biofabrication and testing of a fully cellular nerve graft. Biofabrication 5 (4), 45007.

Ozbolat, I.T., Koc, B., 2011a. Modeling of spatially controlled biomolecules in three-dimensional porous alginate structures. ASME Transactions, Medical Devices 4 (4), 041003.

Ozbolat, I.T., Koc, B., 2011b. Multi-function based modeling of 3D heterogeneous wound scaffolds for improved wound healing. Computer-Aided Design and Applications 8 (1), 43–57.

Ozbolat, I.T., Chen, H., Yu, Y., 2014. Development of "Multi-arm Bioprinter" for hybrid biofabrication of tissue engineering constructs. Robotics and Computer-Integrated Manufacturing 30 (3), 295–304.

Ozbolat, I.T., 2015. Bioprinting scale-up tissue and organ constructs for transplantation. Trends in Biotechnology 33 (7), 395–400.

Pardo, L., Wilson, W.C., Boland, T., 2003. Characterization of patterned self-assembled monolayers and protein arrays generated by the ink-jet method. Langimur 17, 1462–1466.

Pati, F., et al., 2015. Biomimetic 3D tissue printing for soft tissue regeneration. Biomaterials 62, 164–175.

Perkins, J.D., 2007. Are we reporting the same thing?: Comments. Liver Transplantation 13, 465–466.

Pfister, A., et al., 2004. Biofunctional rapid prototyping for tissue-engineering applications: 3D bioplotting versus 3D printing. Journal of Polymer Science, Part A: Polymer Chemistry 42, 624–638.

Poldervaart, M.T., et al., 2013. Sustained release of BMP-2 in bioprinted alginate for osteogenicity in mice and rats. PLoS One 8 (8), e72610.

Rai, B., et al., 2005. Novel PCL-based honeycomb scaffolds as drug delivery systems for rhBMP-2. Biomaterials 26 (17), 3739–3748.

Richardson, J.F., Harker, J.H., Backhurst, J., 1991. Coulson and Richardson's chemical engineering volume 2: particle technology and separation processes. Chemical Engineering Science 2, 1183.

Rinaudo, M., 2006. Chitin and chitosan: properties and applications. Progress in Polymer Science 31, 603–632.

Rücker, M., et al., 2006. Angiogenic and inflammatory response to biodegradable scaffolds in dorsal skinfold chambers of mice. Biomaterials 27, 5027–5038.

Sato, M., et al., 2010. Nozzleless EHD spraying for fine droplet production in liquid-in-liquid system. IEEE Transactions on Industry Applications 46 (6), 2190–2195.

Schek, R.M., et al., 2006. Combined use of designed scaffolds and adenoviral gene therapy for skeletal tissue engineering. Biomaterials 27 (7), 1160–1166.

Skardal, A., et al., 2012. Bioprinted amniotic fluid-derived stem cells accelerate healing of large skin wounds. Stem Cells Translational Medicine 792–802.

Skardal, A., et al., 2010a. Dynamically crosslinked gold nanoparticle - hyaluronan hydrogels. Advanced Materials 22 (42), 4736–4740.

Skardal, A., Zhang, J., McCoard, L., Xu, X., et al., 2010b. Photocrosslinkable hyaluronan-gelatin hydrogels for two-step bioprinting. Tissue Engineering-Part A 16 (8), 2675–2685.

Skardal, A., Atala, A., 2014. Biomaterials for integration with 3-D bioprinting. Annals of Biomedical Engineering 43 (3), 730–746.

Smith, C.M., et al., 2004. Three-dimensional BioAssembly Tool for generating viable tissue-engineered constructs. Tissue Engineering 10 (9), 1566–1576.

Snyder, J.E., et al., 2011. Bioprinting cell-laden matrigel for radioprotection study of liver by pro-drug conversion in a dual-tissue microfluidic chip. Biofabrication 3, 034112.

Soler-Illia, G.J.D.A.A., Louis, A., Sanchez, C., 2002. Synthesis and characterization of mesostructured titania-based materials through evaporation-induced self-assembly. Chemistry of Materials 14 (17), 750–759.

Tan, Y., et al., 2014. 3D printing facilitated scaffold-free tissue unit fabrication. Biofabrication 6 (2), 024111.

Tocchio, A., et al., 2015. Versatile fabrication of vascularizable scaffolds for large tissue engineering in bioreactor. Biomaterials 45, 124–131.

Ventola, C.L., 2014. Medical applications for 3D printing: current and projected uses. P&T 39 (10), 704–711.

Wang, X., et al., 2006. Generation of three-dimensional hepatocyte/gelatin structures with rapid prototyping system. Tissue Engineering 12 (1), 83–90.

Wei, X., et al., 2007. Rapid prototyping three-dimensional cell/gelatin/fibrinogen constructs for medical regeneration. Journal of Bioactive and Compatible Polymers 22, 363–377.

Wu, W., DeConinck, A., Lewis, J., 2011. Omnidirectional printing of 3D microvascular networks. Advanced Materials 23 (24), H178–H183.

Xu, T., et al., 2013. Complex heterogeneous tissue constructs containing multiple cell types prepared by inkjet printing technology. Biomaterials 34 (1), 130–139.

Ye, K., et al., 2014. Chondrogenesis of infrapatellar fat pad derived adipose stem cells in 3D printed chitosan scaffold. PLoS One 9 (6).

Yeong, W.-Y., et al., 2004. Rapid prototyping in tissue engineering: challenges and potential. Trends in Biotechnology 22 (12), 643–652.

Yu, Y., Ozbolat, I.T., 2014. Tissue strands as "bioink" for scale-up organ printing. In: Conference Proceedings of IEEE, Engineering in Medicine and Biology Society, 2014, pp. 1428–1431.

Yoshimoto, H., et al., 2003. A biodegradable nanofiber scaffold by electrospinning and its potential for bone tissue engineering. Biomaterials 24, 2077–2082.

Yu, Y., Moncal, K.K., et al., 2016. Three-dimensional bioprinting using self-assembling scalable scaffold-free "tissue strands" as a new bioink. Sceintific Reports 6, 28714.

Yu, Y., Zhang, Y., et al., 2013. Evaluation of cell viability and functionality in vessel-like bioprintable cell-laden tubular channels. Journal of Biomechanical Engineering 135 (9), 91011.

Yu, Y., Zhang, Y., Ozbolat, I.T., 2014. A hybrid bioprinting approach for scale-up tissue fabrication. Journal of Manufacturing Science and Engineering 136, 061013.

Zein, I., et al., 2002. Fused deposition modeling of novel scaffold architectures for tissue engineering applications. Biomaterials 23 (4), 1169–1185.

Zhang, L., et al., 2012. Coaxial electrospray of microparticles and nanoparticles for biomedical applications. Expert Review of Medical Devices 9 (6), 595–612.

Zhang, W., et al., 2014. Cartilage repair and subchondral bone migration using 3D printing osteochondral composites: a one-year-period study in rabbit trochlea. BioMed Research International 2014, 746138.

Zhang, Y., Yu, Y., Ozbolat, I.T., 2013. Direct bioprinting of vessel-like tubular microfluidic channels. Journal of Nanotechnology in Engineering and Medicine 4 (2), 21001.

Further Reading

Lopes, A.J., et al., 2014. Laser curing of silver-based conductive inks for in situ 3D structural electronics fabrication in stereolithography. Journal of Materials Processing Technology 214 (9), 1935–1945.

Ma, M., et al., 2014. Core-shell hydrogel microcapsules for improved islets encapsulation. Advanced Healthcare Materials 2 (5), 667–672.

5 Droplet-Based Bioprinting*

CHAPTER OUTLINE

The only merit of which I personally am conscious was that of having pleased myself by my studies, and any results that may be due to my researches were owing to the fact that it has been a pleasure for me to become a physicist
John William Strutt, 3rd Baron Rayleigh

*With contributions by Hemanth Gudupati and Madhuri Dey, The Pennsylvania State University.

5.1 Introduction

Droplet-based bioprinting (DBB) has its roots in inkjet printing technology, which has its beginning in the 1950s when Elmqvist of Siemens patented the first practical inkjet device in 1951 (Le, 1998). Later, Sweet from Stanford University spearheaded the development of continuous inkjet (CIJ) printing system in 1960s. In 1970s, Zoltan, Kyser, and Sears pioneered the development of drop-on-demand (DOD) inkjet printing system. Their invention was licensed in the first commercial DOD inkjet printer, the Siemens PT-80, in 1977.

The idea of printing biologics was first introduced by Klebe in 1987 when he used a commercially available Hewlett–Packard (HP) thermal DOD inkjet printer to deposit a bioink solution comprising collagen and fibronectin (Klebe, 1988). Afterward, the first inkjet-based 3D printer was developed by Objet Geometries in 2000 (Wohlers and Gornet, 2014). In 2003, Boland demonstrated the feasibility of using a modified thermal DOD inkjet printer to deposit living cells in a viable form (Wilson and Boland, 2003) and introduced the concept of inkjet bioprinting (Boland et al., 2007). Subsequently, Nakamura's group successfully fabricated viable 3D tubular tissue constructs using a commercially available electrostatic DOD inkjet printer (Nishiyama et al., 2008). Later, several research groups have successfully adopted DBB technologies for bioprinting of a wide array of cells for various purposes, including, but not limited to, bioprinting for stem cell research (Faulkner-Jones et al., 2015; Gurkan et al., 2014; Xu et al., 2013a; Lee et al., 2010), tissue engineering (Xu et al., 2013a,b; Fang et al., 2012), controlled release (Cooper et al., 2010), transplantation (Xu et al., 2013b, 2010), drug screening (Rodríguez-Dévora et al., 2012), high-throughput arrays (Suntivich et al., 2014), and cancer research (Xu et al., 2011; Fang et al., 2012).

Despite the commonly used extrusion-based bioprinting (EBB) (Ozbolat and Hospodiuk, 2016) and the high-precision laser-based bioprinting (LBB) (Odde and Renn, 1999; Barron et al., 2004; Koch et al., 2010), DBB (Xu et al., 2005, 2010; Eagles et al., 2006; Demirci and Montesano, 2007b) offers several advantages due to its simplicity, agility, versatility, and the great control over the deposition pattern. It enables bioprinting with controlled volumes of bioink deposition at predefined locations (Murphy and Atala, 2014) facilitating spatially heterocellular constructs with well-defined positioning of cells (Xu et al., 2012). DBB, as shown in Fig. 5.1, comprises inkjet (Klebe, 1988; Xu et al., 2005, 2012; Murphy and Atala, 2014), electrohydrodynamic (EHD) jet (Jayasinghe et al., 2006; Onses et al., 2015; Gasperini et al., 2013; Eagles et al., 2006), acoustic-droplet-ejection (or simply acoustic) (Tasoglu and Demirci, 2013), and microvalve bioprinting (Faulkner-Jones et al., 2013, 2015; Lee et al., 2009a; Xu et al., 2011; Gurkan et al., 2014). Inkjet bioprinting is classified into two: (1) CIJ and (2) DOD bioprinting. CIJ bioprinting leverages Rayleigh–Plateau instability to break bioink jets into droplets. DOD bioprinting, on the other hand, uses thermal or piezoelectric actuators or electrostatic forces to generate droplets. In contrast, EHD jet bioprinting uses high ranges of electric voltage to eject droplets. Whereas acoustic bioprinting uses acoustic waves to produce droplets, microvalve bioprinting uses a solenoid pump to eject droplets.

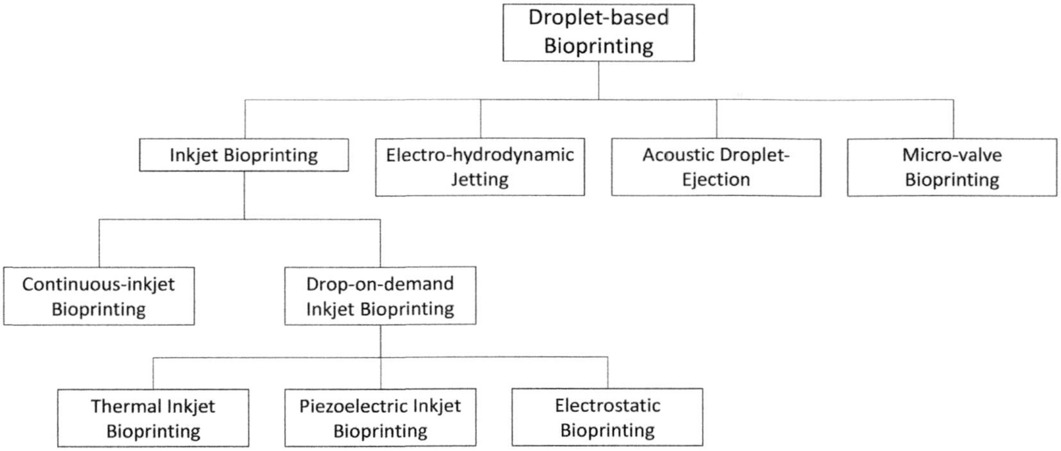

FIGURE 5.1 Classification of droplet-based bioprinting modalities.

5.2 Inkjet Bioprinting

Inkjet bioprinting physically manipulates a bioink solution to generate droplets. It leverages gravity, atmospheric pressure, and the fluid mechanics of the bioink solution to eject droplets onto a receiving substrate. To dispense the bioink, the following relations should be satisfied for a set of physical properties (Saunders and Derby, 2014):

$$Z = \frac{\sqrt{\sigma\rho l}}{\eta} = \frac{\sqrt{\mathrm{We}}}{\mathrm{Re}} = \frac{1}{\mathrm{Oh}} \tag{5.1}$$

where σ, ρ, and η are the surface tension, density, and dynamic viscosity of the bioink, respectively. In Eq. (5.1), l is a characteristic length (the diameter of the nozzle tip), Re is the Reynolds number, We is the Weber number, and Oh is the Ohnesorge number. Reis et al. suggested a limited range for inkjet printing ($1 < Z < 10$). If $Z < 1$, the bioink is too viscous to eject, and if $Z > 10$, inkjet printing generates satellite formation accompanying the main droplet (Reis et al., 2005). Other experimental work reported slightly larger range of limits ($1 < Z < 14$) (Derby, 2011; Jang et al., 2009).

5.2.1 Continuous Inkjet Bioprinting

In CIJ bioprinting, the bioink solution is forced under pressure through a nozzle, which subsequently breaks up into a stream of droplets owing to Rayleigh–Plateau instability (Derby, 2008) as illustrated in Fig. 5.2. The Rayleigh–Plateau instability is a physical phenomenon, where a thread of jet breaks up into droplets to minimize its surface tension. It occurs when the length of a cylindrical volume of liquid jet surrounded by a gas exceeds its radius by a certain limit (Rayleigh, 1878; Cardoso and Dias, 2006; Atkins and Escudier, 2013). During equilibrium state, the jet flows with a radius R_0 and pressure P_0 (where $P_0 = \frac{\sigma}{R_0}$) assuming no external pressure and the influence of gravity is

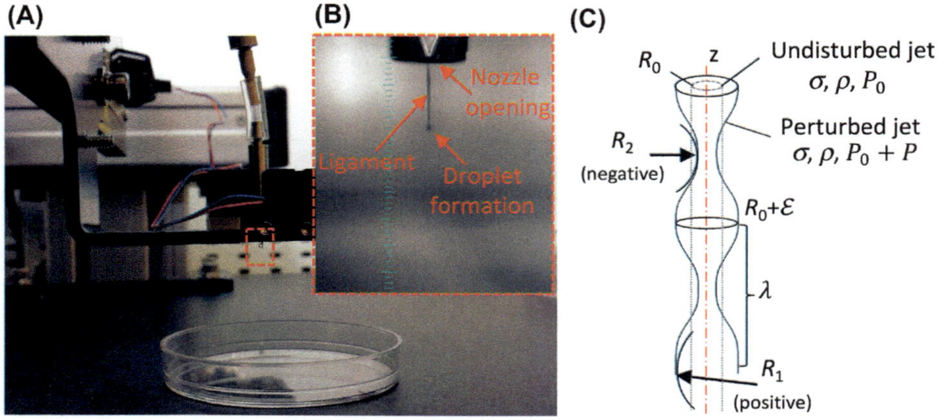

FIGURE 5.2 (A) Inkjet bioprinter with (B) the droplet formation. (C) An illustration of the intermediate stage of jet breaking up into droplets.

neglected (see Fig. 5.2C). Under perturbed conditions, the jet radius (R) can be represented as a wave function:

$$R = R_0 + \varepsilon e^{\omega t + ikz} \tag{5.2}$$

where ε is the perturbation amplitude ($\varepsilon << R$), ω is the growth rate and k is the wave number of the disturbance in z-direction. The wavelength (λ) can be represented as $\lambda = 2\pi/k$. The radial (u_r) and the axial (u_z) component of the perturbation velocity, and the perturbation pressure (P) can be represented as:

$$u_r = R(r)e^{\omega t + ikz} \tag{5.3}$$

$$u_z = Z(r)e^{\omega t + ikz}$$

$$P = P(r)e^{\omega t + ikz}$$

Substituting the previously mentioned perturbation fields into the cylindrical Navier–Stokes equations, one can obtain the following momentum (r,z) and continuity (m) equations:

$$r\colon \omega R = -\frac{1}{\rho}\frac{dP}{dr} \tag{5.4}$$

$$z\colon \omega Z = -\frac{ik}{\rho}P$$

$$m\colon \frac{\partial R}{\partial r} + \frac{R}{r} + ikz = 0$$

By eliminating P and Z to get a differential equation for R, the following equation can be obtained:

$$r^2\frac{d^2R}{dr^2} + r\frac{dR}{dr} - (1 + k^2r^2)R = 0 \tag{5.5}$$

The solution of Eq. (5.5) is a Bessel function of the first kind, which yields the following equation:

$$R(r) = CI_1(kr) \tag{5.6}$$

In Eq. (5.6), C is a constant. Using the relation between P and R given in Eq. (5.4) and the Bessel function identity $I_0^{'}(\zeta) = I_0(\zeta)$, the perturbation pressure can be obtained as the following:

$$P(r) = -\frac{\omega \rho C}{k} I_0(kr) \tag{5.7}$$

To find C, equations for boundary conditions should be further developed. The first boundary condition is the normal stress balance on the free surface:

$$P_0 + P = \sigma \nabla \cdot n = \sigma \left[\frac{1}{R_1} + \frac{1}{R_2} \right] \tag{5.8}$$

In Eq. (5.8), R_1 and R_2 are the principle radii of curvature of the jet and perturbation, respectively (see Fig. 5.2C). R_1 can be approximated as: $\frac{1}{R_1} = \frac{1}{R_0 + \varepsilon e^{\omega t + ikz}} \cong \frac{1 - \frac{(\varepsilon e^{\omega t + ikz})}{R_0}}{R_0}$. The second radius of curvature can be obtained using the second derivative definition as $R_2 = \frac{1}{\varepsilon k^2 e^{\omega t + ikz}}$. The second boundary condition is the kinematic condition on the free surface energy:

$$\frac{\partial R}{\partial t} = u \cdot n \cong u_r \tag{5.9}$$

By substituting Eqs. (5.3) and (5.6) into Eq. (5.9), the constant C can be obtained as $C = \frac{\varepsilon \omega}{I_1(kR_0)}$. Then, by combining Eqs. (5.3) and (5.7) and inserting into Eq. (5.8), the growth rate can be reformulated as:

$$\omega^2 = \left(1 - k^2 R_0^2\right) \frac{k\sigma}{\rho R_0^2} \frac{I_1(kR_0)}{I_0(kR_0)} \tag{5.10}$$

From Eq. (5.10), it can be concluded that unstable modes can be obtained when $kR_o < 1$, and the perturbation grows exponentially and eventually the jet distorts itself to minimize its potential energy and breaks up into a stream of droplets. The condition $kR_o < 1$ can be reformulated as $2\pi R_o < \lambda$, which draws the conclusion that unstable modes can be achieved when the perimeter of the perturbation is less than its wavelength.

5.2.2 Drop-on-Demand Inkjet Bioprinting

DOD inkjet bioprinting is preferred over CIJ bioprinting for tissue bioprinting purposes. DOD inkjet bioprinters generate droplets when required, which makes them more economical, handy to control, and easy to pattern biologics (Derby, 2010). DOD inkjet bioprinters rely on three different mechanisms to generate droplets including (1) thermal inkjet (TIJ), (2) piezoelectric inkjet (PIJ), and (3) electrostatic bioprinting. TIJ bioprinters generate droplets using a thermal actuator whereas PIJ bioprinters generate droplets using a piezoelectric actuator (Wijshoff, 2010). The two techniques are identical in other aspects. Electrostatic bioprinting, in contrast, ejects droplets using an electrostatic force (Kamisuki et al., 1998; Nishiyama et al., 2008).

DOD bioprinters consist of a single or multiple printheads. Each printhead contains a fluid chamber and a single or multiple nozzles. Fig. 5.3 demonstrates a sample DOD bioprinter for high-throughput fabrication of mini–tissue models. The bioink stored in the fluid chamber is held in place by the surface tension at the nozzle orifice (Derby, 2010). Pressure pulses are introduced in the fluid chamber through means of a thermal or a piezoelectric actuator such that a droplet is ejected when the bioink overcomes the surface tension. Some printhead assemblies may require pneumatic pressure (static pressure through means of pressurized air) commonly referred to as the back pressure to supplement the pressure pulses to overcome the surface tension.

5.2.2.1 Thermal Inkjet Bioprinting

The thermal actuator in TIJ bioprinting locally heats the bioink solution when a voltage pulse is applied. The localized heating forms a vapor bubble as shown in Fig. 5.4A. Subsequently, the bubble expands rapidly and collapses (explodes), which generates a pressure pulse inside the fluid chamber (Cui and Boland, 2009; Mohebi and Evans, 2002). Consequently, the bioink overcomes the surface tension at the nozzle orifice and a droplet is ejected.

TIJ bioprinters are capable of dispensing various biologics such as proteins (Roth et al., 2004) and mammalian cells. Bioprinted biologics include Chinese hamster ovary cells (Xu et al., 2005), rat aortic smooth muscle cells (Roth et al., 2004), canine smooth muscle cells (Xu et al., 2013a), rat neural cells (Xu et al., 2005, 2006), bovine aortal endothelial cells (bECs) (Xu et al., 2013a), beta-TC6 cells (Xu et al., 2008), feline cardiomyocytes (Xu et al.,

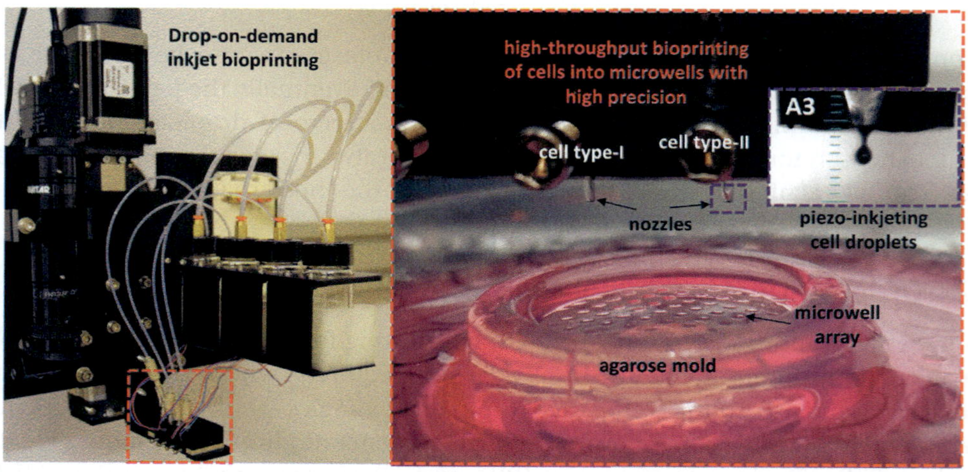

FIGURE 5.3 A drop-on-demand (DOD) bioprinter with multiple printhead is used for high-throughput fabrication of mini–tissue models in an agarose mold with an array of microwells.

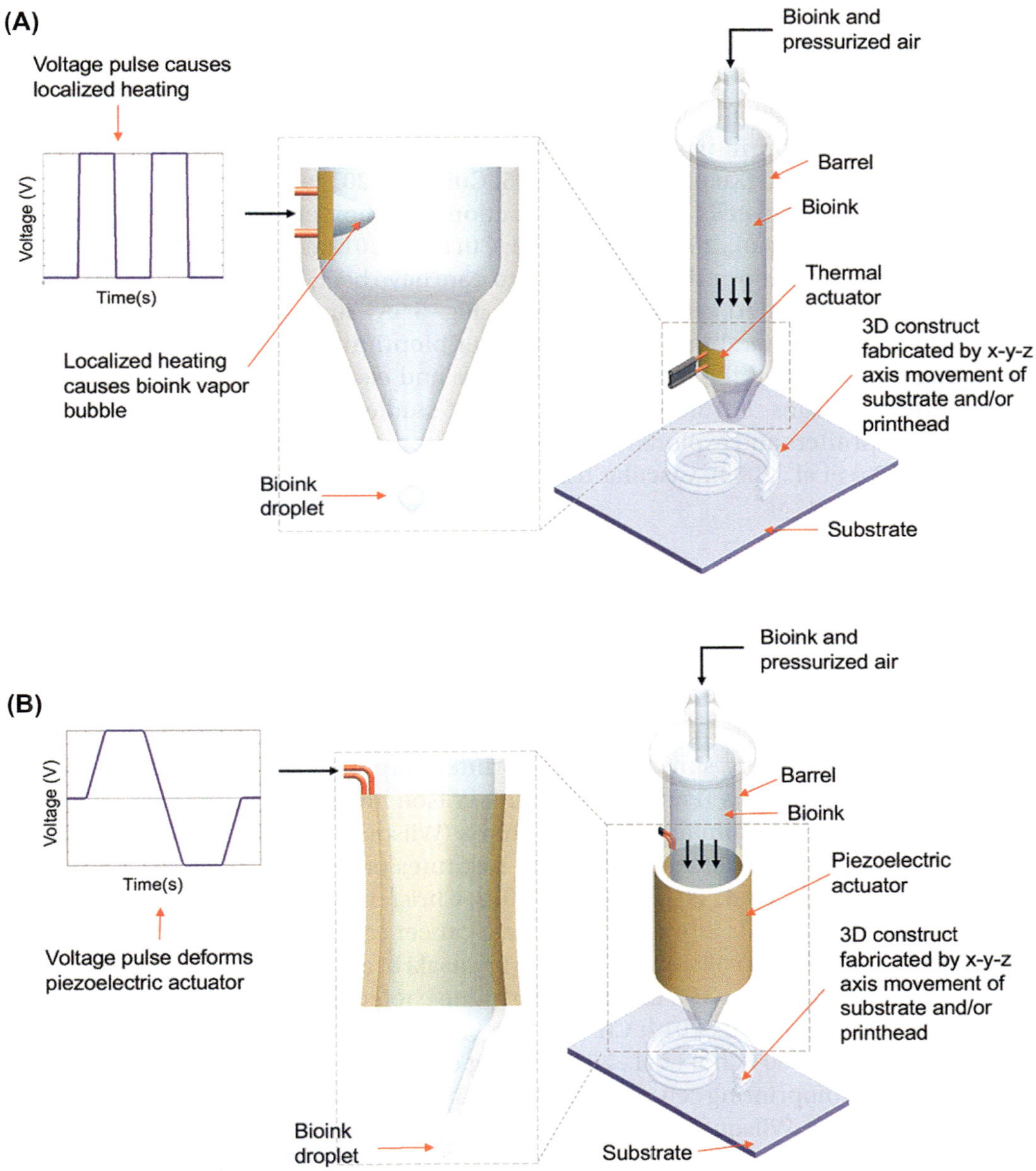

FIGURE 5.4 The mechanism of (A) thermal and (B) piezoelectric drop-on-demand bioprinting.

2009), H1 cardiomyocytes (Xu et al., 2009), human microvascular endothelial cells (HMVECs) (Yanez et al., 2014; Cui and Boland, 2009), neonatal human dermal fibroblasts (NHDFs) (Yanez et al., 2014), neonatal human epidermal keratinocytes (Yanez et al., 2014), human articular chondrocytes (Cui et al., 2012a,b), human mesenchymal stem cells (hMSCs) (Gao et al., 2014, 2015), and human amniotic fluid-derived stem cells (hAFSCs) (Xu et al., 2013a). The bioink temperature during bubble formation reaches 200–300□C for a few milliseconds (ms) (Roth et al., 2004). Moreover, the orifice diameter, in general, is about 50 μm (Xu et al., 2006) and the diameter of the ejected droplets is around 30–60 μm (Xu et al., 2008). Postbioprinting cell viability ranges from 75% to 90% at cell concentrations from 10^5 to 10^7 cells/mL (Xu et al., 2013a, 2005; Cui et al., 2012a,b; Gao et al., 2014, 2015). Furthermore, bioprinted cells retain their functional phenotype and genotype, and proliferation capacity (Xu et al., 2006, 2008, 2013a; Cui et al., 2012a). In summary, bioprinting studies pertaining TIJ bioprinting technology to date have been to assess its impact on the functionality of bioprinted cells. For example, Fig. 5.5A1 and A2 shows TIJ-bioprinted neurons tagged with neural markers 15 days after bioprinting. As seen in the figure, TIJ bioprinting did not affect the neuronal phenotype and electrophysiological functions of the bioprinted neurons. Furthermore, a myriad of studies have utilized modified commercial 2D TIJ printers and explored their role in tissue regeneration such as cardiac tissue (see Fig. 5.5B; Xu et al., 2009), vascular tissue (Cui and Boland, 2009), and in situ cartilage repair (Cui et al., 2012a).

5.2.2.2 Piezoelectric Inkjet Bioprinting

The piezoelectric actuator in PIJ bioprinting changes its shape when a voltage pulse is applied, as depicted in Fig. 5.4B. This deforms the fluid chamber (Wijshoff, 2010) in which a sudden change in the volume of the fluid chamber causes a pressure wave. As a result, the surface tension at the nozzle orifice is overcome and a droplet of the bioink is ejected (Singh et al., 2010).

Piezoelectric bioprinters, similar to TIJ bioprinters, are suitable for bioprinting various biologics including proteins (Pataky et al., 2012; Wilson and Boland, 2003), and bacterial (Choi et al., 2011) and mammalian cells [i.e., bECs (Wilson and Boland, 2003), HeLa cells (Arai et al., 2011; Yusof et al., 2011), National Institutes of Health 3T3 mouse fibroblasts (NIH 3T3 cells) (Pataky et al., 2012; Xu et al., 2012; Christensen et al., 2015), C2C12 mouse myoblasts (Matsusaki et al., 2013), MCF-7 breast cancer cells (Cheng et al., 2014), human umbilical vein endothelial cells, and NHDFs (Matsusaki et al., 2013)]. Generally, the nozzle orifice diameters range from 21.5 μm (for bioprinting bacteria) (Choi et al., 2011) to 120 μm (Xu et al., 2012; Cheng et al., 2014; Christensen et al., 2015) whereas the ejected droplet diameters range from 50 (Choi et al., 2011; Cheng et al., 2014) to 100 μm (Xu et al., 2012). Meanwhile, a postbioprinting cell viability of 70–95% was observed for cell concentrations of 10^5–10^7 cells/mL (Wilson and Boland, 2003; Xu et al., 2012; Matsusaki et al., 2013; Christensen et al., 2015). Overall, studies on PIJ bioprinting technology have thus far investigated the feasibility and possibility of fabricating 3D tissue constructs (Arai et al., 2011; Xu et al., 2012; Christensen et al., 2015; Matsusaki et al., 2013). For example, Fig. 5.5C depicts a PIJ-bioprinted vascularlike tissue construct with horizontal and vertical bifurcations. The tissue construct comprising alginate and NIH 3T3 cells was fabricated by a single nozzle PIJ bioprinter. Moreover, some studies optimized process parameters, including the bioink constituents (Pataky et al., 2012), piezoelectric element actuation

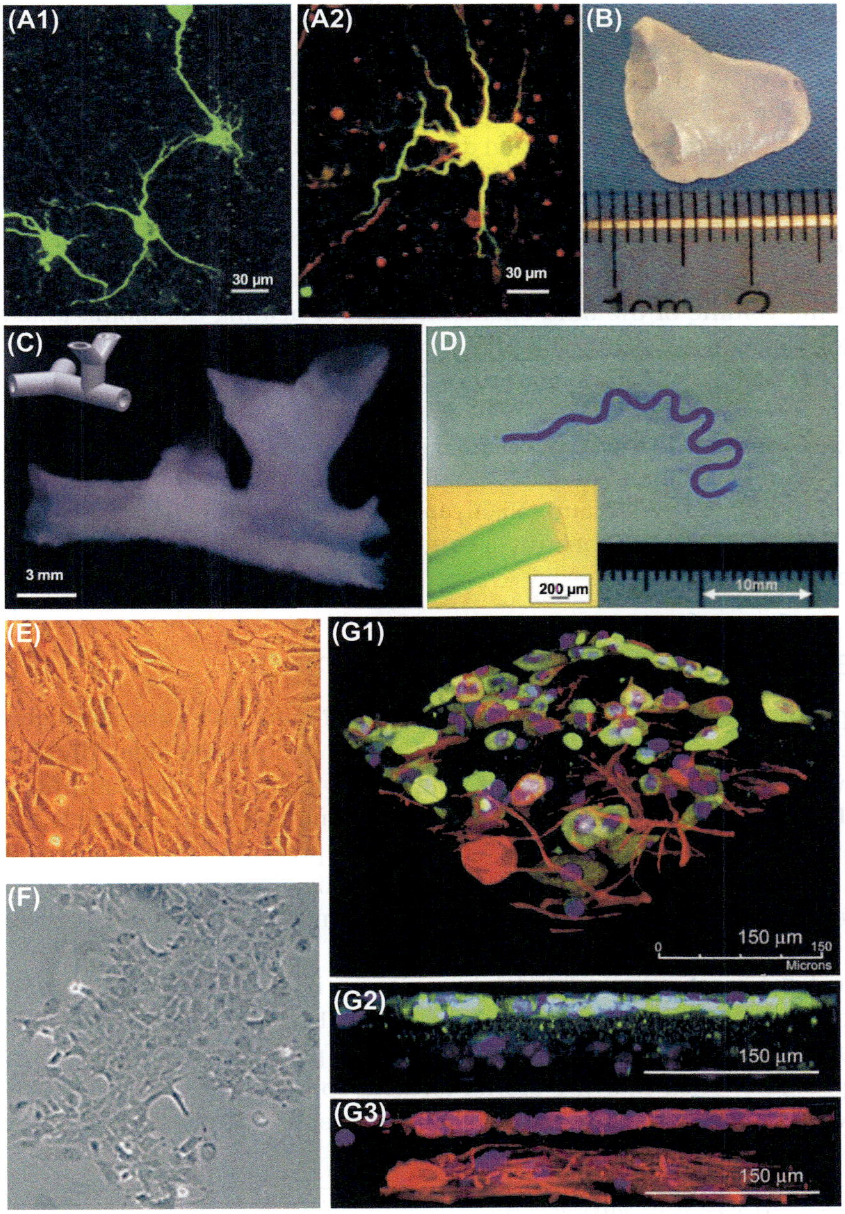

FIGURE 5.5 Droplet-based bioprinting of cells and biologics. Thermal drop-on-demand bioprinting of neurons tagged with neuronal markers after 15 days of culture, (A1) immunostaining of dendrites of rat embryonic cortical neurons with MAP2 monoclonal antibodies (green), (A2) immunostaining of dendrites of rat embryonic hippocampal with anti-MAP2 monoclonal antibodies (green) and axons of the neurons with antineurofilament monoclonal antibodies (red) *(Reproduced/adapted with permission from Xu et al. (2006))*; (B) thermal inkjet bioprinting of 3D cardiac tissue *(Reproduced/adapted with permission from Xu et al. (2009))*; (C) piezoelectric inkjet bioprinting of tissue constructs (NIH 3T3 cells with sodium alginate) with bifurcations *(Reproduced/adapted with

modes (pull–push and push–pull) (Yamaguchi et al., 2012), and voltage pulse characteristics (amplitude, rise and fall times, dwell time, echo time, and frequency) (Xu et al., 2012; Christensen et al., 2015), to improve process efficiency. Furthermore, few other studies attempted to improve process reliability (Cheng et al., 2014) and control the number of encapsulated cells in ejected droplets for potential applications in the areas of diagnostics, therapeutics, and cell biology (Yusof et al., 2011; Yamaguchi et al., 2012).

5.2.2.3 Electrostatic Bioprinting

Electrostatic bioprinters, identical to PIJ bioprinters, generate droplets by temporarily increasing the volume of the fluid chamber, without heating the bioink unlike TIJ bioprinters (Kamisuki et al., 1998). The brief increase in the volume of the fluid chamber as well as the bioink solution is achieved through the means of a pressure plate as shown in Fig. 5.6. The pressure plate deflects when a voltage pulse is applied between the plate itself and an electrode. The pressure plate regains its original shape in the absence of the voltage pulse and subsequently ejects droplets. Electrostatic bioprinters have been primarily used by Nakamura's group (Nishiyama et al., 2008) to fabricate 3D acellular (see Fig. 5.5D) as well as cellular constructs comprising of HeLa cells (6×10^6 cells/mL with 70% postbioprinting viability).

5.3 Electrohydrodynamic Jet Bioprinting

DOD bioprinters generate droplets by propelling bioink solutions through a nozzle. Hence, a very high level of pressure is required when ejecting cell-laden droplets through a nozzle with an extremely small orifice diameter, which is at times harmful to cells. In contrast, EHD bioprinters use an electric field to pull the bioink droplets through the orifice obviating the need for a substantially high pressure (Onses et al., 2015). As a result, EHD bioprinters are ideal for bioprinting applications requiring nozzles with very small orifice diameters ($\leq$100 μm) and highly concentrated bioink solutions (up to 20% weight by volume) (Jayasinghe et al., 2006).

The working mechanism of EHD bioprinting is illustrated in Fig. 5.7 (Sutanto et al., 2012; Gasperini et al., 2015; Onses et al., 2015), where a bioink solution is fed through a metallic nozzle using a certain back pressure (i.e., pneumatic or mechanical pressure) such that the bioink forms a spherical meniscus at the tip of the nozzle owing to the surface tension (Poellmann et al., 2011). A high voltage range

permission from Christensen et al. (2015)); (D) electrostatic bioprinting of alginate tubular construct *(Reproduced/adapted with permission from Nishiyama et al. (2008));* (E) Electrohydrodynamic jet bioprinting of porcine vascular smooth muscle cells after 40 days postbioprinting *(Reproduced/adapted with permission from Jayasinghe (2007));* (F) acoustic bioprinting of AML-12 cells after 12 days postbioprinting *(Reproduced/adapted with permission from* Demirci and Montesano, 2007b)); microvalve bioprinting of fibroblasts and keratinocytes, (G1) immunostained 3D image of the cells and its side views, (G2) keratin layer of KC, (G3) β-tubulin of keratinocytes and fibroblasts *(Reproduced/adapted with permission from Lee et al. (2009a)).*

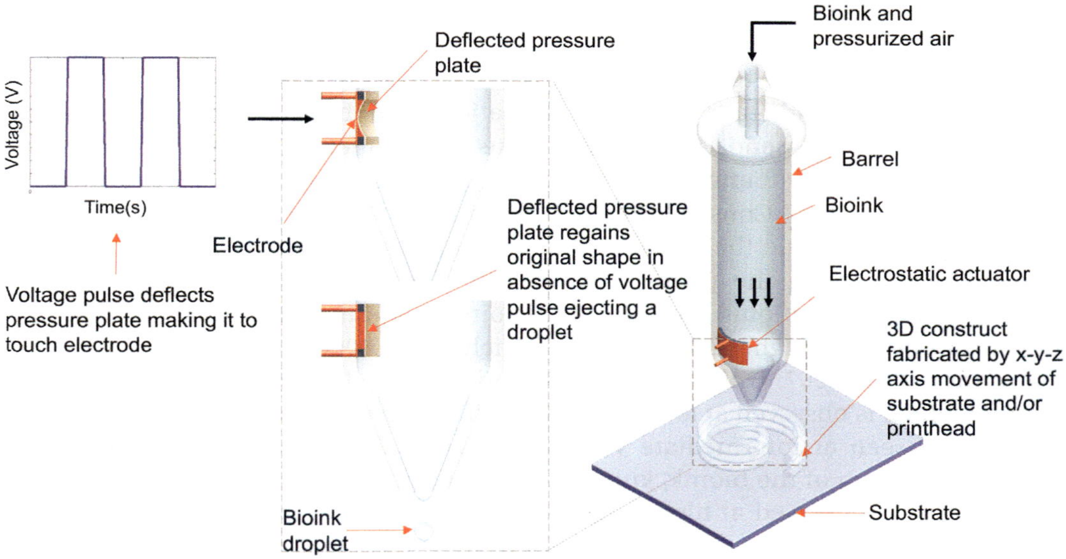

FIGURE 5.6 The mechanism of electrostatic bioprinting.

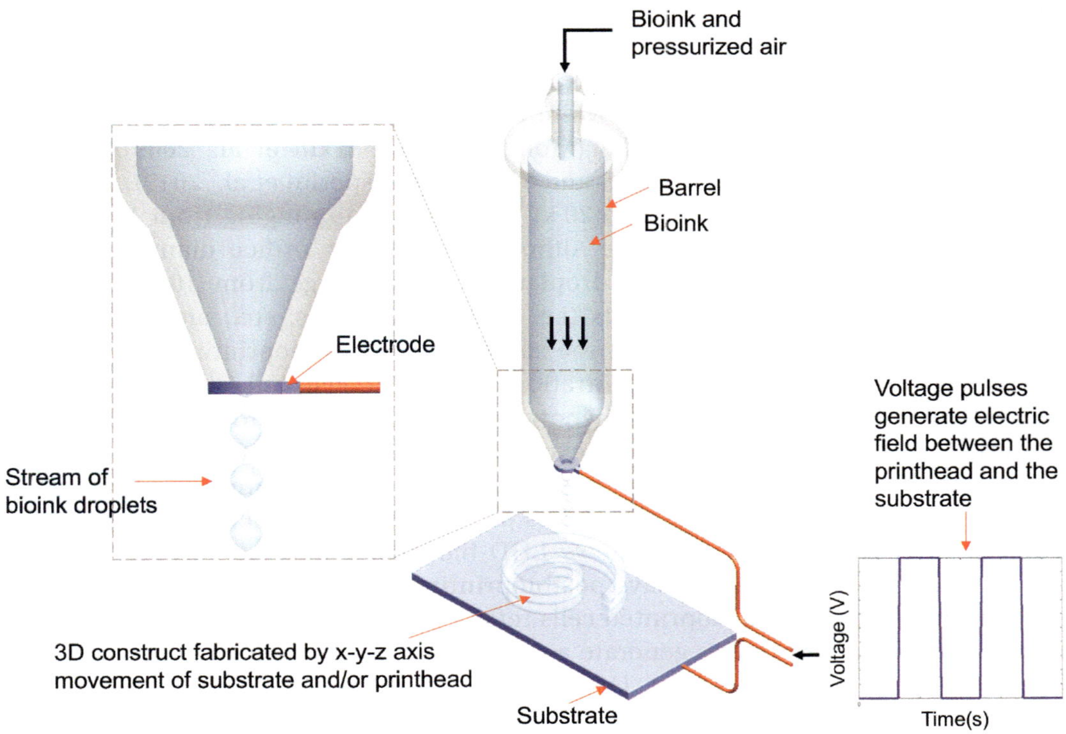

FIGURE 5.7 The mechanism of electrohydrodynamic jet bioprinting.

(0.5–20 kV) (Hayati et al., 1986; Gasperini et al., 2015) is applied between the nozzle and the substrate, which generates an electric field (as a function of the applied voltage and the distance between the nozzle and the substrate) between them. As a result, the electric field leads to the accumulation of mobile ions in the bioink near the surface of the suspended bioink meniscus. Subsequently, the Columbic or the electrostatic repulsions between the ions deform the meniscus into a conical shape called a "Taylor cone." Consequently, bioink droplets are ejected when the electrostatic stresses overcome the surface tension at the orifice under a sufficiently high voltage depending on the process parameters. The strength of the electric field (applied voltage), the bioink flow rate, and bioink properties (including cell type and concentration (Jayasinghe and Townsend-Nicholson, 2006)) determine the jetting mode (Kim et al., 2007; Onses et al., 2015) and cell viability (Workman et al., 2014). Dripping mode is observed at low voltages and flow rates, whereas streams of distinct droplets are seen at intermediate voltages and/or flow rates. At the same time, a continuous stream of the bioink, known as cone-jet-mode (continuous presence of a Taylor cone), is observed at high voltages.

EHD jet bioprinters are suitable for bioprinting proteins, such as collagen (Kim et al., 2007) and antibody immunoglobulin G (IgG) (Poellmann et al., 2011), without any loss of their functionality. In addition, EHD bioprinters are capable of bioprinting mammalian cells including Jurkat cells (Jayasinghe et al., 2006), human astrocytoma cells (Jayasinghe and Townsend-Nicholson, 2006), mouse CAD (Cath.a-differentiated) cells (Eagles et al., 2006), hepatocytes G2 cells (Xie and Wang, 2007), THP-1 cells (Workman et al., 2014), white blood cells (Mongkoldhumrongkul et al., 2009), erythrocytes (red blood cells) (Mongkoldhumrongkul et al., 2009), B50 rat neuronal cells (Gasperini et al., 2013), and 3T3 cells (Gasperini et al., 2015). At times, the applied voltage ranges from 3 to 20 kV for a flow rate ranging from 10^{-10} m^3/s (0.36 mL/h) to 10^{-8} m^3/s (36 mL/h). Although the nozzle orifice diameter ranges from 100 to 1000 μm, the ejected droplet diameters range from 10 to 2000 μm depending on the bioink constituents (i.e., media, hydrogels, etc.) and the process parameters (i.e., applied voltage). At the same time, a postbioprinting cell viability over 90% was reported for cell concentrations of 10^6–10^7 cells/mL, where bioprinted cells retained their functionality, phenotype and genotype, and proliferation capacities (Jayasinghe et al., 2006; Mongkoldhumrongkul et al., 2009). EHD jet bioprinting studies to date have investigated the practicality of bioprinting living cells and for understanding the effect of process parameters on characteristics of ejected droplets. For example, Fig. 5.5E shows EHD-bioprinted porcine vascular smooth muscle cells (PVSMCs) after 40 days postbioprinting. Subsequently, flow cytometric analysis indicated that the bioprinted cells retained their viability (Jayasinghe, 2007). In summary, EHD bioprinters generate a continuous jet or a stream of droplets at a time rather than a single droplet. Hence, they are not suitable for bioprinting applications requiring very accurate placement of cells.

5.4 Acoustic Bioprinting

Acoustic bioprinting, as illustrated in Fig. 5.8, employs a gentle acoustic field to eject droplets from an open pool unlike inkjet or EHD bioprinting, which ejects droplets through a nozzle (Demirci and Montesano, 2007b). As a result, the bioink and the constituent living cells are not exposed to detrimental stressors such as heat, high pressure, large voltage, and significant shear stress during droplet ejection. Typically, an acoustic bioprinter consists of a single or an array of 2D microfluidic channels, in which the bioink is held in place owing to the surface tension at the small channel exit. Further, the bioprinter setup generally consists of a piezoelectric substrate and interdigitated gold rings placed on the substrate to generate surface acoustic waves on demand. The waves are circular in geometry and form an acoustic focal point at the interface between the air and the bioink near the channel exit. The droplets are ejected when the force, exerted by the acoustic radiation at the focal point, exceeds the surface tension at the exit of the channel (Demirci, 2006; Demirci and Montesano, 2007b).

Bioprinting often involves printhead and/or substrate movement; however, a moving printhead and/or a substrate can introduce undesirable disturbances in acoustic-based bioprinting when compared to nozzle-based systems including inkjet and EHD bioprinters. Consequently, the disturbances can bring loss of control over the droplet ejection. In addition, gentle acoustic fields may not be capable of ejecting droplets of viscous bioinks such as hydrogels with high cell concentrations. Sadly, studies investigating acoustic-based bioprinting are very few to date. Acoustic-based bioprinting has

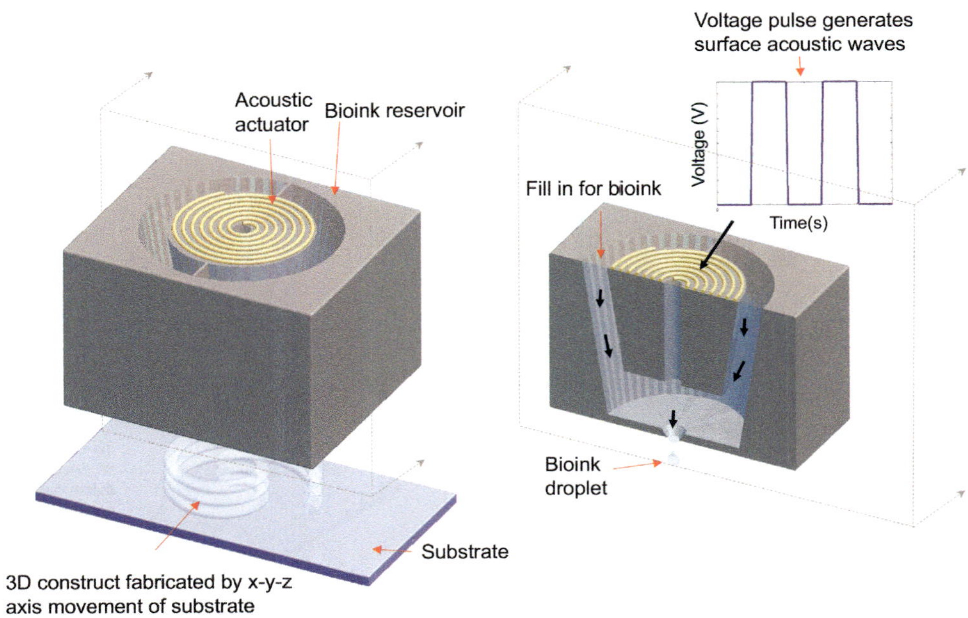

FIGURE 5.8 The mechanism of acoustic-droplet-ejection bioprinting.

enabled bioprinting of a myriad of cell types including mouse embryonic stem cells, 3T3 fibroblasts, AML-12 hepatocytes, Raji cells (a lymphocyte-like B-cell line), HL-1 cardiomyocytes, C2C12 myofibroblasts, MDA MB 231 breast cancer cells, and HEK 293 cells (Demirci and Montesano, 2007b; Fang et al., 2012). Further, the droplet diameter range is specific to the bioink composition and the bioprinter, and is usually between 10 and 500 μm. At the same time, the observed postbioprinting cell viability was above 90% for cell concentrations of 10^5–10^7 cells/mL. For example, Fig. 5.5F shows acoustically bioprinted AML-12 cells after 12 days postbioprinting (Demirci and Montesano, 2007b). The bioprinted cells were viable and became confluent in 12 days.

5.5 Microvalve Bioprinting

Microvalve bioprinting uses an electromechanical valve to generate droplets as shown in Fig. 5.9 (Moon et al., 2010; Lee et al., 2009a; Faulkner-Jones et al., 2013). The bioink in the fluid chamber is pressurized (back pressure) and the nozzle orifice is gated by a microvalve. A typical microvalve consists of a solenoid coil and a plunger, which blocks the orifice. The valve coil generates a magnetic field when a voltage pulse is applied and the magnetic field pulls the plunger upward. As a result, the nozzle is unblocked and the bioink is ejected out when the back pressure is sufficiently large enough to overcome the surface tension at the orifice. The back pressure and the valve-gating time determine the mode of the droplet generation, either CIJ or DOD.

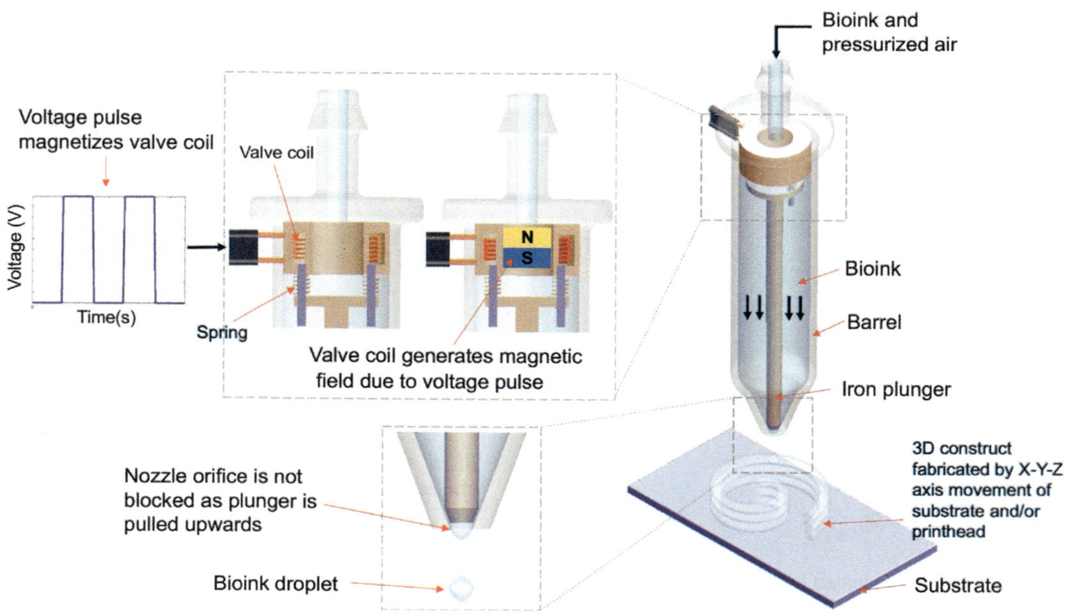

FIGURE 5.9 The mechanism of microvalve (solenoid) bioprinting.

Microvalve bioprinters are favorable for bioprinting various proteins such as collagen (Lee et al., 2009a, 2009b; Moon et al., 2010; Xu et al., 2010), bone morphogenetic protein-2 (BMP-2), and transforming growth factor-β1 (TGF-β1) (Gurkan et al., 2014). Additionally, they are suitable for bioprinting various cell types, including, but not limited to, AML-12 cells (Demirci and Montesano, 2007a), rat embryonic astrocytes, rat embryonic neurons (Lee et al., 2009b), human fibroblasts (Lee et al., 2009a; Xu et al., 2011), human keratinocytes (Lee et al., 2009a), rat primary bladder SMCs (Moon et al., 2010; Xu et al., 2010), epithelial human ovarian cancer cells (OVCAR-5) (Xu et al., 2011), C2C12 cells (Ferris et al., 2013), human embryonic stem cells (hESCs) (Faulkner-Jones et al., 2013, 2015), hMSCs (Gurkan et al., 2014), and human-induced pluripotent stem cells (hiPSCs) (Faulkner-Jones et al., 2015). Process parameters, such as pneumatic pressure, nozzle geometry, cell concentration, and the bioink constituents, determine the droplet volume as well as the cell viability (Faulkner-Jones et al., 2015).

Process parameters, including a nozzle orifice diameter of 150 μm, a pneumatic pressure ranging 6.89–20.7 kPa, and a valve open/close duration of 200 μs, generate droplets of 250 μm in diameter (Lee et al., 2009a, 2009b). Whereas process parameters, including an orifice diameter of 101.6 μm, a pneumatic pressure of 13.79 kPa, and a valve open/close duration of 100 μs, generate droplets of 300 μm in diameter (Faulkner-Jones et al., 2013). At the same time, a postbioprinting cell viability of 90% or greater was reported for cell concentrations of 10^5–10^7 cells/mL (Demirci and Montesano, 2007a; Lee et al., 2009a,b; Moon et al., 2010; Xu et al., 2010, 2011; Ferris et al., 2013; Faulkner-Jones et al., 2013, 2015; Gurkan et al., 2014). Also the bioprinted cells retained their functionality, phenotype and genotype, and proliferation capacity (see Fig. 5.5G1 and G3) (Lee et al., 2009a). In addition, the differentiation capacity of human stem cells was not affected by the bioprinting process (Gurkan et al., 2014; Faulkner-Jones et al., 2015).

In summary, studies pertaining microvalve bioprinting technology to date have examined the impact of bioprinting process on cell viability and functionality. Indeed, studies demonstrating the fabrication of complex 3D tissue constructs, similar to PIJ studies (Christensen et al., 2015; Xu et al., 2012), are lacking. Overall, microvalve bioprinters require low range of pneumatic pressure compared to that of PIJ bioprinters and hence they are less prone cell injury and damage (Lee et al., 2009a). However, microvalve bioprinters dispense larger droplets than other DBB modalities (including TIJ, PIJ, and EHD bioprinters) when identical nozzles are used (Tasoglu and Demirci, 2013). Thus the resolution of microvalve bioprinters is lower than that of TIJ and PIJ bioprinters.

Each DBB modality has its own strengths and limitations, and its use should be carefully considered according to the desired application area and tissue type to be bioprinted. Table 5.1 compares different DBB modalities according to their bioprinting parameters (i.e., nozzle size, cell viability, droplet size, operating conditions, etc.) and present their advantages and disadvantages.

Table 5.1 Comparison of Droplet-Based Bioprinting Modalities

				Bioink Printability					
DBB Modality	**Nozzle Size**	**Droplet Diameter**	**Cell Viability**	**Material**	**Maximum Concentration (w/v)**	**Maximum Viscosity (mPa.s)**	**Operating Conditions**	**Advantages**	**Disadvantages**
Thermal DOD	50 μm (Xu et al., 2006)	30–60 μm (Xu et al., 2008, 2006)	75–90% (Xu et al., 2013a,b, 2005; Cui et al., 2012a,b; Gao et al., 2014, 2015)	Alginate (NaAlg) (Xu et al., 2009, 2008; Boland et al., 2007)	2.3% (Xu et al., 2009, 2008; Boland et al., 2007)	N/A	10^5–10^7 cells/mL (Xu et al., 2013a,b, 2005; Cui et al., 2012a,b; Gao et al., 2014, 2015) exposed to 200–300°C for few milliseconds (ms) (Roth et al., 2004)	Low cost, ideal for feasibility studies	Limited cell types and clogging issues owing to smaller nozzle diameter, thermal and mechanical stress on cells during droplet ejection, difficult to clean as cartridges are designed for 2D paper printing, limited range of orifice diameters, and not available in single nozzle configuration
				PEG (Gao et al., 2015)	10% (Gao et al., 2015)	1.85 (Gao et al., 2015)			
				PEG-GelMA (Gao et al., 2015)	10% PEG and 5% GelMA (Gao et al., 2015)	4 (Gao et al., 2015)			
				Thrombin (Cui and Boland, 2009)	200 unit/mL (Cui and Boland, 2009)	N/A			
Piezoelectric DOD	21.5–120 μm (Xu et al., 2012; Cheng et al., 2014; Christensen et al., 2015; Choi et al., 2011)	50–100 μm (Herran and Huang, 2012; Xu et al., 2012; Choi et al., 2011; Cheng et al., 2014)	70–95% (Wilson and Boland, 2003; Matsusaki et al., 2013; Xu et al., 2012; Christensen et al., 2015)	Alginate (NaAlg from Sigma–Aldrich) (Herran and Coutris, 2013; Xu et al., 2012)	2% (Herran and Coutris, 2013; Xu et al., 2012)	140 (η_0) (Herran and Coutris, 2013; Xu et al., 2012)	10^5–10^7 cells/mL (Wilson and Boland, 2003; Xu et al., 2012; Matsusaki et al., 2013; Christensen et al., 2015)	Control over droplet generation and placement, wide range of nozzle diameters, available in single nozzle configuration, cleanable as long as bioink materials are not dried out	Nozzle clogging, satellite droplets, mechanical stress on cells during droplet ejection, made of glass that is not suitable for certain bioink materials such as fibrinogen

Electrostatic DOD	N/A	10–60 μm (Nishiyama et al., 2008)	70% (Nishiyama et al., 2008)	Alginate (Nishiyama et al., 2008)	1% (Nishiyama et al., 2008)	10 (Nishiyama et al., 2008)	10^6–10^7 cells/mL (Nishiyama et al., 2008)	Low cost, ideal for feasibility studies	Limited cell types and clogging issues owing to smaller nozzle diameter, mechanical stress on cells during droplet ejection, difficult to clean as cartridges are designed for 2D paper printing, limited range of orifice diameters, and not available in single nozzle configuration
Electrohydrodynamic jetting	2–1000 μm (Gasperini et al., 2013; Workman et al., 2014; Jayasinghe and Townsend-Nicholson, 2006; Xie and Wang, 2007; Poellmann	5–2000 μm (Gasperini et al., 2013; Workman et al., 2014; Jayasinghe and Townsend-Nicholson, 2006; Xie and Wang, 2007; Poellmann	>90% (Workman et al., 2014; Xie and Wang, 2007; Gasperini et al., 2015)	Alginate (NaAlg from Sigma–Aldrich) (Workman et al., 2014)	2% (Workman et al., 2014)	>2000 (Workman et al., 2014)	Applied voltage of 0.250–20 kV (Gasperini et al., 2013; Workman et al., 2014; Jayasinghe and Townsend-Nicholson, 2006; Xie and Wang, 2007;	Droplets smaller than nozzle orifice diameter, low mechanical stress on cells during droplets ejection, viscous bioink materials are dispensable	Expensive, unavailability of commercial complete systems, unsafe for operators, not capable of ejecting single droplet at a time
				Collagen (Kim et al., 2007)	3% in 3% acetic acid (Kim et al., 2007)	N/A			

Continued

Table 5.1 Comparison of Droplet-Based Bioprinting Modalities—cont'd

DBB Modality	Nozzle Size	Droplet Diameter	Cell Viability	Bioink Printability			Operating Conditions	Advantages	Disadvantages
				Material	Maximum Concentration (w/v)	Maximum Viscosity (mPa.s)			
	et al., 2011; Gasperini et al., 2015; Kim et al., 2007)	et al., 2011; Gasperini et al., 2015; Kim et al., 2007)					Poellmann et al., 2011; Gasperini et al., 2015; Kim et al., 2007), flow rate from 10^{-10} (0.36 mL/h) to 10^{-8} m^3/s (36 mL/h) (Gasperini et al., 2013; Workman et al., 2014; Jayasinghe and Townsend-Nicholson, 2006; Xie and Wang, 2007; Poellmann et al., 2011; Gasperini et al., 2015; Kim et al., 2007), 10^6 -10^7 cells/mL		

							(Gasperini et al., 2013; Workman et al., 2014; Jayasinghe and Townsend-Nicholson, 2006; Xie and Wang, 2007; Poellmann et al., 2011; Gasperini et al., 2015; Kim et al., 2007)		
Acoustic bioprinting	n/a	5–300 μm (Demirci and Montesano, 2007b; Fang et al., 2012)	>90% (Demirci and Montesano, 2007b; Fang et al., 2012)	Ethylene glycol (Demirci and Montesano, 2007b)	N/A	18 (Demirci and Montesano, 2007b)	10^5–10^7 cells/mL (Demirci and Montesano, 2007b; Fang et al., 2012)	No mechanical stress on cells during droplet ejection, easy to fabricate	Viscous bioinks are not dispensable, unavailability of commercial complete systems
Microvalve bioprinting	100–300 μm (Lee et al., 2009b; Faulkner-Jones et al., 2013; Horváth et al., 2015)	100–600 (Lee et al., 2009b; Faulkner-Jones et al., 2013; Horváth et al., 2015)	>90% (Demirci and Montesano, 2007a; Lee et al., 2009a,b; Moon et al., 2010; Xu et al., 2010, 2011; Ferris et al., 2013; Gurkan et al., 2014;	Collagen type I (Zhao et al., 2012)	0.9% (Zhao et al., 2012)	N/A	10^5–10^7 cells/mL (Demirci and Montesano, 2007a; Lee et al., 2009a,b; Moon et al., 2010; Xu et al., 2010, 2011; Ferris et al., 2013; Faulkner-	Low cost, viscous bioink materials are dispensable, cleanable as long as bioink materials are not dried out, interchangeable nozzles	Significantly larger droplet diameters than nozzle orifice diameter, greater shear stress on cells during droplet ejection as nozzles are not available in tapered configuration

Continued

Table 5.1 Comparison of Droplet-Based Bioprinting Modalities—cont'd

				Bioink Printability					
DBB Modality	**Nozzle Size**	**Droplet Diameter**	**Cell Viability**	**Material**	**Maximum Concentration (w/v)**	**Maximum Viscosity (mPa.s)**	**Operating Conditions**	**Advantages**	**Disadvantages**
			Faulkner-Jones et al., 2015, 2013; Faulkner-Jones et al., 2013)				Jones et al., 2013, 2015; Gurkan et al., 2014)		
				Fibrinogen (Lee et al., 2010)	6.2% (Lee et al., 2010)	N/A			
				Thrombin (Lee et al., 2010)	133 unit/mL (Lee et al., 2010)	N/A			

DOD, drop-on-demand; *GelMA*, methacrylated gelatin; *PEG*, polyethylene glycol.

5.6 Droplet-Substrate Interactions

In addition to jet formation, impingement of a droplet onto the substrate is also crucial during DBB as it affects the fidelity and spreading of the droplet. While the ultimate goal of bioprinting is to pattern the cells and fabricate 3D tissue constructs, the ideal placement of droplets should accommodate the preservation of the droplet integrity as splashing or spreading of the droplet results in displacement of the deposited cells from their desired position or structural failure in 3D bioprinting. For viscoelastic hydrogels used in DBB, there exist two major impingement characteristics including splashing and spreading of the droplet. In splashing, the droplet disintegrates into secondary droplets after colliding with a substrate. In spreading, on the other hand, the droplet spreads over the surface and expands its surface area. According to Worthington, the droplet shape highly depends on the velocity of the droplet, where higher velocity generates splashing and lower velocity leads to spreading (Worthington, 1876). According to Weber, the critical number (We) of droplet splashing is formulated as:

$$\mathrm{We} = \frac{\rho d U^2}{\sigma} \tag{5.11}$$

where d is the characteristics length that corresponds to the diameter of the droplet and U is the velocity. In general, larger Weber numbers generate splashes and lower ones lead to spreading. As these properties are important for the droplet formation (Son et al., 2008; Stringer and Derby, 2009; Rioboo et al., 2002), properties of the substrate are also important as the factors including but not limited to wettability of the surface, surface roughness as well as viscous forces (Roisman et al., 2002). Furthermore, the spreading of the droplet occurs faster than its polymerization in a typical bioprinting setup (Pataky et al., 2012) and the parameters associated with the crosslinking mechanism (i.e., ionic crosslinker solution concentration) influence the spreading behavior of the droplet (Xu et al., 2008). Droplet–substrate interactions broadly consist of two regimes from a fluid mechanics perspective (Saunders and Derby, 2014; Stringer and Derby, 2009). The first is the dynamic regime during which the kinetic energy of the droplet is dissipated. The second is the viscous dissipation regime during which surface energy interactions between the droplet and the substrate determine the spreading of the droplet to an equilibrium shape. In addition, gravity has minimal influence on landing and spreading of the droplet (Schiaffino and Sonin, 1997).

Transitioning from 2D (on a substrate) to 3D bioprinting necessitates a 3D-printing mechanism, which enables fabrication of 3D constructs through deposition of droplets in a layer-by-layer fashion. Depending on the utilized hydrogel and its crosslinking mechanisms, four types of 3D-printing schemes have been utilized in fabrication of tissue constructs including (1) alternating printing of the bioink and the crosslinker solutions (Fig. 5.10A), (2) bioprinting of the bioink solution into a reservoir filled with the crosslinker solution (Fig. 5.10B), (3) bioprinting of the bioink solution followed by spraying the crosslinker solution on top (Fig. 5.10C), and (4) bioprinting of the bioink

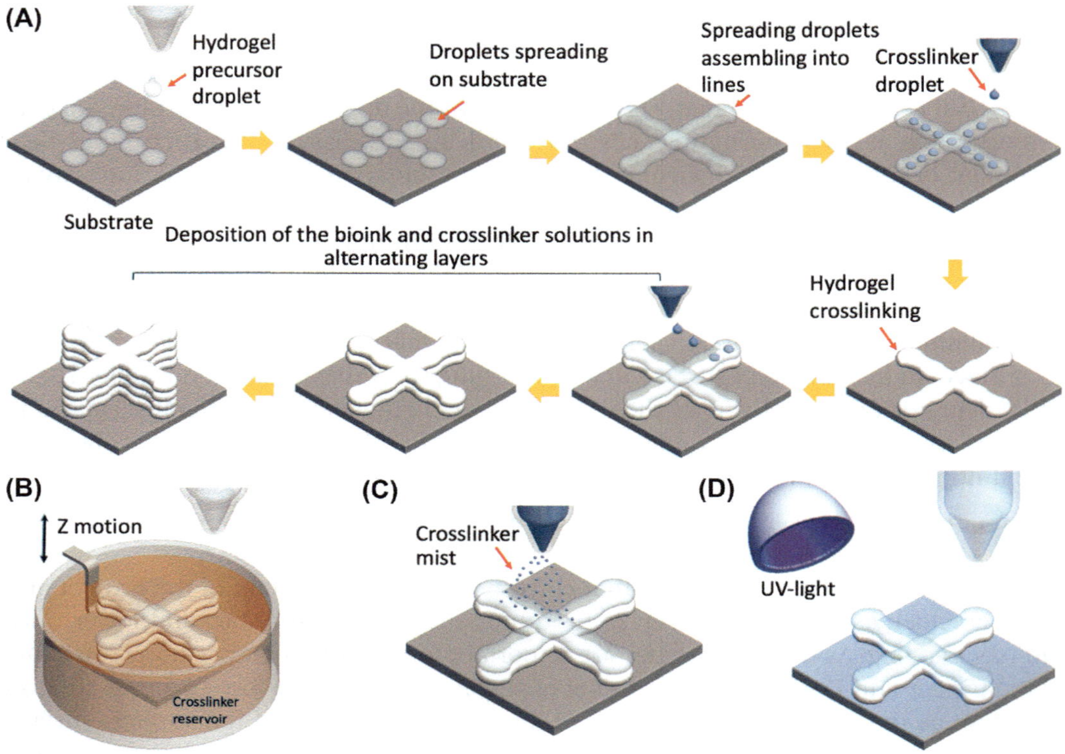

FIGURE 5.10 Droplet–substrate interactions and fabrication of 3D constructs through layer-by-layer deposition. (A) Droplets of a cell-laden hydrogel precursor solution are deposited at specific locations on the lateral plane by controlling the movement of the printhead and/or the substrate. The deposited droplets spread and coalesce to form lines on the substrate. The coalesced lines in turn assemble to form the first layer of the desired 3D pattern, which is subsequently polymerized by depositing the droplets of crosslinking (ionic or enzymatic) solution. This cycle is repeated until the fabrication of the entire construct is completed. (B) Alternatively, each layer of the bioprinted hydrogel precursor solution is polymerized by lowering the substrate into a reservoir of the crosslinker and raising it again before a new layer is bioprinted. (C) Each layer of the bioprinted hydrogel precursor solution is polymerized by spraying the crosslinking solution. (D) Each layer of the bioprinted hydrogel precursor solution (photocurable bioink) is polymerized using ultraviolet (UV) light.

solution followed by exposing it to a UV source (Fig. 5.10D). As fabricating scale-up tissue constructs necessitate the integration of vascular networks, such vascularization can be generated by printing thermally crosslinking sacrificial materials (i.e., gelatin) and liquefying them thereafter.

The resolution at which the 3D construct is fabricated depends on various factors including the volume and velocity of ejected droplets, droplet–substrate and droplet–droplet interactions, and the applied crosslinking mechanism. The volume of ejected droplets is mediated by several operating parameters such as the bioink material characteristics, the printhead geometry (orifice diameter), and its actuation voltage pulse characteristics (Herran and Huang, 2012; Lee et al., 2009a,b; Faulkner-Jones et al., 2015;

Demirci and Montesano, 2007a; Fang et al., 2012; Workman et al., 2014; Gasperini et al., 2013; Nishiyama et al., 2008). For example, the width of each coalesced line in Fig. 5.10A depends on several fabrication parameters including the volume of droplets, the spacing between droplets, and the printing speed, which consequently control the bioprinting resolution (Xu et al., 2012; Nishiyama et al., 2008; Soltman and Subramanian, 2008). In addition, how droplets interact with the substrate affects the spreading behavior of the droplet, which consequently affects the bioprinting resolution (Son et al., 2008; Schiaffino and Sonin, 1997; Stringer and Derby, 2009).

5.7 Biomaterials Used in Droplet-Based Bioprinting

A bioprintable material comprising various biologics (i.e., cells, growth factors, deoxyribonucleic acid (DNA), or drugs loaded in a delivery medium such as media or hydrogels) that is employed to fabricate 3D constructs with or without the use of external stimulations is rightfully referred to as "bioink," as introduced earlier in Chapter 3. Essential characteristics of bioink include low viscosity, suitable biodegradability and biocompatibility, enhanced cell adhesive properties, bioprintability, and high mechanical strength. However, such characteristics limit the range of exploitable biomaterials for DBB. Therefore, a limited range of hydrogels are available as bioink in DBB. Alternatively, hydrogels are also used as a substrate material when their viscosity is higher and/or the nozzle orifice diameter is extremely small. Hence, cells and other biologics are directly bioprinted into them.

5.7.1 The Bioink Consideration

A limited range of hydrogels including alginate, collagen, fibrin, methacrylated gelatin (GelMA), and polyethylene glycol (PEG) have been used in DBB due to their own or their crosslinkers' ease of ejectability and the compatibility of their crosslinking mechanism with different DBB modalities. This section discusses the bioink within the context of DBB and provides the reader with examples of bioprinted tissue constructs using the previously mentioned bioink materials. The reader is referred to Chapter 3 for a comprehensive discussion on a myriad of bioink materials used in bioprinting technologies.

Alginate undergoes ionic crosslinking, through the negatively charged carboxylate (COO^-) group that is present in its polymeric backbone. When the negatively charged COO^- group is exposed to positively charged ions such as divalent calcium cations (Ca^{2+}), it yields a crosslinked hydrogel network. Exploiting this crosslinking mechanism of alginate with $CaCl_2$, Atala's group fabricated heterogeneous tissue constructs comprising AFSCs, dSMCs, and bECs (Xu et al., 2013a). Alginate was also combined with several other materials to enhance the mechanical and functional properties of the fabricated constructs. Blaeser's group, for instance, fabricated a bifurcated vascular tissue construct using a composite blend of 3% (w/v) low-melting agarose and 3% (w/v) low-viscosity alginate (Blaeser et al., 2013). The bioprinting process was performed under nontoxic fluorocarbon, which provided the necessary buoyancy forces needed to support the soft tissue structure. Additionally, Boland and his coworkers bioprinted the crosslinking solution ($CaCl_2$) using a modified HP DeskJet inkjet printer to fabricate a heart-like tissue construct with connected ventricles (Xu et al., 2009). In another study, Huang's group mixed 3T3 fibroblast cells in 1% sodium alginate solution and bioprinted it into the crosslinker pool to fabricate zigzag cellular constructs (Xu et al., 2012). Similarly, alginate comprising hepatocyte-like cells, which were obtained through directed differentiation of hiPSCs, was bioprinted to fabricate a 3D mini–liver tissue model (Faulkner-Jones et al., 2015).

Collagen type I has been extensively exploited in tissue engineering for fabrication of tissue constructs due to its biocompatibility and cell adhesive properties (Roth et al., 2004); however, it has a limited use in DBB due to its fibrous nature as fibers can likely to clog the nozzle. In one study Boland's group used it as a bioink constituent to investigate adhesion and proliferation of cells on collagen-coated cell repellant substrates (Roth et al., 2004). Also, Boland's group fabricated a bilayer skin graft, which generated neoskin identical to native skin with microvessels (Yanez et al., 2014). In another study, fibrin–collagen bioink comprising one of the two cell types, AFSCs or MSCs, was bioprinted into wound sites for treating skin burns (Skardal et al., 2012).

Methacrylated gelatin forms a biomimetic (Nichol et al., 2010) as well as an enzymatically degradable (Hutson et al., 2011) hydrogel that is mechanically strong when photo-crosslinked with UV in presence of a photoinitiator providing a suitable material for DBB. For example, Demirci's group incorporated GelMA and growth factors (BMP-2 and TGF-β1) as bioink constituents to imitate native fibrocartilage microenvironments that differentiated bioprinted hMSCs toward osteogenic and chondrogenic lineages spatially (Gurkan et al., 2014).

Fibrin, a hydrogel formed by the reaction of thrombin with fibrinogen, supports extensive cell growth and proliferation (Cui and Boland, 2009). Boland's group used fibrin to engineer microcapillaries by bioprinting HMVECs-laden thrombin and Ca^{2+} solution on a fibrinogen substrate (Cui and Boland, 2009). Employing TIJ bioprinting, HMVECs were precisely bioprinted on crosslinked fibrin. Bioprinted HMVECs aligned well in fibrin and formed into an extensive capillary network after 21 days of culture. In another study, the same group bioprinted alternating layers of neural cells and fibrin gel to fabricate viable neural constructs for potential neural engineering applications (Xu et al., 2006). In another study, Atala's group used fibrin to engineer cartilage tissue with enhanced mechanical and functional properties employing a hybrid method involving electrospinning and microvalve bioprinting (Xu et al., 2013b). In general, it is more convenient to bioprint thrombin instead of fibrinogen due to the fibrous nature of fibrinogen leading to clogging issues.

Polyethylene glycol has greater mechanical properties compared to naturally derived polymers, such as alginate, fibrin, agarose, and collagen type I, making it an appealing bioink material for DBB. Altering the composition of PEG-based hydrogels in tandem with photo-crosslinking them in presence of a photoinitiator enables the control of structural, functional, and mechanical properties of fabricated tissues. Using TIJ bioprinting, Cui et al. 2012a,b bioprinted human articular chondrocytes in PEGDMA in a layer-by-layer fashion concurrent UV crosslinking of each layer, which yielded 3D construct with homogenous distribution of cells and supported neocartilage formation. In a similar study, acrylated PEG was bioprinted with acrylated peptide containing the Arg-Gly-Asp (RGD) sequence (essential for cell adhesion), followed by photopolymerization of the bioprinted layer (Gao et al., 2015). Bone marrow–derived hMSCs were suspended in PEGDMA in conjunction with bioactive glass and hydroxyapatite nanoparticles, and bioprinted using a TIJ bioprinter (Gao et al., 2014). This approach allowed control over the spatial delivery of hMSCs and bioactive ceramic materials in the fabricated bone tissue constructs.

There are a limited number of hydrogels that can be employed in DBB owing to very fine nozzle diameters. Therefore, it is essential to use bioink materials with low viscosity to obviate nozzle clogging issues. Bioprintability, cost, crosslinking mechanisms, and viscosity are some of the factors that are essential to consider while selecting a bioink for DBB.

5.7.2 The Substrate Consideration

In addition to bioprinting hydrogels, a myriad of endeavors has been made to bioprint macromolecules (i.e., growth factors, proteins, or even cells in media) directly onto hydrogel substrates. By controlling the spatial distribution of growth factors on hydrogel substrate, differentiation of stem cell into specific lineages has been widely attempted. Phillippi et al. (2008) used cyanin-3–labeled BMP-2 in media as a bioink solution and bioprinted it on fibrin-coated glass slides using a piezoelectric DOD bioprinter (Phillippi et al., 2008). They spatially immobilized BMP-2 with a varying concentration according to a predesigned pattern and cultured primary muscle-derived stem cells (MDSCs) on the BMP-2 patterned surface. This led to the differentiation of MDSCs into multiple lineages, namely osteogenic and myogenic in that study. Another study conducted by Ilkhanizadeh et al. (2007) showed that the fate and differentiation ability of neural stem cells could be effectively controlled by inkjet bioprinting of various macromolecules, such as fibroblast growth factor-2, ciliary neurotrophic factor, and fetal bovine serum, on neural stem cell–seeded polyacrylamide-based hydrogel substrates.

Demirci's group fabricated co-culture cancer models by bioprinting human ovarian cancer cells and fibroblasts in a controlled manner on Matrigel-coated glass culture dish (Xu et al., 2011). Collagen type I and fibrinogen has also been used as gel substrates for spatially controlled bioprinting of HMVECs mixed in thrombin for fabricating skin grafts (Yanez et al., 2014). This bilayered skin graft comprising of keratinocytes and fibroblasts in collagen (as the top layer and bottom layer, respectively), and HMVECs encapsulated in fibrin network as the middle layer resulted in a portable construct, which was eventually placed on full thickness wounds in mice model for in vivo studies. Polyacrylamide gel substrates have also been employed for micropatterning proteins and cells by peeling off the protein from functionalized glass slides coated with PA substrates (Tang et al., 2012). Poly(allylamine hydrochloride)/poly(styrene sulfonate) (PAH/PSS) based films were patterned on alginate gels for vascular tissue engineering by peeling off from the substrate as well (Kerdjoudj et al., 2011). These studies reveal the feasibility of bioprinting cells on gel substrates, and depending on the application, these substrates can be engineered to be peeled off for further studies.

5.8 Comparison of Droplet-Based Bioprinting With Other Bioprinting Techniques

DBB has several advantages and disadvantages with respect to other bioprinting techniques, including EBB (mechanical (Skardal et al., 2010; Jakab et al., 2008; Gaetani et al., 2012; Hockaday et al., 2012; Owens et al., 2013), pneumatic (Khalil et al., 2005; Fedorovich et al., 2008; Ozbolat et al., 2014; Marchioli et al., 2015; Yu et al., 2014), or valve-based (Snyder et al., 2011; Markstedt et al., 2015; Chang et al., 2008, 2010)) or LBB (stereolithography (Salonitis, 2014) and its modifications (Lin et al., 2013), laser-guidance direct writing (Odde and Renn 1999, 2000), and laser-induced forward transfer (Mézel et al., 2010; Xiong et al., 2015; Barron et al., 2004)).

DBB technology is a multifaceted technology. Highly complex heterocellular tissue constructs with different compositions of biologics (i.e., biomaterials, cells, growth factors, drugs, and genes) can be easily patterned when compared to EBB and LBB techniques as it is highly challenging to incorporate multiple types of biologics in LBB and generating heterogeneity in a delicate manner is difficult using EBB. While DBB has a process resolution higher than that of EBB and possesses a greater versatility in incorporating multiple biologics, DBB has attracted several researchers in the bioprinting community as well as researchers adopting bioprinting technology in other field of studies such as regenerative medicine and pharmaceutics (Horváth et al., 2015; Rodríguez-Dévora et al., 2012). Moreover, it has a reasonable resolution comparable to LBB, which allows better control on the geometry and size of bioprinted constructs by mediating the gelation process precisely as crosslinker and precursor hydrogel solutions can be selectively deposited. This enables mighty control on swelling and shrinkage properties of the bioprinted constructs.

Droplet-based bioprinters are highly versatile and affordable, where a simple HP printer can be easily modified and used as a bioprinter (Cui et al., 2014). A wide range of droplet-based bioprinters are commercially available within affordable price band (Mironov et al., 2009). If the reproducibility and flexibility becomes a concern, extra capabilities can be easily implemented with a reasonable additional cost. For example, printheads in DBB may not be suitable for certain bioink materials such as fibrous bioink (i.e., fibrinogen and collagen) and generate inconsistent results due to nozzle clogging or accumulation of cell debris or fibers anywhere in the line from reservoir to the nozzle in the tubing system. A commercial droplet-based bioprinter can be modified to overcome such issues by replacing the original dispenser with dispensers having larger nozzles or dispensers with different droplet generation mechanisms as the rest of bioprinter subcomponents are common for all DBB modalities.

DBB technology is also user-friendly and easy to implement. It can be readily used by operators, who have limited exposure to the technology while generated computer-aided design (CAD) models can be easily transferred to print out by simply pressing "bioprint." In other words, it has a non-steep learning curve circumventing the need for extensive experimentation, which is a major impediment in EBB as the operator needs to understand the shear-thinning behavior of hydrogels as well as their bioprintability on the printing stage.

The other advantage of DBB is that it facilitates rapid bioprinting through an array of nozzles in a highly reproducible manner. This capability enables rapid fabrication of an array of samples, which is highly desirable in high-throughput screening applications such as drug testing and cancer screening (Fang et al., 2012; Xu et al., 2011; Yusof et al., 2011). Producing high-throughput arrays using EBB or LBB, on the other hand, is highly challenging and not practical. In addition to its appealing features, DBB has a great translational potential in clinical use for tissue bioprinting. It is highly convenient for in situ bioprinting purposes as defects (i.e., cranio- or maxilla-facial defects, skin burns or deep wounds) on human body can be easily reconstructed using DBB as DBB operates in a noncontact manner. The defects can be easily filled by jetting droplets from a distance into the defect. This feature also enables bioprinting of growth factors or other biologics on existing tissue constructs as biologics can be selectively sprayed over the tissue constructs (Cooper et al., 2010). The noncontact nature of DBB processes alleviates other major issues observed in EBB such as collision between the printhead and the bioprinted constructs, or unexpected increase in clearance between the orifice and the receiving substrate.

5.9 Recent Achievements in Droplet-Based Bioprinting

Recent achievements in DBB are in the areas of stem cell research, organs-on-chip models and regenerative medicine including tissue regeneration using in situ bioprinting. DBB does not affect stem cells functionality and differentiation capacity (Faulkner-Jones et al., 2015; Gurkan et al., 2014; Xu et al., 2013a; Gao et al., 2015). For example, Shu's group engineered 3D liver tissue models with hepatocytes derived from hiPSCs and hESCs (Faulkner-Jones et al., 2015). The group bioprinted a bioink solution (comprising hepatocytes and sodium alginate) using a microvalve bioprinter to fabricate 3D tissue model (see Fig. 5.11A1 and A2). During the bioprinting process, alternating layers of the bioink and crosslinker solutions [calcium chloride ($CaCl_2$)] were bioprinted to enable the crosslinking of alginate. After 17 days postbioprinting (after 23 days post-differentiation), bioprinted cells maintained their differentiated phenotype, which was

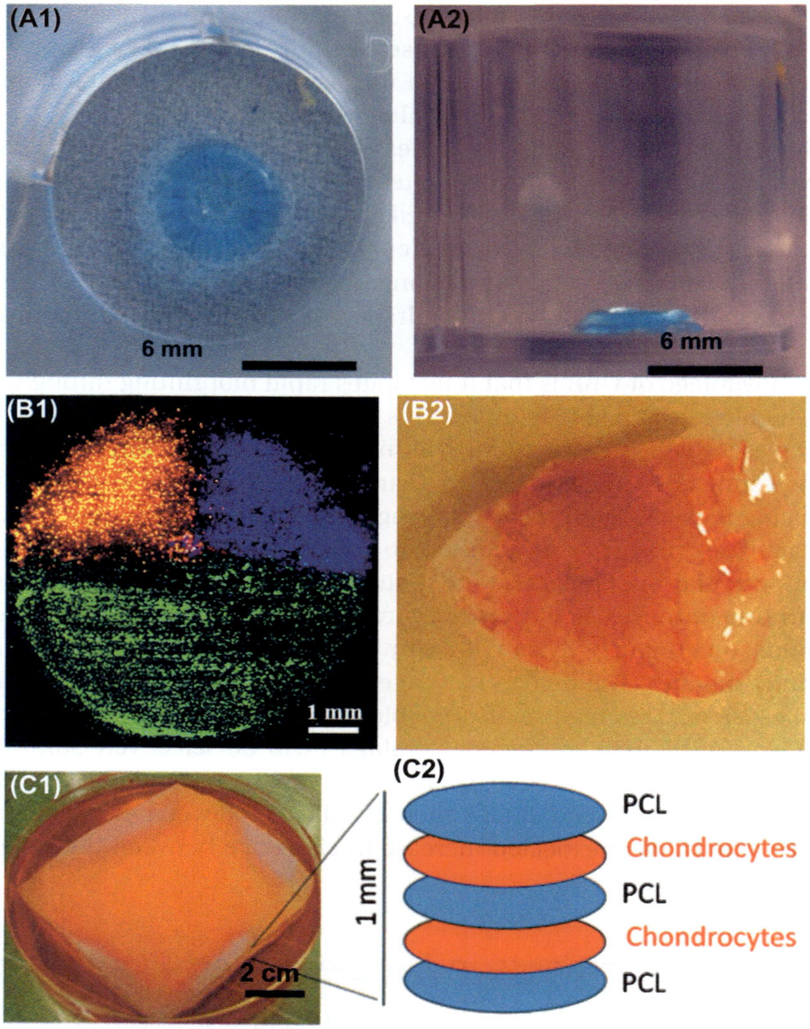

FIGURE 5.11 Recent achievements in droplet-based bioprinting. (A1) Three-dimensional (3D) liver tissue model (top view) comprising of 40 layers of bioprinted alginate and HLCs acquired through differentiation of hiPSCs and hESCs and the side view (A2) *(Reproduced/adapted with permission from Faulkner-Jones et al. (2015))*; (B1) 3D heterogeneous tissue model consisting of bioprinted dSMCs (red) labeled with PKH 67 dye, hAFSCs (blue) labeled with CMHC dye, and bECs (green) labeled with PKH 26 dye that retained its functionality and the differentiation capacity both in vitro and in vivo, (B2) vascularization of the bECs constructs 8 weeks after implantation *(Reproduced/adapted with permission from Xu et al. (2013a))*; Bioprinted 3D cartilage tissue transplants (C1) maintained their biological functions both in vitro and in vivo, (C2) cartilage tissue construct fabrication by layer-by-layer deposition of chondrocytes-fibrinogen-collagen into a previously electrospun layer of PCL fibers *(Reproduced/adapted with permission from Xu et al. (2013a))*.

confirmed through the presence of hepatic markers such as hepatocyte nuclear factor 4 alpha (HNF4α) and albumin. In another study, Atala's group demonstrated that bioprinted stem cells retained their functionality and the differentiation capacity both in vitro and in vivo (Xu et al., 2013a). The group bioprinted three different cell types, hAFSCs, dSMCs, and bECs, along with $CaCl_2$ solution using a TIJ bioprinter. Consecutive layers of cell-laden $CaCl_2$ crosslinker solution were bioprinted into a sodium alginate-collagen solution to fabricate 3D pie-shaped heterogeneous tissue constructs. The pie-shaped constructs were comprised of three distinct sections each with a particular cell type as shown in Fig. 5.11B1. Similarly, 3D cuboidal homogenous tissue constructs of each cell type were also fabricated. Later, bioprinted constructs were cultured for 1 week and subcutaneously implanted into outbred athymic nude mice. Afterward, the constructs were surgically retrieved either after 4 or 8 weeks (see Fig. 5.11B2). Subsequent analysis showed that biological functions (i.e., viability, proliferation, phenotypic expression, and physiological properties) of the bioprinted cells of each type were not affected significantly both in vitro and in vivo. Another notable observation was the vascularization of implanted bEC constructs with substantial blood vessels compared to that of control groups.

Achievements in regenerative medicine include tissue transplants (Xu et al., 2013b; Yanez et al., 2014) and in situ bioprinting (Cui et al., 2012a) for improved wound healing. In a recent study (Xu et al., 2013b), Atala's group engineered hybrid cartilage tissue by employing microvalve bioprinting and electrospinning. In that study, a bioink solution comprising chondrocytes, fibrinogen, and collagen was bioprinted into previously electrospun layers of poly-ε-caprolactone (PCL) fibers as illustrated in Fig. 5.11C1 and C2. In addition, thrombin was bioprinted on each bioprinted layer of the bioink solution to facilitate crosslinking. Afterward, the constructs were cultured in vitro to evaluate cell proliferation and organization. Additionally, some constructs were cultured in vitro for 2 weeks and implanted subcutaneously in immunodeficient mice. Subsequently, the constructs were surgically retrieved after 2, 4, and 8 weeks for characterization. The characterization study indicated that cartilage constructs maintained their biological functions both in vitro and in vivo. At the same time, the cartilage constructs possessed enhanced biological and mechanical characteristics than the cartilage constructs fabricated without incorporating the electrospun PCL fibers. Further, the constructs supported formation of a new cartilage-like tissue.

In situ bioprinting is an alternative approach to two-step bioprinting (bioprinting followed by implantation), where cells and other biologics are directly bioprinted into lesion sites (Skardal et al., 2012; Cui et al., 2012a). In one study (Cui et al., 2012a), Lima's group engineered a cartilage tissue with comparable characteristics of the native cartilage. Using a TIJ bioprinter, human articular chondrocytes were bioprinted within photopolymerizable PEGDMA into 2–5 mm deep defects in osteochondral explants. The explants were previously harvested from bovine femoral condyles using an 8-mm-diameter stainless steel punch. The defects in explants were repaired by bioprinting layers of chondrocytes and PEGDMA while crosslinking each bioprinted layer through photopolymerization. Afterward, the repaired explants were cultured in vitro for 2, 4, and 6 weeks postbioprinting. After 4 weeks, more chondrocytes with higher glycosaminoglycan (GAG) and collagen type II production were observed in tissue constructs bioprinted into the osteochondral explants than the constructs bioprinted in vitro (control group). Thus in situ bioprinting leveraged the presence of native cartilage tissue to accelerate chondrogenesis and extracellular matrix (ECM) production. Similarly, Skardal et al. (2012) employed in situ bioprinting to regenerate skin tissue with AFSCs and MSCs. To compare their healing properties, the two cell types were separately bioprinted over surgical skin wounds (2.0 × 2.0 cm) on the back (middorsal region) of nude mice using a microvalve bioprinter. Overall, three layers of thrombin solution and two layers of cell-laden collagen-fibrinogen solution were alternatively bioprinted over the wounds resulting in 5×10^6 AFSCs or SMCs in each wound. Photographic images were taken immediately as well as 7 and 14 days postbioprinting to monitor wound healing. Furthermore, regenerated skin was harvested from animals at 7 and 14 days for histological analysis. Results indicated that AFSCs were comparable to MSCs in skin regeneration and in situ bioprinting of cells overall accelerated the wound healing process.

5.10 Limitations

Despite the great advantages of DBB, the technology possesses considerable limitations and drawbacks. One of the major limitations of DBB is the clogging of orifice during bioprinting process as highly small fragments in the bioink can accumulate within the orifice and obstruct the flow. This can sometimes necessitate the replacement of the entire orifice if the clogged material does not dissolve or cannot be removed. Because of the small orifice diameter ranging from 10 to 150 μm, as discussed earlier, a limited number of biomaterials are available for DBB such as low-viscosity hydrogels or their components. Thus a wide majority of the bioink materials used in EBB, including cell aggregates, microcarriers, and highly viscous hydrogels (Ozbolat and Hospodiuk, 2016), cannot be used in DBB. Due to this issue, researchers have preferred to create substrates of hydrogels and bioprint cells or other biologics on them using cell media as a delivery medium (Gurkan et al., 2014). This approach has been widely employed for bioprinting arrays of droplets for high-throughput screening (Suntivich et al., 2014). Although the noncontact nature of DBB provides great advantages as discussed earlier, gelation characteristics of printed droplets should be well experimented as ejected droplets can quickly gel in the air and do not assemble to the bioprinted substrate easily.

The other limitation of DBB is the inability to fabricate mechanically strong and structurally well-integrated constructs due to the limited range of available bioink materials, particularly in high concentrations (Dababneh and Ozbolat, 2014). This can be however alleviated to some extent by infiltrating the bioprinted constructs within another biomaterial as a postprocess. Alternatively, a reinforcement approach can also be employed, where nanofibers of stronger polymers can be reinforced into the inkjet bioprinted hydrogels using a hybrid fabrication setup (Xu et al., 2013b). While DBB facilitates fabrication of constructs in a discontinuous manner, where discrete droplets are assembled in 3D, it is highly challenging to fabricate porous tissue constructs. Porous tissue constructs are favorable for perfusion purposes to facilitate sufficient media exchange and can be easily bioprinted using EBB or LBB (only stereolithography and its modifications) techniques. Using DBB, porous architecture can be created either using a plotting medium as a support material with the help of buoyancy or utilizing a two-step approach such as applying porogens or fugitive hydrogels. Lastly, as the resolution of DBB is higher than that of EBB, it takes a longer time to fabricate scalable tissue constructs, where some minor issues can be experienced such as change in the size of the construct due to swelling, contraction, or dehydration (when not bioprinted into the medium).

5.11 Future Directions

Different bioprinting modalities, including DBB, are envisioned to fabricate functional replacement human organs in the future (Ozbolat and Yu, 2013); however, several challenges have yet to be overcome to make it a reality. The first challenge is the printhead design for DBB. The physical characteristics of currently available printheads limit the control over several parameters including droplet volume, the number of cells to be encapsulated in each droplet, the precise placement of droplets, cell concentration, bioink material properties (viscosity), and the long-term reliability of the entire system. Printhead design constraints arise because of the current microfabrication processes, which impose several restrictions including the nozzle geometry. Hence, new nano- or microfabrication techniques are required to overcome the physical limitations with novel nozzle and printhead designs.

The second challenge is associated with materials that constitute the bioink. Each human organ is comprised of several billions of cells of various types (Bianconi et al., 2013). Hence, acquiring cells such as stem cells in such quantities for autologous transplantation applications is constrained by cell cycle times, which may take several weeks to months (Cooper, 2000; Bruce et al., 2002). Hence, new strategies for accelerating the cell cycle time are required. Another bioink-related challenge is the availability of biomimetic materials with controlled degradability and signaling cues to stimulate the proliferation and differentiation of cells (Murphy and Atala, 2014). For example, matrix material properties, such as elasticity, impact the differentiation of bioprinted cells into specific phenotypes (Engler et al., 2006). Thus development of new materials or mechanisms that instill the bioink material with specific biomimetic characteristics, particularly after bioprinting, is desired as the nozzle geometry imposes material constraints. Growth factors and other signaling molecules could partially reduce the necessity of biomimetic materials; however, transporting them to specific bioprinted cells in a sustained manner over time imposes its own set of challenges. Perhaps, the transport of targeted growth factors and signaling molecules is possible by controlling the micropore geometry of bioprinted hydrogels such that of molecules of particular conformation (shape) are selectively transported.

The third challenge is the fabrication of 3D tissue constructs of complex conformations at submicrometer to micrometer resolution. For example, fabrication of complete vascular network at the single–cell level is challenging because DBB at high resolution is limited by the nozzle geometry, which constraints the droplet volume (size) and the bioink viscosity. Moreover, available bioprintable materials or hydrogels are characterized by weak mechanical strength and hence simultaneous codeposition of degradable and biocompatible support materials is essential for counteracting gravity. Although, strategies such as support by means of liquid buoyancy have been proposed (Christensen et al., 2015), leveraging natural mechanisms of cells is potentially most effective of all as it addresses several challenges at once. For instance, angiogenesis of microcapillaries (Lee et al., 2014) obviates the codeposition of support materials and the development of novel printheads with extremely small orifice diameter.

Currently, DBB is not capable of fabricating functional replacement human organs at clinically relevant dimensions; however, it can improve drug discovery and disease modeling as it enables fabrication of spatially patterned multicellular microenvironments in a high-throughput and reproducible manner. Further, only a tiny tissue model can be sufficient for drug screening. At present, many drugs are not effective. For example, 97% of the patients see no benefits from antihypertensives (McCormack, 2014) given for high blood pressure whereas 98% of the patients see no benefits from statins given for high cholesterol (Newman, 2015). The low efficacy of prescription drugs can be attributed to the low numbers of human test subjects (Friedman et al., 2010), which may not account for the genetic diversity among millions of patients. Bioprinted organ-on-a-chip models based on hiPSCs derived from diverse groups can account for the genetic variations and improve the drug discovery. Further, genomic analysis tools and individual genetic tests are becoming inexpensive and they can be used to personalize treatment plans or drug doses. Moreover, 3D tissue models are better at mimicking human physiology and pathology than currently used 2D cell culture models (Wüst et al., 2011; Billiet et al., 2012) as well as the animal models (Shanks et al., 2009). Hence, DBB in combination with targeted genome editing tools such as CRISPR (clustered regularly interspaced short palindromic repeats)/CAS9 (Barrangou and Marraffini, 2014; Hsu et al., 2014) can improve disease modeling (Hinson et al., 2015; Liu et al., 2016).

5.12 Summary

DBB offers great advantages due to its simplicity, agility, and versatility with great control on the deposition pattern. Although the technology currently enables fabrication of heterocellular tissue constructs in a high-throughput and reproducible manner, and has been widely used in several application areas such as tissue engineering and regenerative medicine, transplantation, drug testing and high-throughput screening, and cancer research, the technology currently faces several limitations such as weak structural and mechanical properties of bioprinted tissue and organ constructs as well as their lack of vascularization and perfusability, and the limited translation of the technology into clinics. Despite these limitations, novel breakthroughs such as angiogenesis and in situ bioprinting, which leverage nature-driven mechanisms, make the eventual clinical translation of DBB technology inevitable.

References

Arai, K., et al., 2011. Three-dimensional inkjet biofabrication based on designed images. Biofabrication 3 (3), 034113.

Atkins, T., Escudier, M., 2013. A Dictionary of Mechanical Engineering, first ed. Oxford University Press, Oxford.

Barrangou, R., Marraffini, L.A., 2014. CRISPR-Cas systems: prokaryotes upgrade to adaptive immunity. Molecular Cell 54 (2), 234–244.

Barron, J.A., et al., 2004. Application of laser printing to mammalian cells. Thin Solid Films 453–454, 383–387.

Bianconi, E., et al., 2013. An estimation of the number of cells in the human body. Annals of Human Biology 40 (6), 463–471.

Billiet, T., et al., 2012. A review of trends and limitations in hydrogel-rapid prototyping for tissue engineering. Biomaterials 33 (26), 6020–6041.

Blaeser, A., et al., 2013. Biofabrication under fluorocarbon: a novel freeform fabrication technique to generate high aspect ratio tissue-engineered constructs. BioResearch Open Access 2 (5), 374–384.

Boland, T., et al., 2007. Drop-on-demand printing of cells and materials for designer tissue constructs. Materials Science and Engineering: C 27 (3), 372–376.

Bruce, A., et al., 2002. An overview of the cell cycle. In: Molecular Biology of the Cell. Garland Science, New York.

Cardoso, V., Dias, O.J.C., 2006. Rayleigh-Plateau and Gregory-Laflamme instabilities of black strings. Physical Review Letters 96 (18), 181601.

Chang, R., et al., 2010. Biofabrication of a three-dimensional liver micro-organ as an in vitro drug metabolism model. Biofabrication 2 (4), 045004.

Chang, R., Nam, J., Sun, W., 2008. Direct cell writing of 3D microorgan for in vitro pharmacokinetic model. Tissue Engineering Part C: Methods 14 (2), 157–166.

Cheng, E., Ahmadi, A., Cheung, K.C., 2014. Investigation of the hydrodynamics of suspended cells for reliable inkjet cell printing. In: ASME Proceedings of the 12th International Conference on Nanochannels, Microchannels, and Minichannels, Chicago, pp. 1–8.

Choi, W.S., et al., 2011. Synthetic multicellular cell-to-cell communication in inkjet printed bacterial cell systems. Biomaterials 32 (10), 2500–2507.

Christensen, K., et al., 2015. Freeform inkjet printing of cellular structures with bifurcations. Biotechnology and Bioengineering 112 (5), 1047–1055.

Cooper, G.M., et al., 2010. Inkjet-based biopatterning of bone morphogenetic protein-2 to spatially control calvarial bone formation. Tissue Engineering Part A 16 (5), 1749–1759.

Cooper, G.M., 2000. The eukaryotic cell cycle. In: The Cell: A Molecular Approach. Sinauer Associates, Sunderland.

Cui, X., et al., 2012a. Direct human cartilage repair using three-dimensional bioprinting technology. Tissue Engineering Part A 18 (11–12), 1304–1312.

Cui, X., Breitenkamp, K., Lotz, M., et al., 2012b. Synergistic action of fibroblast growth factor-2 and transforming growth factor-beta1 enhances bioprinted human neocartilage formation. Biotechnology and Bioengineering 109 (9), 2357–2368.

Cui, X., et al., 2014. Human cartilage tissue fabrication using three-dimensional inkjet printing technology. Journal of Visualized Experiments: JoVE (88), e51294.

Cui, X., Boland, T., 2009. Human microvasculature fabrication using thermal inkjet printing technology. Biomaterials 30 (31), 6221–6227.

Dababneh, A.B., Ozbolat, I.T., 2014. Bioprinting technology: a current state-of-the-art review. Journal of Manufacturing Science and Engineering 136 (6), 061016.

Demirci, U., 2006. Acoustic picoliter droplets for emerging applications in semiconductor industry and biotechnology. Journal of Microelectromechanical Systems 15 (4), 957–966.

Demirci, U., Montesano, G., 2007a. Cell encapsulating droplet vitrification. Lab on a Chip 7 (11), 1428–1433.

Demirci, U., Montesano, G., 2007b. Single cell epitaxy by acoustic picolitre droplets. Lab on a Chip 7 (9), 1139–1145.

Derby, B., 2008. Bioprinting: inkjet printing proteins and hybrid cell-containing materials and structures. Journal of Materials Chemistry 18 (47), 5717.

Derby, B., 2011. Inkjet printing ceramics: from drops to solid. Journal of the European Ceramic Society 31 (14), 2543–2550.

Derby, B., 2010. Inkjet printing of functional and structural materials: fluid property requirements, feature stability, and resolution. Annual Review of Materials Research 40 (1), 395–414.

Eagles, P.A., Qureshi, A.N., Jayasinghe, S.N., 2006. Electrohydrodynamic jetting of mouse neuronal cells. The Biochemical Journal 394 (Pt 2), 375–378.

Engler, A.J., et al., 2006. Matrix elasticity directs stem cell lineage specification. Cell 126 (4), 677–689.

Fang, Y., et al., 2012. Rapid generation of multiplexed cell cocultures using acoustic droplet ejection followed by aqueous two-phase exclusion patterning. Tissue Engineering Part C: Methods 18 (9), 647–657.

Faulkner-Jones, A., et al., 2015. Bioprinting of human pluripotent stem cells and their directed differentiation into hepatocyte-like cells for the generation of mini-livers in 3D. Biofabrication 7 (4), 044102.

Faulkner-Jones, A., et al., 2013. Development of a valve-based cell printer for the formation of human embryonic stem cell spheroid aggregates. Biofabrication 5 (1), 015013.

Fedorovich, N.E., et al., 2008. Three-dimensional fiber deposition of cell-laden, viable, patterned constructs for bone tissue printing. Tissue Engineering Part A 14 (1), 127–133.

Ferris, C.J., et al., 2013. Bio-ink for on-demand printing of living cells. Biomaterials Science 1 (2), 224–230.

Friedman, L.M., Furberg, C.D., DeMets, D.L., 2010. Introduction to clinical trials. In: Fundamentals of Clinical Trials. Springer, New York.

Gaetani, R., et al., 2012. Cardiac tissue engineering using tissue printing technology and human cardiac progenitor cells. Biomaterials 33 (6), 1782–1790.

Gao, G., et al., 2014. Bioactive nanoparticles stimulate bone tissue formation in bioprinted three-dimensional scaffold and human mesenchymal stem cells. Biotechnology Journal 9 (10), 1304–1311.

Gao, G., et al., 2015. Inkjet-bioprinted acrylated peptides and PEG hydrogel with human mesenchymal stem cells promote robust bone and cartilage formation with minimal printhead clogging. Biotechnology Journal 10 (10), 1568–1577.

Gasperini, L., et al., 2015. An electrohydrodynamic bioprinter for alginate hydrogels containing living cells. Tissue Engineering Part C: Methods 21 (2), 123–132.

Gasperini, L., Maniglio, D., Migliaresi, C., 2013. Microencapsulation of cells in alginate through an electrohydrodynamic process. Journal of Bioactive and Compatible Polymers 28, 413–425.

Gurkan, U.A., et al., 2014. Engineering anisotropic biomimetic fibrocartilage microenvironment by bioprinting mesenchymal stem cells in nanoliter gel droplets. Molecular Pharmaceutics 11 (7), 2151–2159.

Hayati, I., Bailey, A.I., Tadros, T.F., 1986. Mechanism of stable jet formation in electrohydrodynamic atomization. Nature 319 (6048), 41–43.

Herran, C.L., Coutris, N., 2013. Drop-on-demand for aqueous solutions of sodium alginate. Experiments in Fluids 54 (6), 1548.

Herran, C.L., Huang, Y., 2012. Alginate microsphere fabrication using bipolar wave-based drop-on-demand jetting. Journal of Manufacturing Processes 14 (2), 98–106.

Hinson, J.T., et al., 2015. Titin mutations in iPS cells define sarcomere insufficiency as a cause of dilated cardiomyopathy. Science (New York, N.Y.) 349 (6251), 982–986.

Hockaday, L.A., et al., 2012. Rapid 3D printing of anatomically accurate and mechanically heterogeneous aortic valve hydrogel scaffolds. Biofabrication 4 (3), 035005.

Horváth, L., et al., 2015. Engineering an in vitro air-blood barrier by 3D bioprinting. Scientific Reports 5, 7974.

Hsu, P.D., Lander, E.S., Zhang, F., 2014. Development and applications of CRISPR-Cas9 for genome engineering. Cell 157 (6), 1262–1278.

Hutson, C.B., et al., 2011. Synthesis and characterization of tunable poly(ethylene glycol): gelatin methacrylate composite hydrogels. Tissue Engineering Part A 17 (13–14), 1713–1723.

Ilkhanizadeh, S., Teixeira, A.I., Hermanson, O., 2007. Inkjet printing of macromolecules on hydrogels to steer neural stem cell differentiation. Biomaterials 28 (27), 3936–3943.

Jakab, K., et al., 2008. Tissue engineering by self-assembly of cells printed into topologically defined structures. Tissue Engineering Part A 14 (3), 413–421.

Jang, D., Kim, D., Moon, J., 2009. Influence of fluid physical properties on ink-jet printability. Langmuir 25 (5), 2629–2635.

Jayasinghe, S.N., 2007. Bio-electrosprays: the development of a promising tool for regenerative and therapeutic medicine. Biotechnology Journal 2 (8), 934–947.

Jayasinghe, S.N., Qureshi, A.N., Eagles, P.A.M., 2006. Electrohydrodynamic jet processing: an advanced electric-field-driven jetting phenomenon for processing living cells. Small 2 (2), 216–219.

Jayasinghe, S.N., Townsend-Nicholson, 2006. Stable electric-field driven cone-jetting of concentrated biosuspensions. Lab on a Chip 6 (8), 1086–1090.

Kamisuki, S., et al., 1998. A low power, small, electrostatically-driven commercial inkjet head. In: Proceedings of the Eleventh Annual International Workshop on Micro Electro Mechanical Systems. IEEE, Heidelberg, pp. 63–68.

Kerdjoudj, H., et al., 2011. Cellularized alginate sheets for blood vessel reconstruction. Soft Matter 7 (7), 3621.

Khalil, S., Nam, J., Sun, W., 2005. Multi-nozzle deposition for construction of 3-D biopolymer tissue scaffolds. Rapid Prototyping Journal 11, 9–17.

Kim, H.S., et al., 2007. Optimization of electrohydrodynamic writing technique to print collagen. Experimental Techniques 31 (4), 15–19.

Klebe, R., 1988. Cytoscribing: a method for micropositioning cells and the construction of two- and three-dimensional synthetic tissues. Experimental Cell Research 179 (2), 362–373.

Koch, L., et al., 2010. Laser printing of skin cells and human stem cells. Tissue Engineering Part C: Methods 16 (5), 847–854.

Le, H.P., 1998. Progress and trends in ink-jet printing technology. Journal of Imaging Science and Technology 42 (1), 49–62.

Lee, V., et al., 2014. Generation of multi-scale vascular network system within 3D hydrogel using 3D bio-printing technology. Cellular and Molecular Bioengineering 7 (3), 460–472.

Lee, W., et al., 2009a. Multi-layered culture of human skin fibroblasts and keratinocytes through three-dimensional freeform fabrication. Biomaterials 30 (8), 1587–1595.

Lee, W., et al., 2009b. Three-dimensional bioprinting of rat embryonic neural cells. NeuroReport 20 (8), 798–803.

Lee, Y.B., et al., 2010. Bio-printing of collagen and VEGF-releasing fibrin gel scaffolds for neural stem cell culture. Experimental Neurology 223 (2), 645–652.

Lin, H., et al., 2013. Application of visible light-based projection stereolithography for live cell-scaffold fabrication with designed architecture. Biomaterials 34 (2), 331–339.

Liu, J., et al., 2016. CRISPR/Cas9 facilitates investigation of neural circuit disease using human iPSCs: mechanism of epilepsy caused by an SCN1A loss-of-function mutation. Translational Psychiatry 6 (1), e703.

Marchioli, G., et al., 2015. Fabrication of three-dimensional bioplotted hydrogel scaffolds for islets of Langerhans transplantation. Biofabrication 7 (2), 025009.

Markstedt, K., et al., 2015. 3D bioprinting human chondrocytes with nanocellulose–alginate bioink for cartilage tissue engineering applications. Biomacromolecules 16 (5), 1489–1496.

Matsusaki, M., et al., 2013. Three-dimensional human tissue chips fabricated by rapid and automatic inkjet cell printing. Advanced Healthcare Materials 2 (4), 534–539.

McCormack, J., 2014. Anti-hypertensives to Prevent Death, Heart Attacks, and Strokes. Available from: http://www.thennt.com/nnt/anti-hypertensives-to-prevent-death-heart-attacks-and-strokes/.

Mézel, C., et al., 2010. Bioprinting by laser-induced forward transfer for tissue engineering applications: jet formation modeling. Biofabrication 2 (1), 014103.

Mironov, V., et al., 2009. Biofabrication: a 21st century manufacturing paradigm. Biofabrication 1 (2), 022001.

Mohebi, M.M., Evans, J.R., 2002. A drop-on-demand ink-jet printer for combinatorial libraries and functionally graded ceramics. Journal of Combinatorial Chemistry 4 (4), 267–274.

Mongkoldhumrongkul, N., et al., 2009. Bio-electrospraying whole human blood: analysing cellular viability at a molecular level. Journal of Tissue Engineering and Regenerative Medicine 3 (7), 562–566.

Moon, S., et al., 2010. Layer by layer three-dimensional tissue epitaxy by cell-laden hydrogel droplets. Tissue Engineering Part C: Methods 16 (1), 157–166.

Murphy, S.V., Atala, A., 2014. 3D bioprinting of tissues and organs. Nature Biotechnology 32 (8), 773–785.

Newman, D., 2015. Statins for Heart Disease Prevention (Without Prior Heart Disease). Available from: http://www.thennt.com/nnt/statins-for-heart-disease-prevention-without-prior-heart-disease/.

Nichol, J.W., et al., 2010. Cell-laden microengineered gelatin methacrylate hydrogels. Biomaterials 31 (21), 5536–5544.

Nishiyama, Y., et al., 2008. Development of a three-dimensional bioprinter: construction of cell supporting structures using hydrogel and state-of-the-art inkjet technology. Journal of Biomechanical Engineering 131 (3), 35001.

Odde, D.J., Renn, M.J., 1999. Laser-guided direct writing for applications in biotechnology. Trends in Biotechnology 17 (10), 385–389.

Odde, D.J., Renn, M.J., 2000. Laser-guided direct writing of living cells. Biotechnology and Bioengineering 67 (3), 312–318.

Onses, M.S., et al., 2015. Mechanisms, capabilities, and applications of high-resolution electrohydrodynamic jet printing. Small 11 (34), 4237–4266.

Owens, C.M., et al., 2013. Biofabrication and testing of a fully cellular nerve graft. Biofabrication 5 (4), 045007.

Ozbolat, I.T., Chen, H., Yu, Y., 2014. Development of 'Multi-arm Bioprinter' for hybrid biofabrication of tissue engineering constructs. Robotics and Computer-Integrated Manufacturing 30 (3), 295–304.

Ozbolat, I.T., Hospodiuk, M., 2016. Current advances and future perspectives in extrusion-based bioprinting. Biomaterials 76, 321–343.

Ozbolat, I.T., Yu, Y., 2013. Bioprinting toward organ fabrication: challenges and future trends. IEEE Transactions on Biomedical Engineering 60 (3), 691–699.

Pataky, K., et al., 2012. Microdrop printing of hydrogel bioinks into 3D tissue-like geometries. Advanced Materials 24 (3), 391–396.

Phillippi, J.A., et al., 2008. Microenvironments engineered by inkjet bioprinting spatially direct adult stem cells toward muscle- and bone-like subpopulations. Stem Cells 26 (1), 127–134.

Poellmann, M.J., et al., 2011. Patterned hydrogel substrates for cell culture with electrohydrodynamic jet printing. Macromolecular Bioscience 11 (9), 1164–1168.

Rayleigh, L., 1878. On the instability of jets. Proceedings of the London Mathematical Society 10, 4–13.

Reis, N., Ainsley, C., Derby, B., 2005. Ink-jet delivery of particle suspensions by piezoelectric droplet ejectors. Journal of Applied Physics 97 (9), 094903.

Rioboo, R., Marengo, M., Tropea, C., 2002. Time evolution of liquid drop impact onto solid, dry surfaces. Experiments in Fluids 33 (1), 112–124.

Rodríguez-Dévora, J.I., et al., 2012. High throughput miniature drug-screening platform using bioprinting technology. Biofabrication 4 (3), 035001.

Roisman, I.V., Rioboo, R., Tropea, C., 2002. Normal impact of a liquid drop on a dry surface: model for spreading and receding. Proceedings of the Royal Society of London A: Mathematical, Physical and Engineering Sciences 458 (2022), 1411–1430.

Roth, E., et al., 2004. Inkjet printing for high-throughput cell patterning. Biomaterials 25 (17), 3707–3715.

Salonitis, K., 2014. Stereolithography. In: Hashmi, S., et al. (Eds.), Comprehensive Materials Processing. Elsevier, Oxford, pp. 19–67.

Saunders, R., Derby, B., 2014. Inkjet printing biomaterials for tissue engineering: bioprinting. International Materials Review 59 (8), 430–448.

Schiaffino, S., Sonin, A.A., 1997. Molten droplet deposition and solidification at low Weber numbers. Physics of Fluids 9 (11), 3172.

Shanks, N., Greek, R., Greek, J., 2009. Are animal models predictive for humans? Philosophy, Ethics, and Humanities in Medicine : PEHM 4, 2.

Singh, M., et al., 2010. Inkjet printing-process and its applications. Advanced Materials 22 (6), 673–685.

Skardal, A., et al., 2012. Bioprinted amniotic fluid-derived stem cells accelerate healing of large skin wounds. Stem Cells Translational Medicine 1 (11), 792–802.

Skardal, A., et al., 2010. Photocrosslinkable hyaluronan-gelatin hydrogels for two-step bioprinting. Tissue Engineering Part A 16 (8), 2675–2685.

Snyder, J.E., et al., 2011. Bioprinting cell-laden matrigel for radioprotection study of liver by pro-drug conversion in a dual-tissue microfluidic chip. Biofabrication 3, 034112.

Soltman, D., Subramanian, V., 2008. Inkjet-printed line morphologies and temperature control of the coffee ring effect. Langmuir 24 (5), 2224–2231.

Son, Y., et al., 2008. Spreading of an inkjet droplet on a solid surface with a controlled contact angle at low Weber and Reynolds numbers. Langmuir 24 (6), 2900–2907.

Suntivich, R., et al., 2014. Inkjet printing of silk nest arrays for cell hosting. Biomacromolecules 15 (4), 1428–1435.

Sutanto, E., et al., 2012. A multimaterial electrohydrodynamic jet (E-jet) printing system. Journal of Micromechanics and Microengineering 22 (4), 045008.

Stringer, J., Derby, B., 2009. Limits to feature size and resolution in ink jet printing. Journal of the European Ceramic Society 29 (5), 913–918.

Tang, X., Yakut Ali, M., Saif, M.T., 2012. A novel technique for micro-patterning proteins and cells on polyacrylamide gels. Soft Matter 8, 7197.

Tasoglu, S., Demirci, U., 2013. Bioprinting for stem cell research. Trends in Biotechnology 31 (1), 10–19.

Wijshoff, H., 2010. The dynamics of the piezo inkjet printhead operation. Physics Reports 491 (4–5), 77–177.

Wilson, W.C., Boland, T., 2003. Cell and organ printing 1: protein and cell printers. The Anatomical Record Part A: Discoveries in Molecular, Cellular, and Evolutionary Biology 272A (2), 491–496.

Wohlers, T., Gornet, T., 2014. History of Additive Manufacturing. Wohlers Report, Fort Collins.

Workman, V.L., et al., 2014. Controlled generation of microspheres incorporating extracellular matrix fibrils for three-dimensional cell culture. Advanced Functional Materials 24 (18), 2648–2657.

Worthington, A.M., 1876. On the forms assumed by drops of liquids falling vertically on a horizontal plate. Proceedings of the Royal Society of London 25 (171–178), 261–272.

Wüst, S., Müller, R., Hofmann, S., 2011. Controlled positioning of cells in biomaterials—approaches towards 3D tissue printing. Journal of Functional Biomaterials 2 (4), 119–154.

Xie, J., Wang, C.H., 2007. Electrospray in the dripping mode for cell microencapsulation. Journal of Colloid and Interface Science 312 (2), 247–255.

Xiong, R., et al., 2015. Freeform drop-on-demand laser printing of 3D alginate and cellular constructs. Biofabrication 7 (4), 045011.

Xu, C., et al., 2012. Scaffold-free inkjet printing of three-dimensional zigzag cellular tubes. Biotechnology and Bioengineering 109 (12), 3152–3160.

Xu, F., et al., 2010. A droplet-based building block approach for bladder smooth muscle cell (SMC) proliferation. Biofabrication 2 (1), 014105.

Xu, F., et al., 2011. A three-dimensional in vitro ovarian cancer coculture model using a high-throughput cell patterning platform. Biotechnology Journal 6 (2), 204–212.

Xu, T., et al., 2013a. Complex heterogeneous tissue constructs containing multiple cell types prepared by inkjet printing technology. Biomaterials 34 (1), 130–139.

Xu, T., et al., 2013b. Hybrid printing of mechanically and biologically improved constructs for cartilage tissue engineering applications. Biofabrication 5 (1), 015001.

Xu, T., et al., 2009. Fabrication and characterization of bio-engineered cardiac pseudo tissues. Biofabrication 1 (3), 035001.

Xu, T., et al., 2008. High-throughput production of single-cell microparticles using an inkjet printing technology. Journal of Manufacturing Science and Engineering 130 (2), 021017.

Xu, T., et al., 2005. Inkjet printing of viable mammalian cells. Biomaterials 26 (1), 93–99.

Xu, T., et al., 2006. Viability and electrophysiology of neural cell structures generated by the inkjet printing method. Biomaterials 27 (19), 3580–3588.

Yamaguchi, S., et al., 2012. Cell patterning through inkjet printing of one cell per droplet. Biofabrication 4, 045005.

Yanez, M., et al., 2014. In vivo assessment of printed microvasculature in a bilayer skin graft to treat full-thickness wounds. Tissue Engineering Part A 21 (1–2), 224–233.

Yu, Y., Zhang, Y., Ozbolat, I.T., 2014. A hybrid bioprinting approach for scale-up tissue fabrication. Journal of Manufacturing Science and Engineering 136 (6), 61013.

Yusof, A., et al., 2011. Inkjet-like printing of single-cells. Lab on a Chip 11 (14), 2447–2454.

Zhao, L., et al., 2012. The integration of 3-D cell printing and mesoscopic fluorescence molecular tomography of vascular constructs within thick hydrogel scaffolds. Biomaterials 33 (21), 5325–5332.

6

Laser-Based Bioprinting*

CHAPTER OUTLINE

Great discoveries are made accidentally less often than the populace likes to think
Wilhelm Conrad Röntgen

6.1 Introduction

Stereolithography (SLA) is the first three-dimensional (3D) printing technology invented by Charles W. Hull and patented in 1985, where ultraviolet (UV) light selectively scans a photocurable material in a vat enabling selective solidification of the material layer by layer to create in 3D structures (Salonitis, 2014). SLA has been utilized in fabrication of tissue scaffolds; however, living cells were generally seeded postfabrication. The process brought various unique qualities to the fabricated scaffolds as SLA enabled construction

*With minor contributions by Hemanth Gudapati, The Pennsylvania State University.

3D Bioprinting.

of high-definition scaffolds with controlled geometry and interconnected porous architecture. Incorporation of living cells had not been attempted until 2004 when Boland and his coworkers at the Clemson University first attempted the use of a commercially available SLA system to bioprint human cells (Dhariwala et al., 2004), which was then further refined by various research groups as it enabled fabrication of highly complex scaffolds that cannot be achieved using droplet-based bioprinting (DBB) or extrusion-based bioprinting (EBB) modalities.

Transferring of living cells using a laser-assisted technology was first introduced by Odde and Renn (1999) to facilitate two-dimensional (2D) patterning of cells, which enabled rapidly formed patterns of viable cells on cover slides within cell media. Several other groups began to print living cells using laser energy from 2000 to 2010 including but not limited to Chickov's group in Germany (Ovsianikov et al., 2007a,b), Guillemot's group in France (Guillemot et al., 2010), and Chrisey's group in the United States (US) (Ringeisen et al., 2004). Although laser-guidance direct writing (LGDW) was first used for 2D patterning of cells, with the invention of laser-assisted bioprinting as an extension of matrix-assisted pulsed-laser evaporation (MAPLE), fabrication of 3D tissue constructs became feasible. All these approaches and techniques utilizing laser energy to pattern cells and fabricate 3D tissue constructs are classified under the technique, referred to as "laser-based bioprinting (LBB)."

Due to its high accuracy and resolution, LBB has been preferred in biofabrication of well-defined tissue constructs; however, its highly intricate setup limited its use in bioprinting domain compared to other commonly available bioprinting modalities, such as EBB or DBB. Although there is only one company in the world utilizing LBB for commercialization of tissues such as skin, there is currently no commercially available laser-assisted bioprinting technology that is applicable to direct cell printing (Roots Analysis Private Ltd, 2014). Researchers, however, can acquire components of the setup and custom build their own platforms. On the other hand, there are various companies commercializing SLA-based 3D printers, which can be modified for fabrication of cell-laden scaffolds. The use of toxic photoinitiators for rapid curing of tissue scaffolds limits the further transition of SLA and its modifications into the bioprinting arena.

With the advent of two-photon polymerization (2PP) and its application in the field of tissue engineering to the fabrication of tissue scaffolds with unprecedented resolution capabilities, and the invention of dynamic projection printing, which increases fabrication speed significantly, utilization of these technologies in the bioprinting has escalated in the last decade.

This chapter presents LBB with a thorough discussion on its modalities including the processes involving photopolymerization and the processes based on cell transfer. A detailed discussion is provided to the reader revealing the advantages and limitations of LBB with respect to other bioprinting modalities including EBB (Chapter 4) and DBB (Chapter 5), recent notable studies are highlighted, and the future prospects are presented to the reader.

6.2 Modalities of Laser-Based Bioprinting

According to their working mechanisms, LBB techniques can be classified into two major submodalities including (1) processes involving photopolymerization and (2) processes based on cell transfer (see Fig. 6.1). Processes involving photopolymerization include SLA, dynamic optical projection stereolithography (DOPsL), and 2PP, and processes based on cell transfer can be further classified into three including LGDW, matrix-assisted pulsed laser evaporation-direct write (MAPLE-DW), and laser-induced forward transfer (LIFT).

6.2.1 Processes Involving Photopolymerization

6.2.1.1 Stereolithography

Photopolymerization-based bioprinting of tissue constructs is performed similar to typical SLA used in 3D printing of objects. In SLA process, as shown in Fig. 6.2A, the

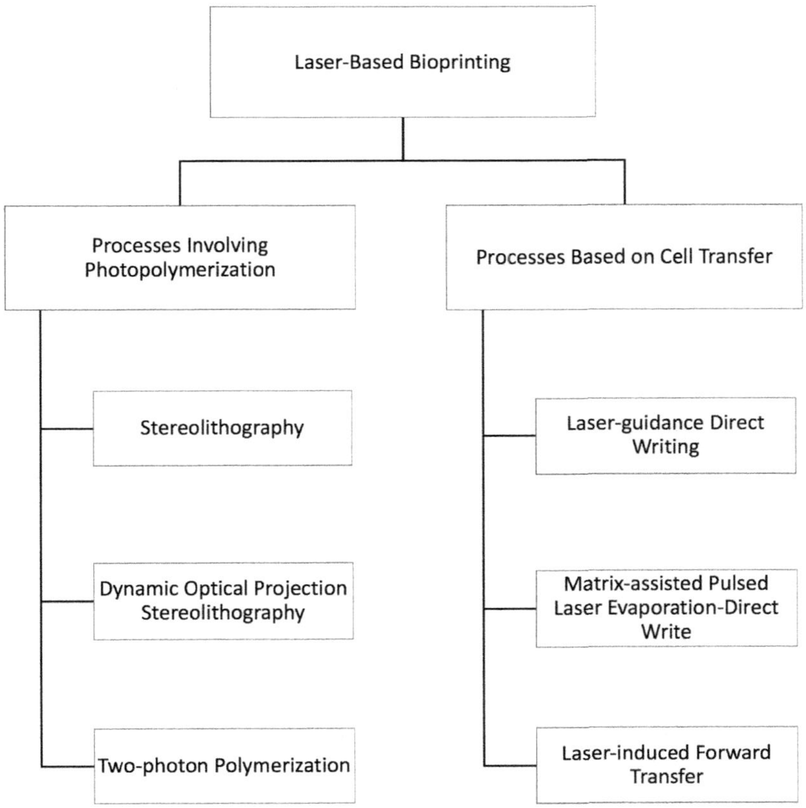

FIGURE 6.1 Classification of laser-based bioprinting modalities.

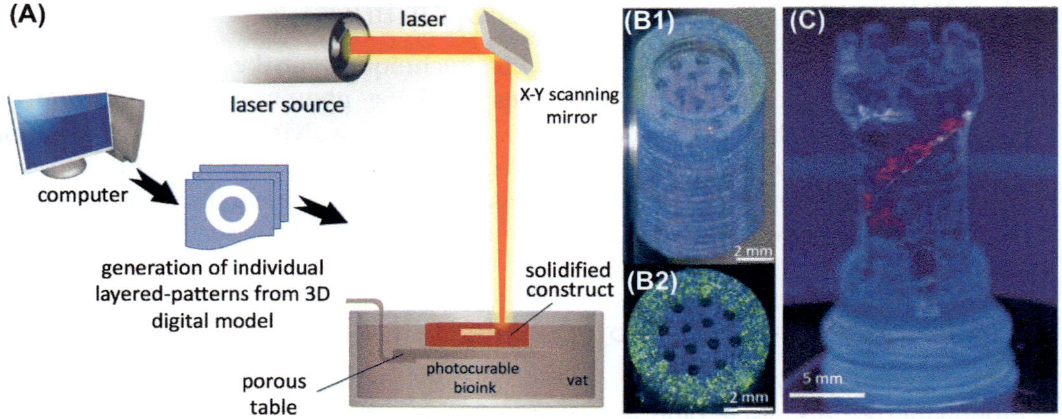

FIGURE 6.2 (A) A typical setup of stereolithography for bioprinting of tissue constructs. Sample 3D-printed tissue constructs including spatially controlled multimaterial bioactive poly(ethylene glycol)-dimethacrylate scaffolds in the form of (B1 and B2) multilumen conduits loaded with two fluorescent particles *(Reproduced/adapted with permission from Arcaute et al. (2006))* and (C) a rook chess piece *(Reproduced/adapted with permission from Arcaute et al. (2010))*.

bioink solution (cells in a photocurable material) is loaded into a vat, which is equipped with a porous table mounted on an elevator apparatus that controls the position of the table in z-axis. For the first layer, the table is positioned to the surface of the bioink solution, which is then exposed to UV; to immediately polymerize the bioink. In photopolymerization, monomers or weakly crosslinked polymers, in either liquid or solid state, interact to form 3D polymeric network. Absorption of a photon by a photoinitiator leads to generation of radicals, which react with monomers and initiates radical polymerization (Ovsianikov and Chichkov, 2012). The photoreaction is terminated when two radicals react, which takes places in regions that are exposed to irradiation. The entire layer is scanned based on the toolpath obtained from the computer-aided design (CAD) model. When the solidification of a layer is completed, the porous table moves down to a distance equal to the layer thickness to print the next layer. The process continues in the same manner until the entire tissue construct is built.

SLA allows bioprinting of tissue constructs ranging in size from a few hundred micrometers to a few millimeters (Bajaj et al., 2014). The application of SLA in bioprinting was first demonstrated by Dhariwala et al. (2004). Using a commercial SLA 3D printer (SLA-250, 3D Systems), they encapsulated Chinese hamster ovary (CHO) cells (cell line CHO-B2) within poly(ethylene oxide) (PEO) and poly(ethylene glycol)-dimethacrylate (PEGDMA) hydrogels to construct tubular geometries. In their study, over 90% cell viability was achieved and the authors showed that increasing the photoinitiator within the hydrogel solution decreased the cell viability in the second day. A similar approach was taken place at the University of Texas El Paso, where Arcaute et al. (2006) used the same 3D printer equipped with a He–Cd laser (325 nm, 40 mW) for encapsulation of 3T3 fibroblasts within PEGDMA hydrogels. They bioprinted cylindrical scaffolds with multiple channels, which could potentially be used in nerve conduit fabrication (see Fig. 6.2B1 and B2). Using a self-aligning minisetup, the same group further demonstrated fabrication of multimaterial scaffolds in highly intricate geometries (see Fig. 6.2C). Jeong et al. then used a similar approach in utilizing a commercial SLA printer and encapsulated 3T3 fibroblasts within microvascular stamps made of poly(ethylene glycol)-diacrylate (PEGDA) and PEGDMA hydrogels to mediate neovascularization within chorioallantoic membrane of chick embryos. The authors demonstrated that treating the printed samples with 12-O-tetradecanoylphorbol-13-acetate, which is a protein kinase C (PKC) activator, enabled cells to express multiple angiogenic factors, including vascular endothelial growth factor (VEGF) and endothelin-1, which in turn mediated the formation of neovessels within chorioallantoic membranes.

In SLA, the photocurable material determines the speed of curing and the resolution of the process. It should possess certain mechanical, biological, and chemical properties to serve for different tissue fabrication purposes. In this regard, the right combination of photocurable materials, curing agent, solvent, bioreagent, and light absorber should be selected to design the optimal process. There are a wide variety of photopolymers used in SLA such as acrylates with urethane units and most dialkylacrylamide (particularly trimethylolpropane triacrylate) (Lu and Chen, 2012). Along with photocurable hydrogels, photoinitiators have been used to speed up the solidification process as well as improve the mechanical stability of the tissue constructs as they have low photodissociation energy. However, photoinitiators are not easily applied to bioprinting as they are toxic and can harm the cells. For example, the least cytotoxic of known photoinitiators, Irgacure 2959 (2-hydroxy-1-[4-(2-hydroxyethoxy)pheny]-2-methyl-1-propanone) is cytotoxic at the concentrations greater than 0.5% (Melchels et al., 2010), where only 25% of the cells were viable after a day in an aqueous PEGDMA resin. Other studies recommend a concentration of <0.1% for Irgacure 2959 (Lu and Chen, 2012; Fedorovich et al., 2009); however, using such low concentration can result in low mechanical properties and hence excessive swelling as well as increased depth of curing, which affects the solidification in other layers and deteriorated the quality of bioprinting.

6.2.1.2 Dynamic Optical Projection Stereolithography

Dynamical optical projection SLA is a digital mask, or maskless, projection printing system that utilizes a digital micromirror device (DMD) available in conventional computer projectors (Hribar et al., 2014). In the literature, various research groups experimented with a dynamic mask system in microstereolithography (μSLA) to accelerate the fabrication process. For example, a liquid crystal display (LCD) was proposed as a dynamic mask for fabrication of double-end collector fluidic parts and springs (Bertsch et al., 2000). Later in 2005, Itoga et al. (2004) demonstrated the use of LCD projectors in μSLA, where micropatterning of PEGDA was achieved enabling attachment of endothelial cells (ECs). As LCD has a limited optical efficiency, Chen and his coworkers utilized the DMD approach as it offers better performance in terms of optical fill factors such as 85% with DMD versus 64% with LCD and light transmission with 71% in

DMD and 21% in LCD (Lu and Chen, 2012). In their approach (see Fig. 6.3A), the general system operates as in traditional SLA system where a UV (365 nm) source can be used to polymerize photocurable materials. The digital mask, generated by a DMD device, enables controllable and interchangeable reflected light patterns rather than static, impractical, and more expensive physical masks used in photolithography process (Hribar et al., 2014). The DMD chip reflects the collimated UV light based on a digital pattern with a resolution of 1920 × 1080. The digital patterns were drawn in series of Microsoft PowerPoint images to generate a dynamic mask (Lu and Chen, 2012). The chip consists of an array of mirrors, which are coated with reflective aluminum and can tilt in two angles either +12 or −12 degrees with respect to the surface. By tilting the mirrors, "on" and "off" states can be obtained at +12 or −12 degrees, respectively, where the pixel appears dark while the illuminated light is reflected away from the projection lens. A motorized z-axis is used to enable fabrication of scaffolds in 3D using a typical layer-by-layer fabrication approach.

The major advantage of using DOPsL approach over other SLA-based bioprinting techniques is that DOPsL is rapid, as each layer can be made at once in seconds, which is a highly complex process using serial writing in single-photon polymerization (Billiet et al., 2012). It allows precise fabrication of scaffolds with complex internal architecture. However, the major limitation of the system compared to single/two-photon polymerization is the lack of high resolution due to the limitations of the projection lens. The other limitation of the system is the substantial use of photocurable materials (containing expensive biological reagents), which needs to be loaded in the vat resulting in loss during loading and unloading of the system. In addition, the thickness of each layer is difficult to control unless a light absorber is added to the bioink material. In this regard, the authors demonstrated the use of perfluorohexane (C_6F_{14}) as a support material, which is an inert liquid with high density (1.685 g/cm^3) and a molecular polarity that is smaller than that of the photocurable material (Lu and Chen, 2012). To use the support material, the authors made a modification in the build platform. In this regard, an automated syringe pump system was used to fill the vat with the photocurable material and perfluorohexane independently. The vat was first filled with perfluorohexane leaving some space at the top of the vat for the photocurable material. Upon solidification of the photocurable material on the top of the vat with exposure to laser energy, the motorized z-stage was submerged into perfluorohexane to clean the uncured material. Next, the stage was elevated to print the second layer. The cycle was repeated until the entire scaffold is built. The authors also tested the effect of oxygen deprivation as oxygen is a strong radical inhibitor and could be detrimental to polymerization at low initiator concentration. In this regard, a nitrogen environment was employed, which increased the gelation speed and hence the bioprinting speed; however, leakage in the system caused some fluctuations in curing process.

Using DOPsL approach, Chen and his coworkers have bioprinted various cell-laden scaffolds. Fig. 6.3B1 and B2 illustrates a bioprinted vascular network to demonstrate cancer cell migration into the printed channels (Huang et al., 2014). High-definition

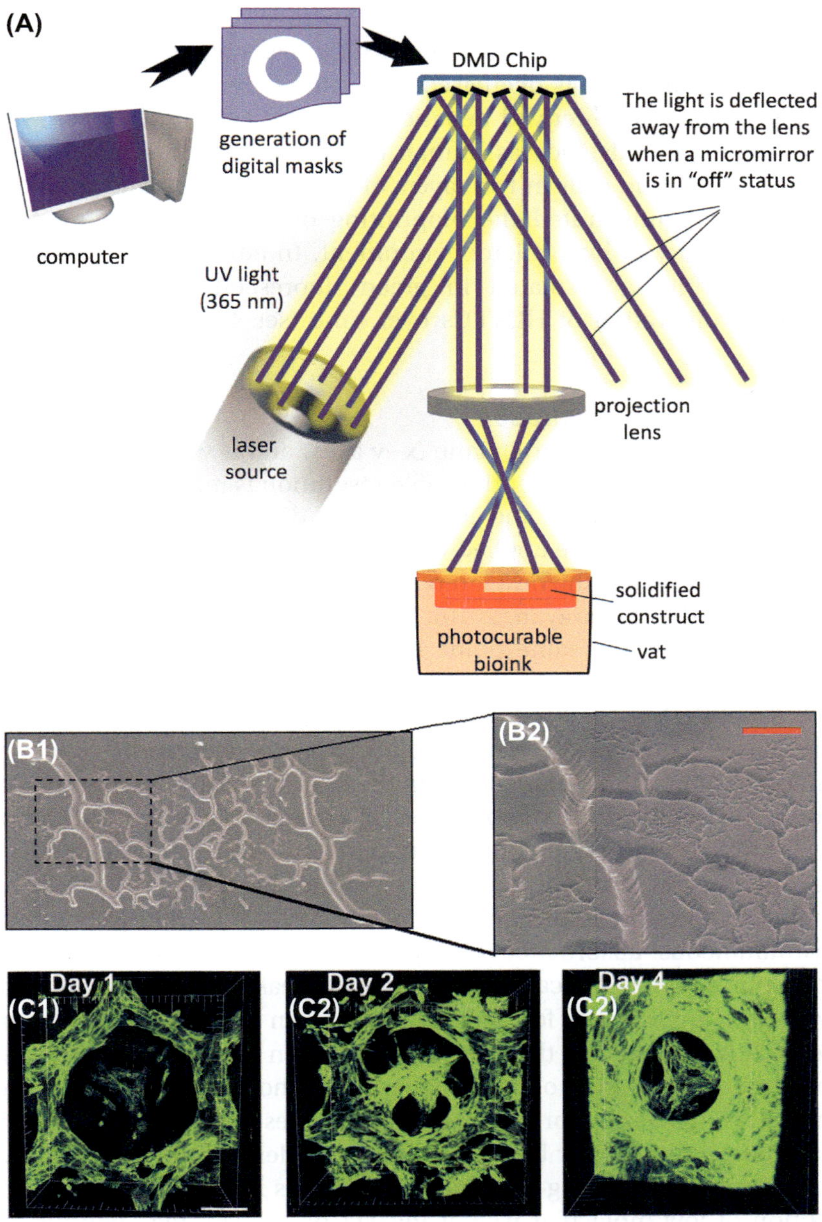

FIGURE 6.3 (A) The schematic of dynamic optical projection stereolithography (DOPsL) system, where digital masks are generated to control the status of micromirrors (on/off) to direct the UV light selectively onto a photocurable material; bioprinted tissue constructs using DOPsL system including (B1) a vasculature in multiscale on poly(ethylene glycol)-diacrylate (B2) with high-definition capillary structures (scale bar = 100 μm) *(Reproduced/adapted with permission from Hribar et al. (2014))* and (C1–C3) hexagonal scaffolds with spreading of green fluorescent protein–labeled human umbilical vein endothelial cellshuman umbilical vein endothelial cells on day 1, 2, and 4 (scale bar = 100 μm) *(Reproduced/adapted with permission from Gauvin et al. (2012)).*

vascular channels were created using PEGDA hydrogel-laded HeLa cells and noncancerous 10 T1/2 fibroblasts. It was shown that HeLa cells migrated significantly when the vascular channel diameter was decreased. Recently, they demonstrated the use of human pluripotent stem cell–derived hepatic progenitor cells (iPSC-HPCs) encapsulated with other supporting cells such as human umbilical vein endothelial cells (HUVECs) and adipose-derived stem cells in two layers of gelatin methacrylate (GelMA) (Ma et al., 2016). Such work demonstrated the bioprinting of a human liver model mimicking anatomical complexity of liver microenvironment. In addition, they bioprinted hexagonal structures with encapsulated in green fluorescent protein–labeled HUVECs demonstrating proliferation of HUVECs over time (see Fig. 6.3C1–C3) (Gauvin et al., 2012).

6.2.1.3 Two-Photon Polymerization

SLA has a high resolution in lateral plane (x–y axes) and is widely used in fabrication of microscale objects; however, its depth profile resolution is inferior. The resolution of SLA depends on the focal spot size and is limited by diffraction resulting in a minimum feature size equal to half of the applied laser wavelength; however, due to technicalities inherent to SLA technology, the best lateral resolution obtained so far is in the range of a few microns (Gittard and Narayan, 2010). Therefore, with the advent of 2PP where two photons are exerted on the same point simultaneously confining the region of polymerization in 3D (Fig. 6.4A), resolution has been increased significantly (Cumpston et al., 1999). In 2PP, the structural resolution beyond the diffraction limit (the limit on collimating a laser beam) has been realized bringing the feature size to less than 50 nm, which is an order of magnitude smaller than the laser wavelength (Emons et al., 2012). In single-photon polymerization, a fluorophore is excited by a single photon of a specific energy level, whereas multiple photos are used to excite the fluorophore with a relatively lower level of energy in multiphoton polymerization (Bajaj et al., 2014). The probability of two-photon absorption is proportional to the square of the laser intensity, which requires simultaneous absorbance of multiple photons (Zipfel et al., 2003). While femtosecond pulsed lasers are capable of very high peak intensities at moderate average laser power, they are suitable for and widely used in 2PP (Ovsianikov and Chichkov, 2012). Use of 2PP is limited in the bioprinting domain as the resolution achieved is far greater than the average size of mammalian cells; however, the technique has been applied in tissue engineering for fabrication of high-resolution scaffolds. Early efforts in use of multiphoton process for biological hydrogels demonstrated spatial patterning of bioactive materials into existing photoactive materials in 3D (Hahn et al., 2006). A precursor solution of low molecular weight PEGDA or acrylate-PEG-peptide containing a photoinitiator was allowed to diffuse into the PEGDA hydrogel, and a multiphoton photopolymerization approach with a digital mask was utilized to solidify the biologically active materials within PEGDA hydrogel. The authors also demonstrated migration of HT-1080 cells within acrylate–PEG–RGDS-patterned sections within the entire construct. In addition to the abovementioned hydrogel, a limited number of materials

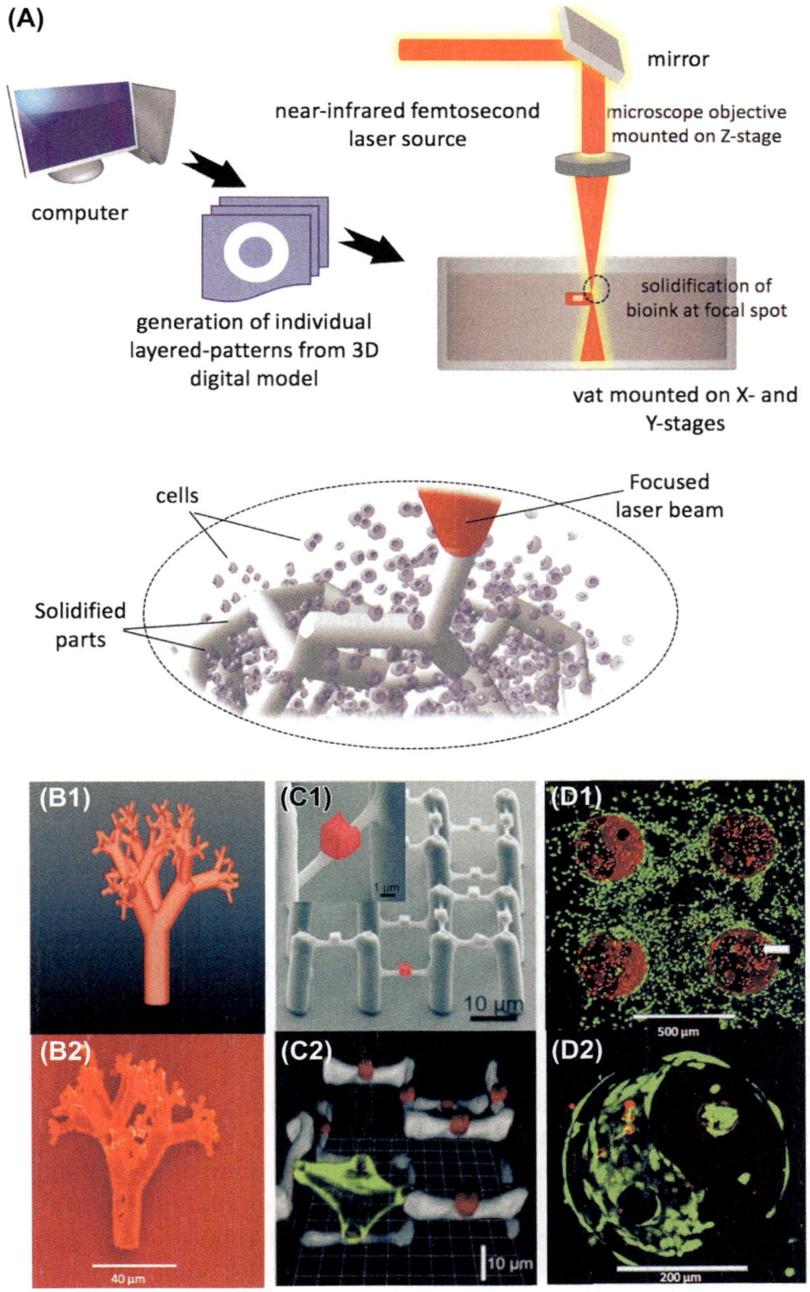

FIGURE 6.4 (A) A schematic of two-photon polymerization (2PP) process for cell encapsulation (bottom image), *(Reproduced/adapted from Ovsianikov et al. (2014))*. Fabrication of 3D pulmonary alveoli-like structures made of SU8: (B1) a computer-aided design model and (B2) a SEM image *(Reproduced/adapted with permission from Ovsianikov et al. (2007a,b))*. (C1) Two-step 2PP of scaffolds with protein repellant poly(ethylene glycol)-diacrylate (as the frame) and protein binding Ormocomp cubes (*red*) and (C2) 3D reconstruction of confocal images showing cell adhesion on different Ormocomp cubes at different heights and stretching of f-actin filaments *(Reproduced/adapted with permission from Klein et al. (2011))*. Bioprinting of MG63 cells in 20% methacrylamide-modified gelatin, (D1) where 2PP was used to generate Yin-Yang symbols (in *dark red*) demonstrating live (*green*) and dead (*red*) cells. (D2) MG63 cells trapped within the voids of the 2PP hydrogel construct proliferated in 3 weeks *(Reproduced/adapted from Ovsianikov et al. (2014))*.

have been used in 2PP including commercially available ORMOCOMP® and SU8, which support cell growth and proliferation as well as facilitate formation of cell–cell junctions (Ovsianikov and Chichkov, 2012). Using these commercial materials, Serbin et al. (2004) fabricated porous tissue scaffolds, 3D pulmonary alveoli-like structures (see Fig. 6.4B1 and B2), and hollow microneedles for transdermal drug delivery (Ovsianikov et al., 2007a,b). One of the greatest advantages of this system is that it operates at room temperature, preventing the denaturation of proteins or biologically active materials. In addition, the system does not require costly clean room facilities. As this technique couples high-definition technology with the nanoscale resolution, it may be beneficial in a hybrid bioprinting platform, where small nanosize features can be built to control adhesion and orientation in 3D. For example, Fig. 6.4C1 and C2 shows multiscale constructs printed using a two-step 2PP process made of protein-repellant PEGDA as the frame and protein-binding Ormocomp cubes to support cell adhesion. Such environment facilitated control on 3D culture of cells with engineered adhesion points. Ovsianikov et al. (2014) recently demonstrated the use of 2PP in bioprinting of living cells. They used water-soluble photoinitiators (two benzylidene cycloketone-based photoinitiators G2CK and P2CK), loaded human osteosarcoma MG63 cells in 20% methacrylamide-modified gelatin (gelMOD), and printed Yin-Yang symbols successfully. The results demonstrated that a significant cell damage was observed due to reactive species generated during 2PP, and only 25.7% of the cells were viable in the voids of Ying-Yang constructs (see Fig. 6.4D1). Interestingly, 95% of the cells were viable outside the laser-exposed regions and cells trapped within the voids of Ying-Yang constructs proliferated in 3-week in vitro culture (see Fig. 6.4D2).

6.2.2 Processes Based on Cell Transfer

In LBB processes based on cell transfer, cells are bioprinted by utilizing the mechanism of transferring living cells from one location to another in either culture medium or viscoelastic hydrogels such as alginate and Matrigel™.

6.2.2.1 Laser-Guidance Direct Writing

LGDW is the first LBB technique used for bioprinting of living cells. It was first demonstrated by Odde and Renn (1999), where living cells were patterned in 2D using laser-induced optical forces. Based on the principle explained by Ashkin and Dziedzic (1987), who pioneered optical force–based particle manipulation, Odde and Renn (1999) used laser-beam focus and successfully manipulated thousands of particles simultaneously. Before attempting deposition of living cells, the authors demonstrated patterning of a wide range of organic and inorganic particles in both gas and liquid phases (Renn et al., 1999). The key parameter that determines the interaction between light and cells is the refractive index of the cells relative to the surrounding fluid, where larger differences promote further interactions. In their work, the authors called the technique “laser-guided direct writing” as there was no guidance, such as a mask, during

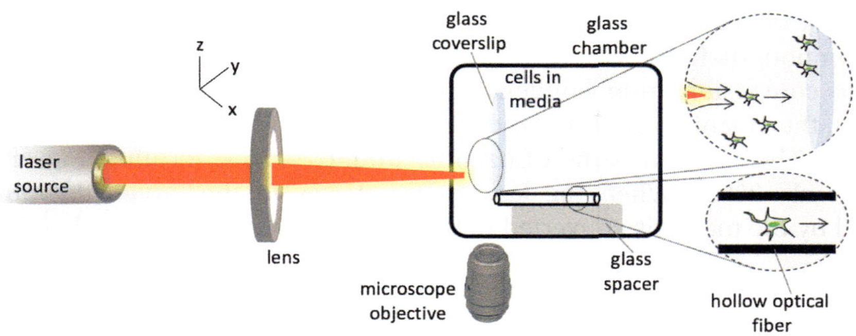

FIGURE 6.5 A schematic of laser-guidance direct write process, where cells are entrapped due to the gradient forces generated by the laser pulse and propelled toward a coverslip. The low numerical aperture lens is attached to a three-axis micromanipulator to print cells sequentially and create patterns. As the distance of cell delivery is limited to 300 μm, a fused silica hollow optical fiber is used to guide the laser beam and cells, which is elevated on a glass coverslip spacer with its long axis aligned coaxially with the laser beam axis and the focal point.

the bioprinting process. In that study, as shown in Fig. 6.5, cells were loaded into the medium and the laser beam was weakly focused. When a cell interacted with the light, it generated a gradient force, which immediately pulled the cell to the center of the light (where the light intensity was maximal) and then pushed the cell axially in the direction of beam and deposited it onto the substrate of interest such as a coverslip. The authors demonstrated bioprinting of embryonic chick spinal cord cells at a velocity of 11.4 μm/s, where a force of 1 pN was exerted on cells (Odde and Renn, 2000). After bioprinting, cells exhibited normal proliferation and spreading characteristics confirming that they were unaffected by the applied laser irradiation. In their study, the authors demonstrated 2D patterning by changing the position of the low numerical aperture focusing lens, which was translated using a micromanipulator to move the focal point to a new spot adjacent to the previous location. Either single cells or cell clusters were printable with an average deposition rate of 2.5 cells/min. This number is quite low compared to what is achieved using current LBB technologies such as LIFT. One of the major limitations in this simple setup was the limited distance when the cells were transferred, which was about 300 μm as the beam divergence and connective fluid flow forces overwhelmed the optical forces (Odde and Renn, 2000). To better guide deposition of cells and achieve longer travel distance of cells in the centimeter range, the authors utilized a hollow optical fiber, which transmitted the light as well as passed the cells through the fiber core. The cells were transferred with a mean velocity of 53 μm/s through fibers with 100 μm inner diameter.

6.2.2.2 Matrix-Assisted Pulsed-Laser Evaporation-Direct Write

MAPLE was developed at the US Naval Research Laboratory in late 1990s to deposit fine layers of functional materials, including but not limited to organic compounds, chemoselective polymers, and biomaterials (Chrisey et al., 2003). Compared to conventional pulsed laser deposition, MAPLE enables deposition of wide range of organic and polymeric compounds from smaller to larger molecular weight with less damage resulting from the conversion from condensed to vapor state (Piqué, 2011). In MAPLE (see Fig. 6.6A), the organic compound is dissolved in a matrix, which is usually a solvent such as alcohol. The solution is then frozen at around −196°C forming a laser target (Fitz-Gerald et al., 2000). When the laser pulse strikes to the target, the photon energy absorbed by the matrix is converted to thermal energy, which is absorbed by the organic

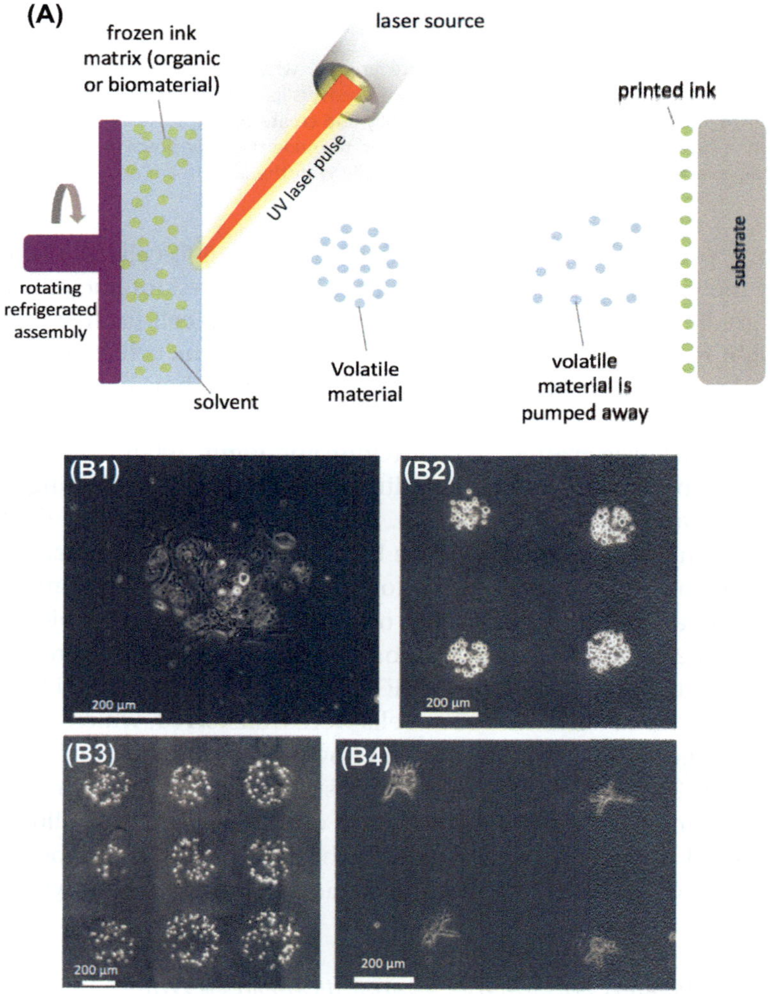

FIGURE 6.6 (A) A schematic of matrix-assisted pulsed-laser evaporation process. Phase-contrast images of bioprinted cells using matrix-assisted pulsed laser evaporation direct write: (B1) human dermal fibroblasts showing normal morphology at 4 h, (B2) bovine pulmonary artery endothelial cells approximately 1 min postbioprinting, (B3) rat neural stem cells approximately 1 min postbioprinting, and (B4) mouse myoblast cells 20 h postbioprinting *(Reproduced with permission from Schiele et al. (2009))*.

molecules within the solvent. These molecules are converted into a gaseous state with increased kinetic energy, resulting in desorption of the compounds from the matrix and selective transfer to the collector based on a user-defined pattern. As a result, a thin film is formed on the collector while the volatile solvent molecules with limited adhesion coefficients are pumped away in the vacuum chamber. MAPLE process enables transfer of compounds in their native chemical structure and biological functionality without denaturation. In the literature, it has been shown that the temperature of the matrix material influenced the morphology and other film characteristics (Sellinger et al., 2008). MAPLE technology, as is, could not be used for bioprinting of living cells as cells cannot be encapsulated within the matrix due to solvent toxicity. In addition, the incompatible nature of the cryogenic setup, heated substrate, and vacuum chamber is not a hospitable environment for living cells. For bioprinting, the setup was further modified to accommodate living cells. Cells are first encapsulated into bioink solution, and a thin coating is formed under a ribbon. Thus, the technology was further adapted and evolved into a viable form for bioprinting of living cells.

MAPLE-DW process utilizes all benefits of MAPLE, where a thin layer of biomaterial (i.e., hydrogels) is coated at the bottom side of a transparent quartz support (print ribbon). The purpose of the quartz material is to absorb the wavelength of the laser. In general, the majority of the laser energy is absorbed by the ribbon as well as the biomaterial–ribbon interface. This reduces the severity of genetic damage caused by the UV light. In this regard, Corr's group conducted DNA damage analysis to determine whether gelatin-based writing induces double-strand DNA breaks (Schiele et al., 2010). In their study, the bioprinted fibroblasts were positive for Hoechst nuclear staining without any colocalization with phosphor-H2AX, indicating that the process did not induce any double-stranded DNA damage to fibroblasts. In MAPLE-DW, a range of laser fluences below the ablation threshold of the coated material is used (Zhang et al., 2015). When the laser beam passes through the support material, it focuses at the interface of the quartz support and the coated material (the sublime part of the coated material), which results in rapid localized heating followed by high-pressure vapor formation, generating a plasma bubble. The resulting bubble expands and ejects the coating material and transfers it to the collector substrate. The formation of the plasma bubble and hence the subsequent jet formation can be tuned by selecting the proper coating material based on its rheological properties as well as thickness and laser fluence. There are only a few hydrogels used as a coating material in LBB, such as alginate (Xiong et al., 2015a), Matrigel™ (Ringeisen et al., 2004), and gelatin (Schiele et al., 2010). Depending on the bioink properties, the laser pulse forms a thin or thick jet, which then breaks into one or more droplets and recoils back to the coating. A typical MAPLE-DW setup utilizes a low-powered UV pulsed laser, where a laser pulse with a short duration around 8 ns is applied to create bubble, transferring the jet from the coating material to the substrate (Riggs et al., 2011). In general, a short distance around 200–7000 μm is appropriate for successful patterning of living cells (Patz et al., 2006). Fig. 6.6B1–B4 shows bioprinting and patterning of various cells types transferred from a ribbon coated in a triazene dynamic release layer or Matrigel™ (Schiele et al., 2009).

6.2.2.3 Laser-Induced Forward Transfer

LIFT is an advanced version of MAPLE-DW, where cells encapsulated in a coating material on an optically transparent quartz support are transferred to a substrate in close proximity or in contact with the coating material. In LIFT, compared to MAPLE-DW, an energy-absorbing IR-transparent interlayer of thin film (in the order of 10–50 nm) of metal (Ag, Ti, Au), metal oxide (TiO_2), or photo-decomposing volatile polymer (triazene) is used (Devillard et al., 2013). With the aid of the intermediate light-absorbing layer, the detrimental effects of intensive UV light could be sufficiently mitigated, which has increased the use of this technique and diminished the use of MAPLE-DW. A laser-induced setup consists of four major components including CAD software, a laser setup, a cartridge, and a substrate (see Fig. 6.7A), where the cartridge design is highly crucial to bioprint cells successfully.

The cartridge consists of three major layers including a supporting transparent quartz that holds the entire cartridge in place. Then, an interlayer thin film, generally gold, is coated on the bottom of the support quartz. Then, a thin layer of bioink solution is coated on the bottom of the gold layer. Techniques such as spin coating or coating with the aid of a blade can be used to generate a uniform layer of bioink material. The quality of the coating is crucial as it can easily influence the layer thickness, which can generate variations in the droplet size. Therefore, the coating needs to be carefully handled, and its viscoelastic properties should be maintained for reproducibility of the LIFT process (Devillard et al., 2013). During the bioprinting process, cells accumulate at the bottom of the bioink solution due to the gravity bringing inconsistencies to cell printing process. When the laser hits the transparent quartz support, the majority of it is absorbed by the intermediate layer, and the laser focuses on the region, where the absorbing layer and the coating intersect, generating thermal increase, which in turn generates a vapor bubble. The vapor bubble expands as the energy accumulates and a jet forms, which then transfers the bioink onto the substrate. In LIFT, there are three possible regimes. In the first regime (subthreshold regime) where the laser intensity is not sufficient, an annular shape is observed, or "coffee-ring" effect, as a result of droplet evaporation on a surface (Guillemot et al., 2010). When the bioink parameters including the laser fluence and the laser pulse energy are altered, the jetting regime can be obtained with proper jet formation. As the laser energy increases significantly, bubble bursting is observed. Concurrently, traces of film detachment become apparent, particularly around the laser spot (Guillemot et al., 2010). Fig. 6.7B represents a detailed schematic of bubble dynamics and jet formation during the LIFT process (Unger et al., 2011). First, the nanosecond laser pulse generates a rapid local vaporization of the region between the intermediate layer and the subliminal region of the bioink solution. As the vapor starts to expand, it can only expand in the direction of the substrate as the quartz support blocks the expansion of the bubble toward it. As the adhesion forces between the bioink and the

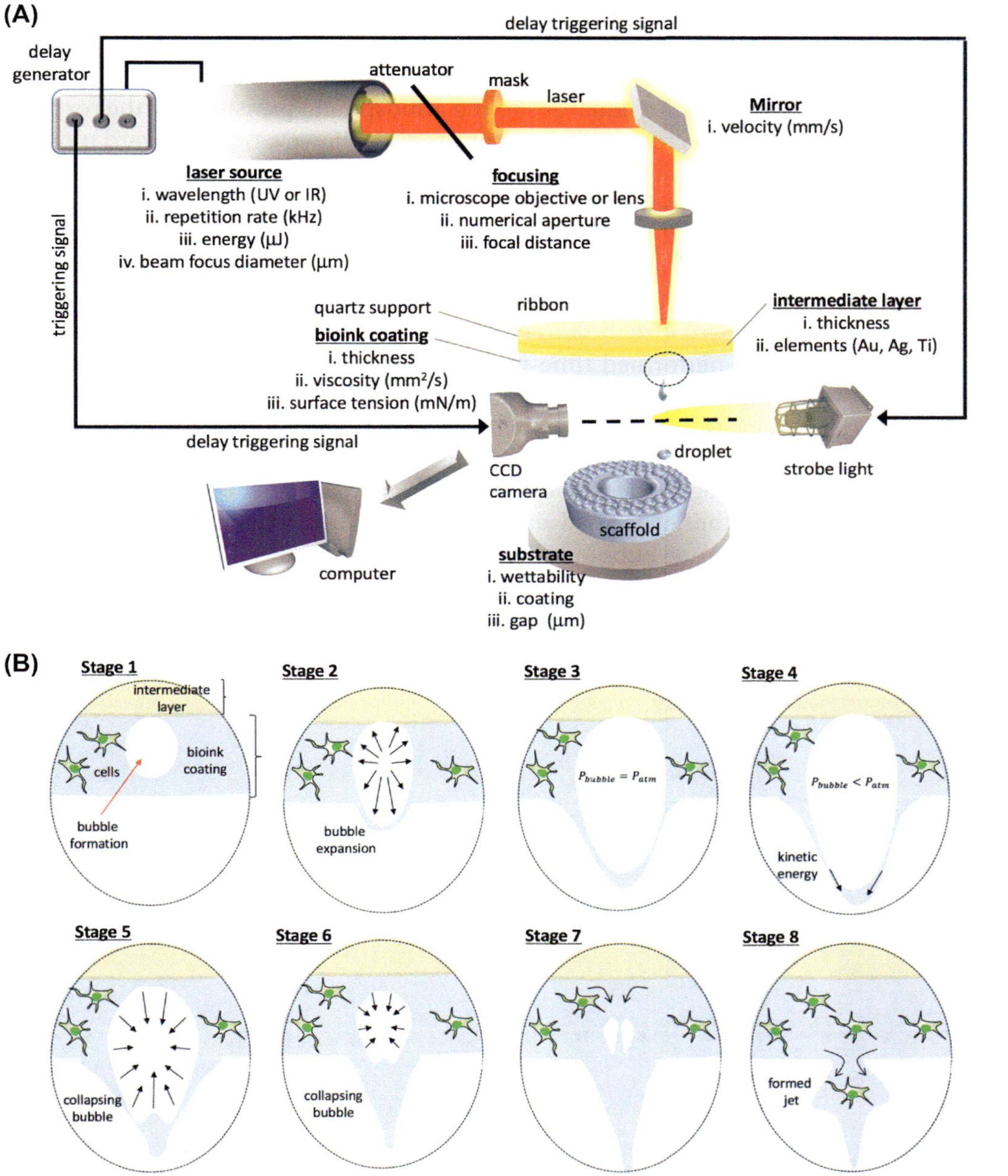

FIGURE 6.7 (A) A schematic of laser-induced forward transfer system, which consists of a laser system (a laser source, an attenuator, a mask, a mirror, and an objective lens), a ribbon (quartz support, intermediate layer, bio-ink coating), image acquisition system (a charged couple device camera, a strobe light, a computer, and a delay generator), and the substrate, where the process parameters influencing bioprinting of cells are highlighted. (B) A step-by-step schematic of physical interactions during bubble and jet formation.

intermediate layer prevent the bubble from detaching from the intermediate layer, the bubble maintains a temporary contact angle of 90 degrees (Unger et al., 2011). The contact angle further increases and the bubble expands in the direction of the substrate until the pressure of the vapor equalizes to the atmospheric pressure. Further expansion of the bubble results in decrease in the vapor pressure; however, the forward moving tip continues to flow due to the inertia, or the momentum gained. With the conversion of the kinetic energy of the vapor to the flow inside the bioink coating, the moving tip pulls the entire protrusion toward the substrate and the vapor bubble collapses. Jet formation begins with a thin tip continuing to elongate until breaking into droplets. As described by the Rayleigh principle (outlined in Chapter 5), droplet formation starts when the perimeter of the jet is larger than the perturbation wavelength.

Unger et al. (2011) performed time-resolved imaging of hydrogel transport without the use of a substrate to understand the dynamics of jet formation. In their study, two different laser fluences were used including 1.6 J/cm^2 (Fig. 6.8A) and 2.7 J/cm^2 (Fig. 6.8B). After 2 μs of laser exposure, a protrusion started to form, elongating further in 5 μs. After 7 μs, the jet began to form and the protrusion diminished in 10 μs. After 20 μs, a bulge at the top of the jet formed due to collision of the hydrogel flow around the ablation spot and the vapor bubble collapsed (Unger et al., 2011). The jet then thinned significantly in 330 μs and broke into droplets; the sublime part of the jet then sprang back. At a larger fluence level (2.7 J/cm^2), the jet formation process demonstrated some

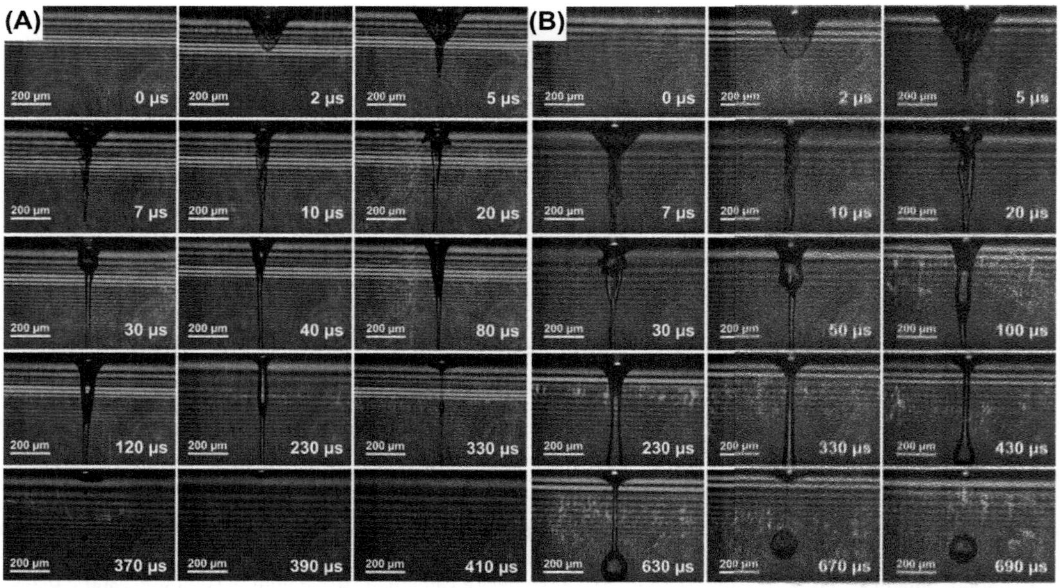

FIGURE 6.8 Time-resolved images of jet formation during laser-induced forward transfer process under a laser fluence of (A) 1.6 J/cm^2 and (B) 2.7 J/cm^2 *(Reproduced/adapted with permission from Unger et al. (2011)).*

differences (see Fig. 6.8B). For example, at the beginning of the protrusion formation, the size of the protrusion was larger and longer at the early phase of jet formation. The diameter of the jet was greater than that formed under lower laser fluence. At 20 μs, a bulge formed at the sublime part of the jet and the bulge gradually diminished into a regular conic shape. The jet profile displayed fluctuations through the lapse time, where the jet thinned from 20 to 50 μs but it then thickened in 330 μs. After 670 μs, the jet broke into a single droplet as the volume of the jet was considerable larger than that under lower laser fluence. In 690 μs, the protrusion disappeared and the process was completed. Compared to the lower fluence at 1.6 J/cm^2, higher laser fluence at 2.7 J/cm^2 generated a thicker jet with a higher velocity and longer process (Unger et al., 2011).

6.2.2.3.1 DROPLET IMPINGEMENT ONTO THE SUBSTRATE

Although LIFT utilizes laser technology, it generates droplets to be deposited onto a substrate similar to DBB techniques presented in Chapter 5. Therefore, impingement of droplets onto the substrate is crucial as it influences the bioprinting accuracy and manufacturability of 3D constructs. For hydrogels used in LBB, there are three main droplet impingement characteristics, such as splashing, spreading, and rebounding. In splashing, the droplet disintegrates into secondary droplets after colliding with a substrate; in spreading, the droplet expands its surface area; and in rebounding, droplets can rebound off the surface. Rebounding is, however, suppressed when viscoelastic hydrogels (i.e., alginate) are used owing to their high elongation viscosity (Bergeron et al., 2000). According to Weber, the critical number (W_e) of droplet splashing or spreading represented as:

$$W_e = \frac{\rho d U^2}{\sigma} \tag{6.1}$$

where ρ is the density of the liquid, d is the characteristics length which corresponds to the diameter of the droplet, U is the velocity, and σ is the surface tension. In general, larger Weber numbers result in splashes and lower ones lead to spreading. While these properties are important for the droplet formation, substrate properties on the collector (i.e., wettability of the surface, surface roughness, and viscous forces) are also critical (Roisman et al., 2002). Zhang et al. (2016) recently performed a study on impingement of alginate droplets using LBB. In their study, the authors showed that the critical Weber number obtained for 2%, 4%, 6%, and 8% alginate solutions are 2993, 3331, 5102, and 13,657, respectively. The corresponding laser influences for these critical Weber numbers are 1300, 1700, 1900, and 2500 mJ/cm^2, respectively. By further understanding droplet impingement into a $CaCl_2$ pool toward larger-scale tissue fabrication, the group later demonstrated bioprinting of 3T3 fibroblasts (loaded in 2% sodium alginate) into $CaCl_2$ pool, resulting in a Y-shaped vascular constructs with a wall thickness greater than a millimeter (see Fig. 6.9) (Xiong et al., 2015a).

In sum, LBB processes involving photopolymerization and based on cell transfer have different advantages and disadvantages with respect to each other. Table 6.1 summarizes

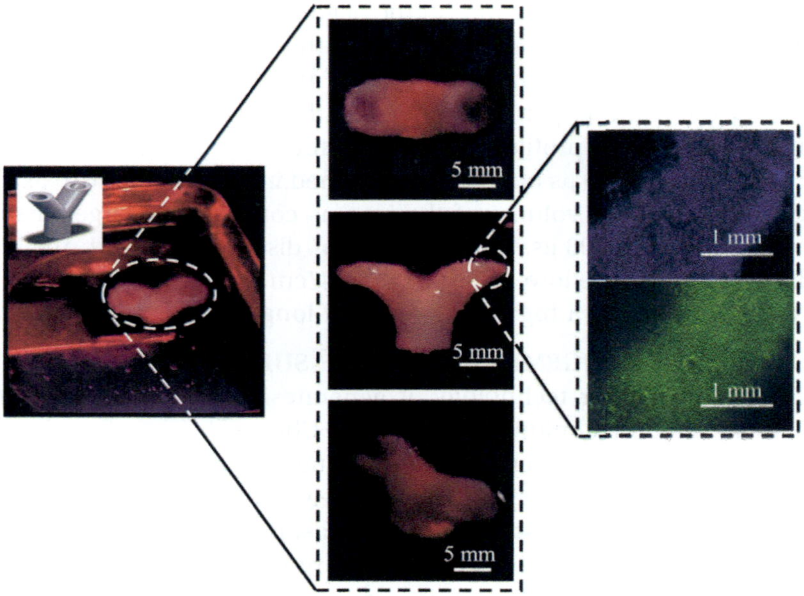

FIGURE 6.9 Bioprinting of 3D thick tissue constructs fabricated using laser-influenced forward transfer. Y-shaped cellular tubes were printed with 2% sodium alginate loaded with 5×10^6 cells/mL, where blue and green shows living cells performed using Hoechst and fluorescein diacetate assays, respectively *(Reproduced with permission from Xiong et al. (2015a))*.

LBB techniques and compares their capabilities and features including their laser spot size, operating conditions, smallest printable feature that can be attained, cell viability, bioink printability along with their strengths and limitations.

6.3 Toward Multimaterial Bioprinting

The majority LBB techniques rely on single bioink material as it is difficult to fabricate multimaterial tissue constructs. As there is only a single bioink type utilized, making heterocellular patterns is thus a challenging task. The vast majority of native tissues are heterocellular with multiple cell types organized in a highly complex pattern (Ozbolat, 2015); therefore, it is vital for future LBB technologies to overcome this problem. In this regard, two major approaches have been proposed, one in SLA and the other in LIFT technology.

For SLA, Wicker's group developed a rotating vat carousel system on a commercial 3D Systems 250/50 SLA machine, which enabled circulation of different materials on a rotational stage (Choi et al., 2011). This way, multiple materials were incorporated into a single object. As discussed before, the authors also demonstrated a similar technology in 2010, where hydrogel-based multimaterial tissue scaffolds were fabricated using PEGDMA or PEGDA as the main biomaterial along with fluorescently labeled dextran

Table 6.1 Comparison of Laser-Based Bioprinting Processes

	Laser Bioprinting Modality	Laser Spot Size (Diameter)	Operating Conditions	Smallest Printable Feature	Cell Viability	Bioink Printability	Strengths	Limitations
Processes involving photopolymerization	Stereolithography	75–250 μm (Arcaute et al., 2006, 2010)	≤350 mJ/cm^2 of laser fluence and (Dhariwala et al., 2004; Arcaute et al., 2006), λ = 325–365 nm (Arcaute et al., 2006; Dhariwala et al., 2004)	250 μm features (Arcaute et al., 2006)	87% (Arcaute et al., 2006)	16.67% (w/v) polyethylene oxide (PEO) (Dhariwala et al., 2004), 20–30% (w/v) poly(ethylene glycol) dimethacrylate (PEGDMA) (Arcaute et al., 2006, 2010), 20% (w/v) (PEGDA) (Arcaute et al., 2010)	Intermediate fabrication times, patterned constructs with high mechanical strength	Low resolution, limited bioink material or material types, photoinitiator cytotoxicity at higher concentrations
	Dynamic optical projection stereolithography	N/A	50 mW/cm^2 of laser (UV) intensity (Gauvin et al., 2012)	Around 50 μm (Hribar et al., 2014)	65–76% (Ma et al., 2016)	10–15% (w/v) gelatin methacrylate (Gauvin et al., 2012), 20% (w/v) PEGDA (Huang et al., 2014)	Shorter fabrication times	Limited bioink materials or material types, limited control on deposited layer thickness
	Two-photon polymerization	N/A	330 mW laser pulses (80 fs, f = 75 MHz, λ = 800 nm) (Ovsianikov et al., 2007a,b)	≤100 nm features (Ovsianikov and Chichkov, 2012)	25.7% in laser-exposed regions and 95% outside the laser-exposed regions (Ovsianikov et al., 2014)	Hybrid organic–inorganic polymers (Ormocers®) (Hadjizadeh and Doillon, 2010), MG63 cells loaded in 20% gelMOD (Ovsianikov et al., 2014)	Very high resolution	Limited biomaterial types, not suitable for cell encapsulation unless water-soluble photoinitiators used, low cell viability around laser-exposed regions

Continued

Table 6.1 Comparison of Laser-Based Bioprinting Processes—cont'd

	Laser Bioprinting Modality	Laser Spot Size (Diameter)	Operating Conditions	Smallest Printable Feature	Cell Viability	Bioink Printability	Strengths	Limitations
Processes based on cell transfer	Laser-guidance direct writing	N/A	200–300 mW of laser power (Renn et al., 1999; Xu et al., 2003; Nahmias et al., 2005), $\lambda = 532$–830 nm (Renn et al., 1999; Xu et al., 2003; Nahmias et al., 2005)	10 μm features (Odde and Renn, 1999; Nahmias et al., 2005)	90% (Nahmias et al., 2005)	Spinal cord cells in media (Odde and Renn, 2000)	High resolution, high cell viability owing to weakly focused laser beam	Limited cell types and biologics because of refractive index constraints, viscous bioink materials are not printable, 3D bioprinting is difficult owing to bioink viscosity constraints
	MAPLE-DW	10–200 μm (Ringeisen et al., 2002; Doraiswamy et al., 2006, 2007; Xiong et al., 2015a)	50–2000 mJ/cm^2 of laser fluence (12–30 ns, $f = 10$ Hz, $\lambda = 193$ nm) (Lin et al., 2009a; Xiong et al., 2015b; Doraiswamy et al., 2007; Ringeisen et al., 2002)	25–50 μm diameter droplets (Lin et al., 2009b; Ringeisen et al., 2002)	50–90% (Gudapati et al., 2014; Lin et al., 2010, 2009a; Xiong et al., 2015a)	8% (w/v) sodium alginate without cells and 2% (w/v) cell-laden alginate (NIH 3T3 cells of concentration 5×10^6 cells/mL) (Gudapati et al., 2014; Xiong et al., 2015a)	Viscous bioink materials of various material types, diverse cell types and biologics, intermediate resolution, nozzle-free transfer of cells	Thermal-induced cell injury, longer fabrication times owing to manual ribbon preparation procedure, low cell viability at higher laser fluence because of focused laser beam, simultaneous deposition of multiple bioink materails is difficult, patterned constructs of low mechanical strength

LIFT	BioLP	100 μm (Barron et al., 2005a,b)	25–400 mJ/cm^2 of laser fluence (2.5 ns, $f = 0.1$ –100 Hz, $\lambda = 248$ nm) (Barron et al., 2004, 2005a,b)	25 μm diameter droplets (Barron et al., 2005a,b)	95–100% (Barron et al., 2005a,b, 2004)	1–20 × 10^7 cells/mL in cell culture media (Barron et al., 2005a,b, 2004)	Minimum-side effects of the laser exposure due to the intermediate energy absorbing layer, viscous bioink materials of various material types, diverse cell types and biologics, intermediate resolution, nozzle-free transfer of cells	Longer fabrication times owing to manual ribbon preparation procedure, low cell viability at higher laser fluence because of focused laser beam, simultaneous deposition of multiple bioink materials is difficult, patterned constructs of low mechanical strength
	LaBP	40–45 μm (Gruene et al., 2011a,b; Koch et al., 2012)	1000–4000 mJ/cm^2 of laser fluence (8 –10 ns, $f = 20$ Hz, $\lambda = 1064$ nm) (Gruene et al., 2011a,b; Koch et al., 2012)	N/A	~100% (Gruene et al., 2011a,b)	1.33% (w/v) hyaluronic acid-fibrinogen (viscosity 120 mPa s) comprising adipose-derived stem cells of concentration 2 × 10^6 cells/mL (Gruene et al., 2011a,b), 4% w/v alginate comprising keratinocytes of concentration 1.5 × 10^6 cells/mL (Koch et al., 2012), 3% (w/v) collagen type I comprising NIH 3T3 fibroblasts of concentration 1.5 × 10^6 cells/mL (Koch et al., 2012)		
	AFA	300 μm (Hopp et al., 2005)	360 mJ/cm^2 of laser fluence (30 ns, $\lambda = 248$ nm) which ejected droplets at an acceleration reaching 10^7 × g (Hopp et al., 2005)	N/A	80–85% (Hopp et al., 2005)	2–6 × 10^6 cells/mL in cell culture media (Hopp et al., 2005)		

λ, wavelength; *AFA-LIFT*, absorbing film assisted LIFT; *BioLP*, biological laser printing; *f*, frequency; *LaBP*, laser-assisted bioprinting; *LGDW*, laser-guided direct writing; *LIFT*, laser-induced forward transfer; *MAPLE-DW*, matrix-assisted pulsed-laser evaporation direct-write; *N/A*, information is not available; *UV*, ultraviolet.

(Arcaute et al., 2010). In their study, a minivat setup was developed that allowed removal and rinsing of the printed scaffolds, and loading and unloading of a new photocurable material. Similar attempts have also been made in mask-image-projection-based SLA, where a prototype setup was developed with a rotational system consisting of two materials, two brushes, a cleaner, and a dryer (Zhou et al., 2013); however, transition of such a technology into biomedical applications has yet to be investigated.

For the LIFT technology, Guillemot et al. (2010) proposed a high-resolution positioning system, which could be placed below a carousel holder with a loading capacity of five different ribbons. During the process, ribbons can rotate on a carousel holder using a motorized system providing additional freedom of motion. This way, different ribbons with different bioink materials can be switched through the process on demand to generate heterocellular tissue constructs. Although the authors envisioned a practical approach, the proposed automated idea has yet to be implemented.

6.4 Comparison of Laser-Based Bioprinting With Other Bioprinting Modalities

LBB is a nozzle-free approach, which circumvents a number of limitations with other bioprinting modalities, which utilize nozzle-based systems such as EBB (Ozbolat and Hospodiuk, 2016) and most of the DBB techniques except acoustic-based bioprinting (Gudapati et al., 2016). First of all, this feature eliminates the issue of shear stress–induced cell injury and death. This is particularly important in DBB and EBB when the nozzle diameter is very small or the bioink is highly viscous. High viscosity is a major problem in DBB as the majority of existing bioink materials used in EBB cannot be used for DBB but can be used in LBB. In general, the bioink material in DBB can easily clog the nozzle or the line from reservoir to the nozzle in the tubing system. This necessitates cleaning of the nozzle tip, reloading of the bioink, and calibration of the bioprinting setup, which is a time-consuming endeavor and sometimes results in permanent failure of expensive nozzles or the cartridge head. Due to high shear stress and the mechanism of droplet formation, a very limited number of cells can be encapsulated in each droplet. LBB, on the other hand, allows for bioprinting of cells in higher numbers, as it does not suffer from the above limitations. This is particularly valuable in generating higher resolution patterns with high cell density, which cannot be achieved using EBB.

The other major advantage of LBB is its high resolution, which is higher than that of DBB and substantially greater than that of EBB (Ozbolat and Yu, 2013). The resolution of DBB depends on the droplet size, which is around 50 μm encapsulating one or two cells; however, with the LBB, one can go down to 10 μm in resolution with this nozzle-free approach. Even with the use of a 20 μm nozzle tip to bioprint living cells, DBB cannot control the precise positioning of cells due to the large nozzle outlet diameter, which dramatically limits control over the distance between deposited cells. Moreover, in DBB, the number of cells encapsulated in each droplet cannot be controlled, where in general one, zero to two cells are encapsulated based on a statistical probability and cannot be repeated a priori (Dababneh and Ozbolat, 2014). These small resolution ranges cannot even be achieved using EBB. The high resolution advantage of LBB enables better control on cell–cell interactions and high-definition patterning of cells.

The other major advantage of LBB, particularly LIFT and MAPLE-DW, is its noncontact nature similar to DBB. This brings great potential for clinical applications of in situ bioprinting of tissues in surgery rooms (i.e., skin reconstruction or cranio- or maxillofacial surgeries). Injuries or defects can be easily filled layer by layer simultaneously patterning cells within the defect without physical contact. This feature has been used by Guillemot and his coworkers (Keriquel et al., 2010) in bioprinting of nano-hydroxyapatite (HA) particles into calvarial defects in mouse models. The noncontact nature of LBB processes alleviates other major issues observed in EBB such as collision between the printhead and the bioprinted constructs, or unexpected increase in clearance between the orifice and the receiving substrate.

In addition to these advantages, some modalities of LBB, such as LIFT and MAPLE-DW, can be also performed horizontally as opposed to DBB and EBB, which are performed vertically. For example, in a few studies, LIFT has been studied with donor substrate oriented vertically and the jet produced horizontally (Barron et al., 2005a,b). This allowed for more convenient imaging with the integration of stroboscopic system for side imaging capabilities and enabled practical analysis of jet formation and the underlying physics. A different orientation has been achieved with direct light processing (DLP)–based bioprinting, which performs bioprinting in a top-down approach. Although the top-down approach is more precise, eliminating shaking of the top surface of the photocurable material, no clear advantage of using top-down approach in DBB or EBB has been identified yet. Perhaps, it may enable fabrication of more intricate geometries which normally needs support material due to gravity but does not need it when bioprinted top-down.

6.5 Recent Achievements in Laser-Based Bioprinting

Although LBB has been around more than a decade, very limited work has been done compared to that of other bioprinting modalities including EBB and DBB. A few seminal works in the domain of LBB have emerged in recent years.

Catros et al. (2011) demonstrated layer-by-layer fabrication of electrospun polycaprolactone along with LIFT-based bioprinting of MG-63 osteosarcoma cells. In their procedure, MG-63 cells were deposited onto electrospun layer (100 μm in thickness) in sodium alginate; the process was repeated three times to get approximately 300-μm-thick tissue constructs implanted into calvarial defects. The cells were proliferated significantly within the bioprinted tissue constructs. Although, the implanted tissue constructs generated fibrous tissue with limited bone regeneration, the work represented the scale-up fabrication of laser-inkjet bioprinted constructs, overcoming one of the most important roadblocks in LIFT.

Gaebel et al. (2011) utilized the LIFT technique to pattern HUVECs and human mesenchymal stem cells in a geometrically defined pattern on polyester urethane urea (PEUU); the fabricated samples were transplanted to the infarcted zone of rat hearts after LAD ligation. Eight weeks posttransplantation, samples with LIFT-derived patterns showed increased vessel formation compared to randomly bioprinted cells and the resulted myocardium patch provided significant functional improvement. Beside primary cells, human cardiac–derived cardiomyocyte progenitor cells (hCMPCs) were also bioprinted in mesh pattern (Gaetani et al., 2012). Bioprinted hCMPCs demonstrated phenotypic properties of cardiac lineage with enhanced expression of early cardiac transcription factors Nkx2.5, Gata-4, and Mef-2c.

A recent work by Phamduy et al. (2015) demonstrated bioprinting of cancer cells, including metastatic breast cancer cells (MDA-MB-231) and nonmetastatic MCF-7 cells, onto ex vivo rat mesenteric tissues. The ex vivo tissue was rich in vascular networks as well as lymphatic vessels. In addition to cancer cells, fibroblasts were also printed as fibroblasts support the metastasis of cancer cells. In their study, it was shown that cancers cells were transferred onto ex vivo tissues successfully in viable form and the metastatic MDA-MB-231 cells proliferated significantly (Burks et al., 2016). Interestingly, bioprinted cancer cells promoted angiogenic sprouting of the vascular network as new capillaries formed compared to unprinted control tissue. The abovementioned work demonstrated bioprinting of cells onto ex vivo tissues, which has great potential for revealing the mechanisms of cancer progression and metastasis; however, it is difficult to bioprint on ex vivo tissues in 3D; very few cells types, such as cancer cells, have the ability to penetrate though the stromal tissue as well as invade into the circulation system. In situ bioprinting, on the other hand, can enhance rebuilding of damaged tissue by bioprinting of cells directly into the defect site. In this regard, Guillemot's group demonstrated a framework study (Keriquel et al., 2010), where nano-HA particles were bioprinted into critical size defects in mouse skulls. Although limited bone regeneration was achieved, this study demonstrated bioprinting using LBB on live animal models for the first time.

6.6 Limitations

LBB systems have high resolution and enable precise patterning of living cells, where cells can maintain registry within $5.6 \pm 2.5\,\mu m$ to the initial pattern in LIFT process (Schiele et al., 2010). This resolution, certainly, cannot be achieved by other bioprinting modalities making LIFT the technology of choice for bioprinting of microcellular features in organs and tissues, i.e., microvasculature. Despite the high resolution, LBB has a number of limitations. Processes involving photopolymerization suffer from prolonged fabrication times, interactions of cell components with laser light, costly setup, and the need for photo-crosslinkable bioink materials. Processes based on cell transfer face with several weaknesses such as laser shock-related thermal- and mechanical-induced cell deformation, gravitational and random settling of cells in the precursor solution, costly laser setup, and limitations in bioprinting in 3D.

SLA has a limitation with the density and uniformity of loaded cells. Due to limited hydrogels used and the cytotoxic nature of photoinitiators, in general, structurally simple and weak constructs (except PEGDA, which can yield rigid constructs) can be built. The elastic modulus of such constructs is typically lower than 1 kPa (Narayan, 2014), which is only applicable to soft tissue engineering. As it takes longer time to build scale-up constructs, which can harm the cells over long print times, the studies are limited to generation of simple geometries. Another limitation with SLA is the nonuniformity of cell distribution as cells are prone to settling within the vat solution due to the gravity. This results in accumulation of large cell numbers at the bottom of the vat and a low cell concentration at the top of the vat. This is particularly problematic when using low concentration hydrogels are necessary to sustain cell viability. In addition, SLA has other limitations; the minimum feature size that can be attained is limited to the laser beam width, which is about 250 μm (Bajaj et al., 2014). As discussed previously, the resolution of SLA depends on the size of the focal spot and the diffraction, and the minimum size cannot be smaller than the half of the laser wavelength. Although these parameters determine the feature size, the resolution also varies among various photocurable polymers as well. Due to the limitations inherent to this technology, the highest resolution that can be attained is on the order of a few micrometers. The resolution in z-axis is even more limited, a problem that has been alleviated by the use of 2PP technique; however, this technique has limited use in bioprinting as only demonstrated in a recent work (Ovsianikov et al., 2014). In this regard, Chichkov's group combined 2PP with LIFT process, where PEGDA was used to 3D print high-definition porous scaffolds made of overlapping rings. Upon fabrication of the scaffold, vascular smooth muscle-like cells (vSMCs) and ovine ECs were bioprinted by changing the donor slide during the process, where vSMCs and ECs were seeded inside and outside the hexagonal borderline in Fig. 6.10, respectively.

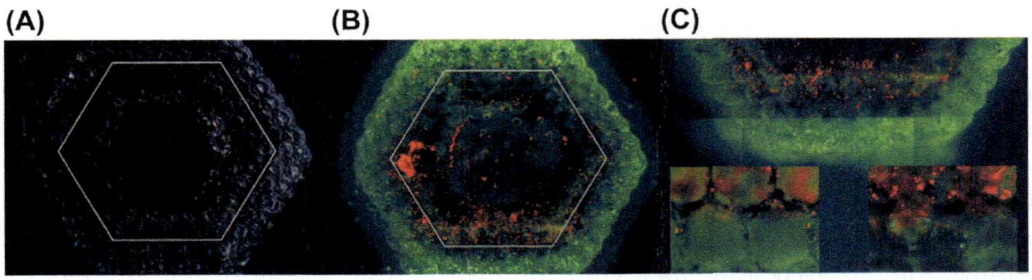

FIGURE 6.10 Scaffolds fabricated via two-photon polymerization were then seeded with vascular smooth muscle-like cells (vSMCs) and endothelial cells (ECs) using laser-induced forward transfer, (A) where vSMC and ECs were deposited inside and outside the hexagonal borderline within scaffolds. (B) A fluorescence image demonstrating the localization of two different cell types with (C) detailed high-resolution images around the borderline.

The effect of UV exposure to cells and photosensitive materials as well as toxic photoinitiators used in the bioink solutions are some of the other major limitations in processes involving photopolymerization. The free radicals generated by the photoinitiators can adversely react with the cell membrane, proteins, and DNA, curtailing use in abovementioned processes. For example, Bryant et al. (2000) investigated the in vitro toxicity of various photoinitiators on dermal fibroblasts and reported that Irgacure 2959 was the least toxic UV-sensitive photoinitiator and triethanolamine was the least toxic visible light-sensitive photoinitiator. A similar work later demonstrated the minimal effect of Irgacure 2959 photoinitiator over a broad range of mammalian cell types and species (Williams et al., 2005). In their work, the authors also reported that different cell types had different responses to the same concentration of the same photoinitiators and the cell lines with shorter cell cycle were prone to photoinitiator-induced cell death.

One of the major limitations of LIFT and MAPLE-DW in bioprinting of tissues is the need for a highly sophisticated setup as well as the obstacles associated with the bioprinting in the third dimension. The majority of LIFT and MAPLE-DW approaches performed in such a way that only 2D patterns have been created. There are only a limited number of studies showing scalable fabrication of tissue constructs using these techniques. For example, Huang and his coworkers developed a vat system within calcium chloride ($CaCl_2$) pool (Xiong et al., 2015b), where deposited alginate droplets were immediately crosslinked upon contact with the pool followed by lowering the table with a distance equal to the layer thickness. Using this approach, vascular constructs were fabricated; however, such capability primarily depends on the crosslinking speed of hydrogels as alginate quickly gels to fabricate such constructs. Other major challenges are the limited speed of printing, reproducibility of similar droplet formation, scaling up from small droplets to a larger tissue construct. In addition, the crosslinking mechanism needs to be integrated within the bioprinting process efficiently. Without successful crosslinking of the ejected droplets, droplets spread easily resulting in insufficient structural integrity necessary for the formation of scale-up tissue constructs.

One of the major limitations of LBB is the incorporation of multiple materials into the bioprinted construct (Choi et al., 2011). The existing technologies both in processes involving photopolymerization and processes based on cell transfer (MAPLE-DW, LIFT-DW, and LGDW) are not amenable to the incorporation of multimaterial bioprinting capabilities. The proposed carousel system by Wicker's group enables rotation of vats of different bioink solutions for the fabrication of multimaterial objects (Choi et al., 2011); however, switching from one material to another is time-consuming and brings about other issues during the fabrication process such as lower resolution of the system. It is highly challenging to remove the scaffold from the built vat and completely replace the photocurable material in it. During the switch from one material to another, it is critical to remove the bioink residue as it contributes to errors in built resolution. Particularly, material contamination needs to be minimized when switching to a different vat as the material accumulating on the bottom and side of the scaffold needs to be removed before building a new layer. The two-step approach proposed by Zhou et al. (2013), where rough cleaning followed by final cleaning slows down the fabrication process. The carousel system in LIFT, on the other hand, does not require any clean-up process as the scaffold is not built within the original bioink solution.

The last, but most important, LBB lacks a wide range of compatible bioink materials. LIFT and MAPLE-DW approaches are limited to a few hydrogels only, and processes involving photopolymerization have a limited choice of compatible bioink materials that are photocurable. Hence, no study so far has demonstrated compatibility of bioink materials other than hydrogels. Particularly, cell aggregate–based bioink materials have not been validated using LBB technologies. This is due to the relatively large size of spheroids and their immobility within hydrogels compared to single cells, which are easily encapsulated during bioprinting.

6.7 Future Directions

For future directions, several advancements should be made to make LBB modalities robust and effective in achieving the ultimate goal of bioprinting functional tissue and organ constructs. In this regard, adaption of DLP into the bioprinting domain will be highly beneficial as it will enable bioprinting of scale-up tissue constructs in a short period of time; use of a single UV light beam that traces the entire region of interest for solidification for each layer is time-consuming. This is, in particular, detrimental to cell viability as cells are encapsulated in monomer solution for an extended period of time without exposure to oxygen. In addition, the use of photoinitiators can also contribute to low cell viability during prolonged fabrication times. Thus, shorter fabrication times (in the order of minutes) will be very beneficial to the bioprinting and tissue engineering process. As photo-crosslinking of each layer takes the same time due to rapid exposure of a thousand of micromirrors, the number of layers required can contribute to extended build time. The number of layers can be easily minimized when the right orientation direction is determined (Ahsan et al., 2015). This, however, may affect the other properties such as surface quality and mechanical properties.

Most of the laser-assisted bioprinting modalities such as MAPLE-DW and LIFT have been used in patterning of living cells in 2D with limited fabrication of 3D constructs. This is highly dependent upon the crosslinking and solidification properties of the bioink materials used in the process. Up to now, a very few bioink types have been used in these processes (Riggs et al., 2011). These hydrogels are mainly thermally crosslinking hydrogels, such as gelatin and Matrigel™, and ionically crosslinking hydrogels such as alginate. In particular, constructs are limited to extremely thin structures when thermally crosslinking hydrogels are used as it is difficult to control the thermal environment confining the scaffold built volume. When thermally controlled substrates are used, the first few layers are easily crosslinked; however, control of the temperature around upper layers is difficult to maintain. Therefore, further advances should be made to assure efficient solidification in 3D.

Since larger-scale tissue construct necessitates the incorporation of macroporosity to support nutrient and oxygen transport, LBB modalities, except processes involving photopolymerization, become a less favorable option as these modalities do not support the generation of porous architecture. In this regard, fugitive or temporary hydrogels can be incorporated into the bioprinting process. For example, when thermally crosslinkable hydrogels are printed, sodium alginate can be printed using a secondary ribbon as previously discussed before. The crosslinker of sodium alginate can be printed within the thermally crosslinkable hydrogel and can crosslink alginate when they contact. Then, a "decrosslinker" of alginate can be used to remove the temporarily printed alginate creating porosity within the 3D construct. Similar architecture can also be constructed using thermally crosslinking hydrogel as a sacrificial support material in a similar manner. For building in z-direction, a movable stage with linear motor can be utilized to control the position of the substrate. As jet and droplet formation dynamics change when the distance between the substrate and ribbon changes, the bioprinting space should be maintained throughout the process.

One of the major advancements needed in LBB is the expansion of the library of photocurable bioink materials as well as the currently available bioink materials used in LIFT. As it is clear that LGDW and MAPLE-DW processes are not currently used in bioprinting field as they were superseded by the LIFT technique, novel materials need to be designed that can achieve uniform spreading of the bioink solution on the ribbon surface and uniform distribution of cells within the bioink coating, possess high viscoelasticity that will prevent bouncing and splashing of the formed droplet and secondary droplet formation, exhibit rapid gelation capabilities enabling bioprinting of thick tissue constructs in the third dimension, and exhibit a high level of biocompatibility that will enable cells to grow and proliferate rapidly without inducing an immunogenic response.

Integrating multiple bioink printing capabilities will be highly beneficial in fabrication of high-definition tissue constructs with multiple cells patterned into a tissuelike unique anatomy. Although some efforts have been made in advancing multimaterial printing capabilities in photopolymerization processes, there is currently no work demonstrating the alternative bioprinting of multiple cell types using cell transfer technologies such as MAPLE-DW or LIFT. The proposed carousal system in LIFT (Guillemot et al., 2010) has not been implemented as manipulations in the position of ribbons during switching influences the bioprinting dynamics of the jet significantly and generates significant variations during the bioprinting process. Therefore, instead of changing the position of the ribbon in the carousal system, multiple ribbons supported by multiple mirror systems that break the main laser beam into a few beams in series will enable bioprinting of the multiple bioink materials in tandem. As this configuration will enable bioprinting of multiple bioink materials, a translational stage is needed to switch the position of the substrate in the lateral plane back and forth. Using this approach, multiple bioink materials can be incorporated into a single platform.

6.8 Summary

LBB has been a powerful method in patterning living cells due to its great resolution and precision, as well as accommodating high cellular density, none of which are possible using low-resolution EBB or DBB with lower cellular density per the deposited droplet size. In addition to LGDW-, LIFT-, and MAPLE-DW-based approaches, processes involving photopolymerization have been of interest to the bioprinting community due to the commercial availability and easy of modification of SLA-based 3D printers. Despite these advantages, LBB has been challenged with its highly complex and costly setup, operational impracticability, low speed, and limited ability in fabrication of scalable heterogeneous tissue constructs; however, with the recent advances and progress in the field, the technology will be more practical for fabrication of 3D tissue constructs for tissue engineering and regenerative medicine practices in the near future.

References

Ahsan, A.N., Habib, M.A., Khoda, B., 2015. Resource based process planning for additive manufacturing. Computer-Aided Design 69, 112–125.

Arcaute, K., Mann, B., Wicker, R., 2010. Stereolithography of spatially controlled multi-material bioactive poly (ethylene glycol) scaffolds. Acta Biomaterialia 6 (3), 1047–1054.

Arcaute, K., Mann, B.K., Wicker, R.B., 2006. Stereolithography of three-dimensional bioactive poly (ethylene glycol) constructs with encapsulated cells. Annals of Biomedical Engineering 34 (9), 1429–1441.

Ashkin, A., Dziedzic, J.M., 1987. Optical trapping and manipulation of viruses and bacteria. Science 235 (4795), 1517–1520.

Bajaj, P., Schweller, R.M., Khademhosseini, A., West, J.L., Bashir, R., 2014. 3D biofabrication strategies for tissue engineering and regenerative medicine. Annual Review of Biomedical Engineering 16, 247–276.

Barron, J.A., Young, H.D., Dlott, D.D., Darfler, M.M., Krizman, D.B., Ringeisen, B.R., 2005a. Printing of protein microarrays via a capillary-free fluid jetting mechanism. Proteomics 5 (16), 4138–4144.

Barron, J.A., Krizman, D.B., Ringeisen, B.R., 2005b. Laser printing of single cells: statistical analysis, cell viability, and stress. Annals of Biomedical Engineering 33 (2), 121–130.

Barron, J.A., Spargo, B.J., Ringeisen, B.R., 2004. Biological laser printing of three dimensional cellular structures. Applied Physics A 79 (4–6), 1027–1030.

Bergeron, V., Bonn, D., Martin, J.Y., Vovelle, L., 2000. Controlling droplet deposition with polymer additives. Nature 405 (6788), 772–775.

Bertsch, A., Bernhard, P., Vogt, C., Renaud, P., 2000. Rapid prototyping of small size objects. Rapid Prototyping Journal 6 (4), 259–266.

Billiet, T., Vandenhaute, M., Schelfhout, J., Van Vlierberghe, S., Dubruel, P., 2012. A review of trends and limitations in hydrogel-rapid prototyping for tissue engineering. Biomaterials 33 (26), 6020–6041.

Bryant, S.J., Nuttelman, C.R., Anseth, K.S., 2000. Cytocompatibility of UV and visible light photoinitiating systems on cultured NIH/3T3 fibroblasts in vitro. Journal of Biomaterials Science, Polymer Edition 11 (5), 439–457.

Burks, H.E., Phamduy, T.B., Azimi, M.S., Saksena, J., Burow, M.E., Collins-Burow, B.M., Chrisey, D.B., Murfee, W.L., 2016. Laser direct-write onto live tissues: a novel model for studying cancer cell migration. Journal of Cellular Physiology 231 (11), 2333–2338.

Catros, S., Guillemot, F., Nandakumar, A., Ziane, S., Moroni, L., Habibovic, P., van Blitterswijk, C., Rousseau, B., Chassande, O., Amédée, J., Fricain, J.C., 2011. Layer-by-layer tissue microfabrication supports cell proliferation in vitro and in vivo. Tissue Engineering Part C: Methods 18 (1), 62–70.

Choi, J.W., Kim, H.C., Wicker, R., 2011. Multi-material stereolithography. Journal of Materials Processing Technology 211 (3), 318–328.

Chrisey, D.B., Pique, A., McGill, R.A., Horwitz, J.S., Ringeisen, B.R., Bubb, D.M., Wu, P.K., 2003. Laser deposition of polymer and biomaterial films. Chemical Reviews 103 (2), 553–576.

Cumpston, B.H., Ananthavel, S.P., Barlow, S., Dyer, D.L., Ehrlich, J.E., Erskine, L.L., Heikal, A.A., Kuebler, S.M., Lee, I.Y.S., McCord-Maughon, D., Qin, J., 1999. Two-photon polymerization initiators for three-dimensional optical data storage and microfabrication. Nature 398 (6722), 51–54.

Dababneh, A.B., Ozbolat, I.T., 2014. Bioprinting technology: a current state-of-the-Art review. Journal of Manufacturing Science and Engineering 136 (6), 061016.

Devillard, R., Correa, M.M., Kériquel, V., Rémy, M., Kalisky, J., Ali, M., Guillotin, B., Guillemot, F., 2013. Cell patterning by laser-assisted bioprinting. Methods in Cell Biology 119, 159–174.

Dhariwala, B., Hunt, E., Boland, T., 2004. Rapid prototyping of tissue-engineering constructs, using photopolymerizable hydrogels and stereolithography. Tissue Engineering 10 (9–10), 1316–1322.

Doraiswamy, A., Narayan, R.J., Lippert, T., Urech, L., Wokaun, A., Nagel, M., Hopp, B., Dinescu, M., Modi, R., Auyeung, R.C.Y., Chrisey, D.B., 2006. Excimer laser forward transfer of mammalian cells using a novel triazene absorbing layer. Applied Surface Science 252 (13), 4743–4747.

Doraiswamy, A., Narayan, R.J., Harris, M.L., Qadri, S.B., Modi, R., Chrisey, D.B., 2007. Laser microfabrication of hydroxyapatite-osteoblast-like cell composites. Journal of Biomedical Materials Research Part A 80 (3), 635–643.

Emons, M., et al., 2012. Two-photon polymerization technique with sub-50 nm resolution by sub-10 fs laser pulses. Optical Materials Express 2 (7), 942–947.

Fedorovich, N.E., Oudshoorn, M.H., van Geemen, D., Hennink, W.E., Alblas, J., Dhert, W.J., 2009. The effect of photopolymerization on stem cells embedded in hydrogels. Biomaterials 30 (3), 344–353.

Fitz-Gerald, J.M., Wu, H.D., Pique, A., Horwitz, J.S., Auyeung, R.C.Y., Chang, W., Kim, W.J., Chrisey, D.B., 2000. Maple direct write: a new approach to fabricate ferroelectric thin film devices in air at room temperature. Integrated Ferroelectrics 28 (1–4), 13–28.

Gaebel, R., Ma, N., Liu, J., Guan, J., Koch, L., Klopsch, C., Gruene, M., Toelk, A., Wang, W., Mark, P., Wang, F., 2011. Patterning human stem cells and endothelial cells with laser printing for cardiac regeneration. Biomaterials 32 (35), 9218–9230.

Gaetani, R., Doevendans, P.A., Metz, C.H., Alblas, J., Messina, E., Giacomello, A., Sluijter, J.P., 2012. Cardiac tissue engineering using tissue printing technology and human cardiac progenitor cells. Biomaterials 33 (6), 1782–1790.

Gauvin, R., Chen, Y.C., Lee, J.W., Soman, P., Zorlutuna, P., Nichol, J.W., Bae, H., Chen, S., Khademhosseini, A., 2012. Microfabrication of complex porous tissue engineering scaffolds using 3D projection stereolithography. Biomaterials 33 (15), 3824–3834.

Gittard, S.D., Narayan, R.J., 2010. Laser direct writing of micro- and nano-scale medical devices. Expert Review of Medical Devices 7 (3), 343–356.

Gruene, M., Pflaum, M., Deiwick, A., Koch, L., Schlie, S., Unger, C., Wilhelmi, M., Haverich, A., Chichkov, B.N., 2011a. Adipogenic differentiation of laser-printed 3D tissue grafts consisting of human adipose-derived stem cells. Biofabrication 3 (1), 015005.

Gruene, M., Pflaum, M., Hess, C., Diamantouros, S., Schlie, S., Deiwick, A., Koch, L., Wilhelmi, M., Jockenhoevel, S., Haverich, A., Chichkov, B., 2011b. Laser printing of three-dimensional multicellular arrays for studies of cell–cell and cell–environment interactions. Tissue Engineering Part C: Methods 17 (10), 973–982.

Gudapati, H., Yan, J., Huang, Y., Chrisey, D.B., 2014. Alginate gelation-induced cell death during laser-assisted cell printing. Biofabrication 6 (3), 035022.

Gudapati, H., Dey, M., Ozbolat, I., 2016. A comprehensive review on droplet-based bioprinting: past, present and future. Biomaterials 102, 20–42.

Guillemot, F., Souquet, A., Catros, S., Guillotin, B., Lopez, J., Faucon, M., Pippenger, B., Bareille, R., Rémy, M., Bellance, S., Chabassier, P., 2010. High-throughput laser printing of cells and biomaterials for tissue engineering. Acta Biomaterialia 6 (7), 2494–2500.

Hadjizadeh, A., Doillon, C.J., 2010. Directional migration of endothelial cells towards angiogenesis using polymer fibres in a 3D co-culture system. Journal of Tissue Engineering and Regenerative Medicine 4 (7), 524–531.

Hahn, M.S., Miller, J.S., West, J.L., 2006. Three-dimensional biochemical and biomechanical patterning of hydrogels for guiding cell behavior. Advanced Materials 18 (20), 2679–2684.

Hopp, B., Smausz, T., Kresz, N., Barna, N., Bor, Z., Kolozsvári, L., Chrisey, D.B., Szabó, A., Nógrádi, A., 2005. Survival and proliferative ability of various living cell types after laser-induced forward transfer. Tissue Engineering 11 (11–12), 1817–1823.

Hribar, K.C., Soman, P., Warner, J., Chung, P., Chen, S., 2014. Light-assisted direct-write of 3D functional biomaterials. Lab on a Chip 14 (2), 268–275.

Huang, T.Q., Qu, X., Liu, J., Chen, S., 2014. 3D printing of biomimetic microstructures for cancer cell migration. Biomedical Microdevices 16 (1), 127–132.

Itoga, K., Yamato, M., Kobayashi, J., Kikuchi, A., Okano, T., 2004. Cell micropatterning using photo-polymerization with a liquid crystal device commercial projector. Biomaterials 25 (11), 2047–2053.

Keriquel, V., Guillemot, F., Arnault, I., Guillotin, B., Miraux, S., Amédée, J., Fricain, J.C., Catros, S., 2010. In vivo bioprinting for computer-and robotic-assisted medical intervention: preliminary study in mice. Biofabrication 2 (1), 014101.

Klein, F., Richter, B., Striebel, T., Franz, C.M., Freymann, G.V., Wegener, M., Bastmeyer, M., 2011. Two-component polymer scaffolds for controlled three-dimensional cell culture. Advanced Materials 23 (11), 1341–1345.

Koch, L., Deiwick, A., Schlie, S., Michael, S., Gruene, M., Coger, V., Zychlinski, D., Schambach, A., Reimers, K., Vogt, P.M., Chichkov, B., 2012. Skin tissue generation by laser cell printing. Biotechnology and Bioengineering 109 (7), 1855–1863.

Lin, Y., Huang, G., Huang, Y., Jeremy Tzeng, T.R., Chrisey, D., 2010. Effect of laser fluence in laser-assisted direct writing of human colon cancer cell. Rapid Prototyping Journal 16 (3), 202–208.

Lin, Y., Huang, Y., Wang, G., Tzeng, T.R.J., Chrisey, D.B., 2009a. Effect of laser fluence on yeast cell viability in laser-assisted cell transfer. Journal of Applied Physics 106 (4), 043106.

Lin, Y., Huang, Y., Chrisey, D.B., 2009b. Droplet formation in matrix-assisted pulsed-laser evaporation direct writing of glycerol-water solution. Journal of Applied Physics 105 (9), 093111.

Lu, Y., Chen, S., 2012. Projection printing of 3-dimensional tissue scaffolds. In: Liebschner, A.K.M. (Ed.), Computer-Aided Tissue Engineering. Humana Press, New York, NY, pp. 289–302.

Ma, X., Qu, X., Zhu, W., Li, Y.S., Yuan, S., Zhang, H., Liu, J., Wang, P., Lai, C.S.E., Zanella, F., Feng, G.S., 2016. Deterministically patterned biomimetic human iPSC-derived hepatic model via rapid 3D bioprinting. Proceedings of the National Academy of Sciences of the United States of America 113 (8), 2206–2211.

Melchels, F.P., Feijen, J., Grijpma, D.W., 2010. A review on stereolithography and its applications in biomedical engineering. Biomaterials 31 (24), 6121–6130.

Nahmias, Y., Schwartz, R.E., Verfaillie, C.M., Odde, D.J., 2005. Laser-guided direct writing for three-dimensional tissue engineering. Biotechnology and Bioengineering 92 (2), 129–136.

Narayan, R. (Ed.), 2014. Rapid Prototyping of Biomaterials: Principles and Applications. Woodhead Publishing.

Odde, D.J., Renn, M.J., 1999. Laser-guided direct writing for applications in biotechnology. Trends in Biotechnology 17 (10), 385–389.

Odde, D.J., Renn, M.J., 2000. Laser-guided direct writing of living cells. Biotechnology and Bioengineering 67 (3), 312–318.

Ovsianikov, A., Chichkov, B., Mente, P., Monteiro-Riviere, N.A., Doraiswamy, A., Narayan, R.J., 2007a. Two photon polymerization of polymer–ceramic hybrid materials for transdermal drug delivery. International Journal of Applied Ceramic Technology 4 (1), 22–29.

Ovsianikov, A., Schlie, S., Ngezahayo, A., Haverich, A., Chichkov, B.N., 2007b. Two-photon polymerization technique for microfabrication of CAD-designed 3D scaffolds from commercially available photosensitive materials. Journal of Tissue Engineering and Regenerative Medicine 1 (6), 443–449.

Ovsianikov, A., Chichkov, B.N., 2012. Three-dimensional microfabrication by two-photon polymerization technique. In: Liebschner, A.K.M. (Ed.), Computer-Aided Tissue Engineering. Humana Press, New York, NY, pp. 311–325.

Ovsianikov, A., et al., 2014. Laser photofabrication of cell-containing hydrogel constructs. Langmuir 30 (13), 3787–3794.

Ozbolat, I.T., 2015. Bioprinting scale-up tissue and organ constructs for transplantation. Trends in Biotechnology 33 (7), 395–400.

Ozbolat, I.T., Hospodiuk, M., 2016. Current advances and future perspectives in extrusion-based bioprinting. Biomaterials 76, 321–343.

Ozbolat, I.T., Yu, Y., 2013. Bioprinting toward organ fabrication: challenges and future trends. IEEE Transactions on Bio-Medical Engineering 60 (3), 691–699.

Patz, T.M., Doraiswamy, A., Narayan, R.J., He, W., Zhong, Y., Bellamkonda, R., Modi, R., Chrisey, D.B., 2006. Three-dimensional direct writing of B35 neuronal cells. Journal of Biomedical Materials Research Part B: Applied Biomaterials 78 (1), 124–130.

Phamduy, T.B., Sweat, R.S., Azimi, M.S., Burow, M.E., Murfee, W.L., Chrisey, D.B., 2015. Printing cancer cells into intact microvascular networks: a model for investigating cancer cell dynamics during angiogenesis. Integrative Biology 7 (9), 1068–1078.

Piqué, A., 2011. The matrix-assisted pulsed laser evaporation (MAPLE) process: origins and future directions. Applied Physics A 105 (3), 517–528.

Renn, M.J., Pastel, R., Lewandowski, H.J., 1999. Laser guidance and trapping of mesoscale particles in hollow-core optical fibers. Physical Review Letters 82 (7), 1574–1577.

Riggs, B.C., Dias, A.D., Schiele, N.R., Cristescu, R., Huang, Y., Corr, D.T., Chrisey, D.B., 2011. Matrix-assisted pulsed laser methods for biofabrication. MRS Bulletin 36 (12), 1043–1050.

Ringeisen, B.R., Kim, H., Barron, J.A., Krizman, D.B., Chrisey, D.B., Jackman, S., Auyeung, R.Y.C., Spargo, B.J., 2004. Laser printing of pluripotent embryonal carcinoma cells. Tissue Engineering 10 (3–4), 483–491.

Ringeisen, B.R., Wu, P.K., Kim, H., Pique, A., Auyeung, R.Y.C., Young, H.D., Chrisey, D.B., Krizman, D.B., 2002. Picoliter-scale protein microarrays by laser direct write. Biotechnology Progress 18 (5), 1126–1129.

Roisman, I.V., Rioboo, R., Tropea, C., 2002. Normal impact of a liquid drop on a dry surface: model for spreading and receding. Proceedings of the Royal Society of London A: Mathematical, Physical and Engineering Sciences 458 (2022), 1411–1430.

Roots Analysis Private Ltd, 2014. 3D Bioprinting Market 2014–2030.

Salonitis, K., 2014. 10.03 – stereolithography. In: Hashmi, S., et al. (Eds.), Comprehensive Materials Processing. Elsevier, Oxford, pp. 19–67.

Schiele, N.R., Koppes, R.A., Corr, D.T., Ellison, K.S., Thompson, D.M., Ligon, L.A., Lippert, T.K., Chrisey, D.B., 2009. Laser direct writing of combinatorial libraries of idealized cellular constructs: biomedical applications. Applied Surface Science 255 (10), 5444–5447.

Schiele, N.R., Chrisey, D.B., Corr, D.T., 2010. Gelatin-based laser direct-write technique for the precise spatial patterning of cells. Tissue Engineering Part C: Methods 17 (3), 289–298.

Sellinger, A.T., Martin, A.H., Fitz-Gerald, J.M., 2008. Effect of substrate temperature on poly (methyl methacrylate) nanocomposite thin films deposited by matrix assisted pulsed laser evaporation. Thin Solid Films 516 (18), 6033–6040.

Serbin, J., Ovsianikov, A., Chichkov, B., 2004. Fabrication of woodpile structures by two-photon polymerization and investigation of their optical properties. Optics Express 12 (21), 5221–5228.

Unger, C., Gruene, M., Koch, L., Koch, J., Chichkov, B.N., 2011. Time-resolved imaging of hydrogel printing via laser-induced forward transfer. Applied Physics A 103 (2), 271–277.

Williams, C.G., Malik, A.N., Kim, T.K., Manson, P.N., Elisseeff, J.H., 2005. Variable cytocompatibility of six cell lines with photoinitiators used for polymerizing hydrogels and cell encapsulation. Biomaterials 26 (11), 1211–1218.

Xiong, R., Zhang, Z., Chai, W., Huang, Y., Chrisey, D.B., 2015a. Freeform drop-on-demand laser printing of 3D alginate and cellular constructs. Biofabrication 7 (4), 045011.

Xiong, R., Zhang, Z., Huang, Y., 2015b. Identification of optimal printing conditions for laser printing of alginate tubular constructs. Journal of Manufacturing Processes 20, 450–455.

Xu, J., Grant, S.A., Pastel, R.L., 2003. Laser-guided direct writing: a novel method to deposit biomolecules for biosensors arrays. IEEE Transactions on Biomedical Engineering 50 (1), 126–128.

Zhang, Z., Xiong, R., Corr, D.T., Huang, Y., 2016. Study of impingement types and printing quality during laser printing of viscoelastic alginate solutions. Langmuir 32 (12), 3004–3014.

Zhang, Z., Xiong, R., Mei, R., Huang, Y., Chrisey, D.B., 2015. Time-resolved imaging study of jetting dynamics during laser printing of viscoelastic alginate solutions. Langmuir 31 (23), 6447–6456.

Zhou, C., Chen, Y., Yang, Z., Khoshnevis, B., 2013. Digital material fabrication using mask-image-projection-based stereolithography. Rapid Prototyping Journal 19 (3), 153–165.

Zipfel, W.R., Williams, R.M., Webb, W.W., 2003. Nonlinear magic: multiphoton microscopy in the biosciences. Nature Biotechnology 21 (11), 1369–1377.

7

Bioprinter Technologies*

CHAPTER OUTLINE

Logic will get you from A to B. Imagination will take you everywhere
Albert Einstein

*With contributions by Hemanth Gudupati and Kazim Moncal, The Pennsylvania State University.

7.1 Introduction

The first bioprinting technology was demonstrated by Klebe in the 1980s (Klebe, 1988), where a bioink solution, comprised of collagen and fibronectin, was bioprinted using a commercially available Hewlett–Packard (HP) thermal drop-on-demand (DoD) inkjet printer. In the late 1990s, Odde and Renn reported the first use of laser technology demonstrating the two-dimensional (2D) patterning of living cells (Odde and Renn, 1999). With this innovative approach, laser energy was used to excite living cells to pattern them for spatial control in their microenvironment, which provided the fundamentals of three-dimensional (3D) laser-based bioprinting (LBB) technology. Later in the early 2000s, Boland further advanced the DoD inkjet printing technology and the concept of inkjet bioprinting was introduced with the demonstration of bioprinting of living cells in viable form and started the development of droplet-based bioprinting (DBB) processes (Xu et al., 2005; Xu et al. 2006, 2009; Boland et al., 2007). In these early efforts, customized commercially available HP and Canon thermal DoD paper printers were utilized to bioprint various proteins and cell types; however, paper printers are not suitable for bioprinting applications due to their closed architecture. The printheads, for example, move along only one axis and are not capable of bioprinting in 2D or 3D. Hence, 2D and 3D construct fabrication requires the introduction of an additional substrate movement, which, at times, is difficult to integrate. As a result, Nakamura's group at University of Toyama built a home-made bioprinter using commercially available stepper motors and EPSON SEA-Jet™ printhead to overcome the limitations of the paper printers. The bioprinter was employed to fabricate hollow cylindrical tissue constructs with improved resolution (Nishiyama et al., 2008). Despite their great versatility and high-throughput ability, a limited number of droplet-based bioprinters are commercially available to the research community and pharmaceutical industry. Similarly, the transfer of LBB technology into the commercial arena has been limited due to the complex, costly, and labor-intensive nature of LBB processes.

In parallel with Boland's efforts, the first extrusion-based bioprinting (EBB) technology, 3D plotting of thermoreversible gels in a liquid medium, was reported by Muelhaupt's group at Freiburg Materials Research Center in the early 2000s (Landers et al., 2002). The technology, named "Bioplotter," was later commercialized by EnvisionTec as "3D-Bioplotter®," which is still commercially available with a number of upgrades and modifications of the bioprinter. The fledgling technology later received enormous attention and advanced rapidly, and several groups utilized the technology by encapsulating cells in hydrogel solutions, extruding filaments, and laying them down layer by layer (Ozbolat and Hospodiuk, 2016). As the field of bioprinting has evolved into its current state, a wide variety of extrusion-based bioprinters has been developed by a myriad of research groups around the globe in addition to the recent emergence of a number of commercial bioprinters (Root Analysis, 2014).

In this chapter, the author presents the bioprinter technologies including the major components of bioprinters and their mechanism classified by three major modalities, EBB, DBB, and LBB. Current bioprinter technologies are reviewed along with a detailed evaluation of commercially available bioprinters. Limitations of bioprinter technologies are discussed and future prospects are provided to the reader.

7.2 Bioprinters

Today, a bioprinter can be built for as low as $50 by modifying a used HP paper printer. Custom-built bioprinters designed to specifications based on ultimate use, may cost up to $1M. As the resolution, motion accuracy, and precision improve, the number of degree-of-freedom and the level of automation of a bioprinter improve, the cost of the bioprinter increases proportionally. According to a recent work (Dababneh and Ozbolat, 2014), the ideal bioprinter meets the following specific requirements:

- *High resolution and accuracy* that enables deposition of bioink solutions with sufficient fidelity to simulate cell placement in native tissues.
- *High degree-of-freedom in motion* that allows deposition of the bioink solution on nonplanar surfaces. This is crucial as bioprinters transition into clinical applications and are used to bioprint cells into a biological lesion site.
- *High speed motion* that enables rapid fabrication of human-scale tissue and organ constructs for clinical transplantation as well as high-throughput production of tissue models for pharmaceutics and cancer research.
- *The ability to dispense various bioink solutions simultaneously* to facilitate fabrication of heterocellular tissues closely mimicking native tissues.
- *Ease of use* that allows operators, with minimum skills and experience, to operate the bioprinter.
- *Compact size* that allows placement under a standard biosafety or a laminar flow hood for bioprinting in sterile conditions.
- *Ease of sterilization* that allows operators to readily sterilize and maintain aseptic conditions during a bioprinting process.
- *Full-automation capability* that facilitates bioprinting of tissue and organ constructs without user intervention.
- *Affordability* that allows researchers to acquire instrumentation and explore new investigative areas.
- *Versatility* that allows operators to modify and expand the instrumentation for multipurpose use.

Not all of the bioprinters possess the aforementioned characteristics; a majority of bioprinters are designed for basic research use only. In the next sections, existing commercial bioprinters are discussed and compared according to their capabilities and features.

7.2.1 Components of Bioprinters

For a typical bioprinting process, computer-aided design (CAD) software is required to generate a toolpath plan, which provides the necessary motion path for the bioprinter to deposit the bioink solutions at the proper time and location on each layer (Ozbolat and Khoda, 2014). The CAD model can be created through various means such as computed tomography or magnetic resonance imaging (as discussed in Chapter 2 in detail) or a freeform design per specifications. Fig. 7.1 illustrates a representative bioprinting system, the Multi-Arm BioPrinter (MABP) (Ozbolat et al., 2014), along with its components. The MABP has dual arms moving in tandem for hybrid tissue fabrication, based on a toolpath sequencing strategy to ensure that the spheroids are deposited between the filament structures in the appropriate timeframe to avoid collision between the two nozzles. As different bioprinters have different bioprinting mechanism, such as the unique simultaneous motion capability of multiple arms in the MABP, the toolpath plan thus varies from bioprinter to bioprinter and bioprinting modality to bioprinting modality. When the toolpath is generated, it is then translated into digital signals by the machine control software. The digital signals control the motion and the dispensing mechanisms, such as actuation of motors and air pressure, respectively.

A typical motion control system consists of a breakout board, power supply, and motor drivers. The breakout board provides access to the individual pins of the parallel port, which are used to connect motor drivers and limit switches. The motor drivers actuate the motors at the desired rotational acceleration, velocity, and distance based on the signal sent from the computer through the parallel port. The motion system provides the bioprinter with the ability to move in x-, y-, and z-axes. This range of motion varies from bioprinter to bioprinter depending on the number of degree-of-freedom of the bioprinter's motion mechanism. For a typical 3D bioprinter, the printhead possesses x-, y-, and z-axis motion freedom; however, this may differ in some cases where the table may assume z-axis motion freedom depending on the bioprinting process. Thus, the Cartesian frame is built according to the bioprinting mission and requirements as well as the mechanical load exerted on the frame. In general, a T-slotted framing system is preferred in bioprinter constructions due to easy of construction and flexibility for reconfigurations (Ozbolat et al., 2014). Each axis has a motor and a linear actuator, where the linear actuator translates the rotational motion of the motor into a linear motion.

The dispensing system controls the deposition of the bioink solution through the printhead in a sufficient accuracy and resolution. The system is triggered by the dispenser control system, which actuates the dispensers using commands contained in the toolpath plan. The dispenser can be pneumatic or mechanical (piston- or screw-driven) or solenoid-based system. In addition to the motion and dispensing systems, vision-based process monitoring technologies can be integrated for calibration, full-automation, and quality inspection of the process. The system presented in Fig. 7.1 is

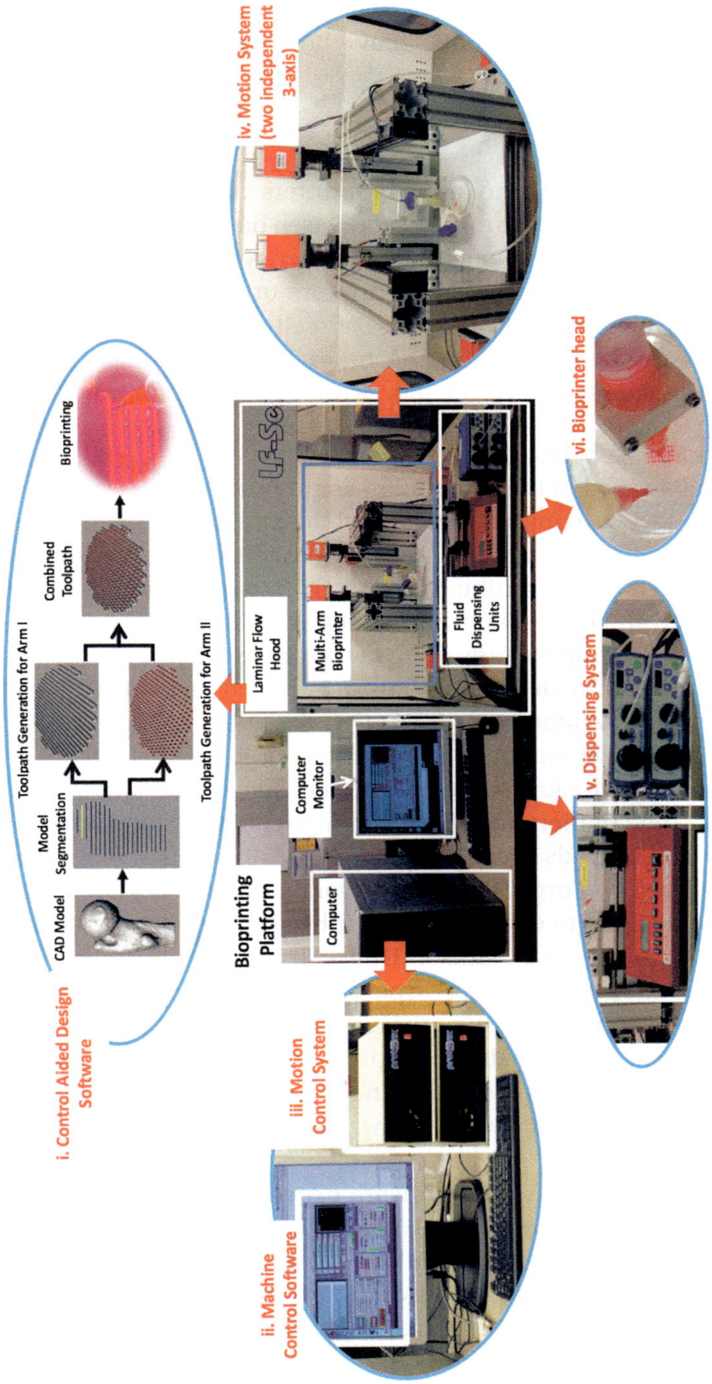

FIGURE 7.1 Components of a bioprinting system.

an EBB system, which is the most common bioprinting modality. Other bioprinting modalities, such as DBB and LBB, may, however, exhibit different motion and dispensing system configurations.

7.2.2 Bioprinter Types

According to their bioprinting modality, bioprinters can be classified under three main groups including extrusion-, droplet-, and laser-based bioprinters. Extrusion-based bioprinters use mechanical- or pneumatic-driven system to deposit cells in the form of a filament, whereas droplet-based bioprinters utilize thermal-, piezo-, or acoustic-driven mechanisms to deposit droplets of cell suspension in a high-throughput manner. Laser-based bioprinters on the other hand utilizes laser energy to deposit cells from a donor slide to a receiver slide without in need for a nozzle.

7.2.2.1 Extrusion-Based Bioprinters

EBB has been widely used in the bioprinting community (Ozbolat and Hospodiuk, 2016). The EBB technique is a combination of a fluid-dispensing system (pneumatic-, mechanical- (piston or screw-driven), or solenoid-based system) and an automated robotic system for extrusion and bioprinting, respectively (Dababneh and Ozbolat, 2014; Ozbolat and Hospodiuk, 2016). During bioprinting, bioink is dispensed by a deposition system, under the control of a computer, resulting in the precise deposition of cells encapsulated in cylindrical filaments of desired 3D custom-shaped structures (Khoda et al., 2011; Ozbolat and Koc, 2011; Zhang et al., 2015; Ozbolat et al., 2014; Ozbolat and Koc, 2010).

Since the first time demonstration of EBB technology by Muelhaupt (Landers et al., 2002), a number of extrusion-based bioprinters have been demonstrated by several research groups; some of them have been commercialized. Some notable ones include a 3D printer with three heads enabling bioprinting of blood vessels and cardiac tissue constructs, developed by Forgacs and his coworkers (Coatnye et al., 2013); the Palmetto printer with the capability to dispense tissue spheroids, developed by Medical University of South Carolina (MUSC) and Clemson University (Jia et al., 2014); a multihead tissue/organ building system possessing six dispensing heads to fabricate heterocellular tissue constructs (i.e., osteochondral tissue), developed by Jin et al. (Shim et al., 2012), and an MABP (Ozbolat et al., 2014) enabling bioprinting of hybrid constructs (scaffold-based and scaffold-free bioink materials) using independent robot arms in tandem. A partial list of noncommercial bioprinters used in academic and research institutions is presented in Table 7.1.

Until 2005, 3D printers, in general, were expensive, proprietary, and in industrial scale, and their high cost and closed nature limited the accessibility of the technology to researchers. With the invention of the Fab@Home printer (Malone and Lipson, 2007), the first open-source low-cost printer was available to the public with versatile and multimaterial printing capabilities that accelerated technology innovation and its migration into the bioprinting space. The emergence of

Table 7.1 Noncommercial Extrusion-Based Bioprinters

	Bioprinter Name	Country	Bioprinting Mechanism	University/ Research Institution	Use	Dual Bioink Printability
Extrusion-Based Bioprinters	Multi-Arm BioPrinter	USA	Mechanical or pneumatic	The University of Iowa, Penn State University	In situ bone printing (Ozbolat, 2015a), vascular tissue (Yu et al., 2014)	+
	Modular tissue printing platform	USA and South Korea	Pneumatic microextrusion	Harvard Medical School and KAIST	Skin (Lee et al., 2009a), fluidic channels (Lee et al., 2010a), vascular network (Lee et al., 2014)	+
	Multihead tissue/organ building system	South Korea	Pneumatic microextrusion	The Catholic University of Korea	Liver (Pati et al., 2015), heart and adipose tissue (Pati et al., 2014), bone and cartilage (Shim et al., 2012)	+
	Three-dimensional (3D) axis bioprinting system	South Korea	Mechanical microextrusion	Korea University	Cell-free scaffold (Song et al., 2010), skin (Hong et al., 2013)	+
	Multinozzle system	USA	Pneumatic, piezoelectric, and solenoid microextrusion	Drexel University	Fibroblasts (Khalil et al., 2005)	+
	Palmetto Printer	USA	Pneumatic microextrusion	Medical University of South Carolina	Adipose-derived stem cells (Jia et al., 2014)	+
	Multimaterial 3D bioprinting	USA	Pneumatic microextrusion	The Wyss Institute, Harvard	Vasculature (Kolesky et al., 2014)	+
	3D Scaffold printer	Germany	Mechanical microextrusion	Fraunhofer Institute for Materials Research and Beam Technology	Acellular Scaffolds (Wu et al., 2011)	N/A
	3D integrated organ printer	USA	Pneumatic microextrusion	Wake Forest Institute for Regenerative Medicine	Keratinocytes (Murphy et al., 2013)	+

N/A, not available; +, capable of bioprinting one or more bioink at a time.

commercially available bioprinters is probably one of the most remarkable developments of the past decade. Examples of those commercially available bioprinters are 3D Bioplotter®, the Alpha and Omega Bioprinters, BioAssemblyBot, BioBot, Biofactory and 3D Discovery®, Bio3D SYN^ and Bio3D Explorer, BioassemblyBot, Fab@Home, Inkredible, NovoGen MMX Bioprinter™, Regemat 3D, Regenovo, and Sciperio/nScrypt (Root Analysis, 2014).

7.2.2.1.1 3D BIOPLOTTER®

3D Bioplotter® was created by a research team at University of Freiburg in Germany (Landers et al., 2002), which was then commercialized by EnvisionTEC company later. 3D Bioplotter® outputs the bioink of various hydrogel solutions ranging from −50 to 150°C and can also print a wider range of biomaterials, including but not limited to ceramics and biodegradable polymers, to structurally and mechanically support tissue constructs (Sheshadri and Shirwaiker, 2015). The first version of the system used compressed air to force cut a liquid- or paste-like plotting medium, where the extruder-head could be heated to control viscosity (Pfister et al., 2004). In bioplotting process, the bioink solution was bioprinted into a plotting medium with compatible viscosities and the deposition characteristics of the dispensed bioink solution can modulate the printing resolution and accuracy. The bioink solidifies when it comes in contact with the substrate or previous layer. The major limitation of bioplotting is the necessity of using similar mediums (matching densities) for the dispensed biomaterial and the plotting media, where hydrogels are generally used in bioplotting process due to their mild properties in maximizing cell growth. The newer version of Bioplotter®, as shown in Fig. 7.2, uses syringe-type pneumatic dispensers without using a plotting medium as it restricts the 3D printing process significantly (EnvisionTEC n.d.). Interchangeable cartridges can be loaded (with up to five materials) for use in one built. For soft-tissue biofabrication and creating 3D biomimetic structures, users can load a dispenser with, but not limited to, living cells, agar, gelatin, chitosan, collagen, alginate, or fibrin. Researchers also utilized Bioplotter® to print inert bioresorbable scaffolds using hard

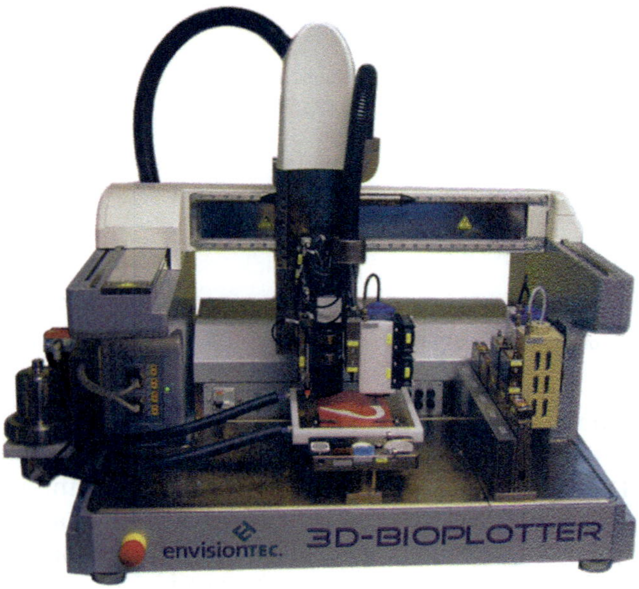

FIGURE 7.2 3D Bioplotter® *(Image courtesy of EnvisionTEC).*

polymeric and inorganic ceramic materials such as polycaprolactone, hydroxyapatite, and tricalcium phosphate (TCP) particles (Sheshadri and Shirwaiker, 2015).

7.2.2.1.2 THE ALPHA AND OMEGA BIOPRINTERS

3Dynamic Systems from the United Kingdom has introduced their commercially available 3D bioprinting systems, the Alpha and Omega Bioprinters, which provide a high degree of accuracy and affordability (3Dynamic Systems n.d.). The company has spun off from Swansea University in the UK and the two bioprinter models are used to develop human tissue constructs for transplantation. The Alpha bioprinter (see Fig. 7.3A) has a single extrusion printhead that is able to bioprint a wide range of biomaterials. This series has an induction heating system available for thermosensitive biomaterials. The Omega bioprinter, on the other hand, possesses further capabilities compared to that of the Alpha bioprinter. As shown in Fig. 7.3B, Omega series has a dual extruder printhead with an optional resistance heating system enabling hybrid bioprinting of complex tissue structures. The size and the work envelope of the Omega bioprinter are larger than that of the Alpha bioprinter. Both bioprinters were designed with a high degree of precision enabling accurate deposition control for bioprinting of anatomically correct, patient-specific scaffolds. The Alpha bioprinter was designed specifically to print bone tissue scaffolds for regenerative medicine and the Omega bioprinter was designed to bioprint soft living tissue structures using bioactive gels, proteins, and hydrogels (3Dynamic Systems n.d.).

7.2.2.1.3 BIOASSEMBLYBOT

Another recent bioprinter development came out from Advanced Solutions from the United States (Advanced Solutions n.d.). A 6-axis robotic bioprinter, called BioAssemblyBot, is capable of moving in six degrees of freedom in its workspace. BioAssemblyBot was designed to assemble different hydrogel solutions encapsulating different cells. Therefore, a unique syringe storage feature has been integrated into the bioprinter, which enables loading and unloading of a standard syringe barrel

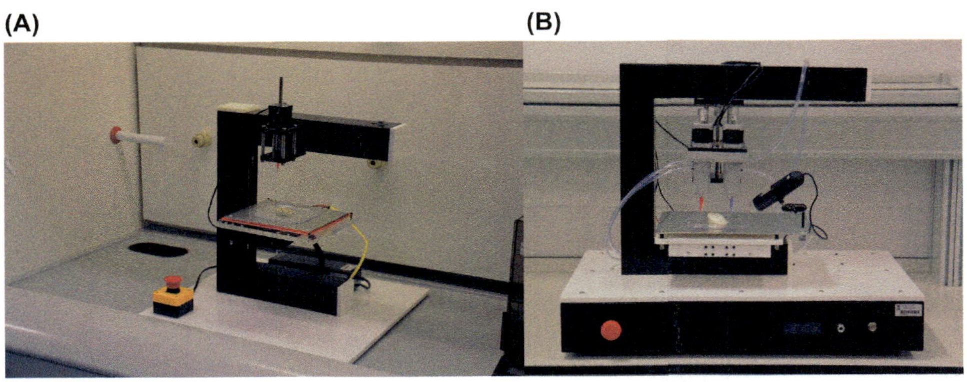

FIGURE 7.3 (A) Alpha and (B) Omega bioprinter *(Image courtesy of 3Dynamic Systems).*

automatically using the robot end effector. The bioprinter is integrated with a human machine interface system that allows loading CAD files and generating a robot path plan for hydrogel deposition. The system was built in an enclosure that can support camera view, and airline or electric or modem cable.

7.2.2.1.4 BIOBOT

Biobots has recently launched in the United States to provide an affordable and versatile, extrusion-based bioprinter to the market as the wide majority of the bioprinters are highly expensive. The first version was delivered to the market in 2014 with a single-nozzle dispensing ability, which has been recently upgraded to a dual-nozzle head version that can bioprint both thermosensitive (with maximum temperature of 100°C) and photocrosslinkable (LED range of 405–410 nm) hydrogels (BioBots n.d.). The new version of their bioprinter, Biobot 1, is shown in Fig. 7.4. The bioprinter is highly compact and occupies a space of 12 x 12 x 12 inches, which is highly smaller than other commercially available bioprinters and can easily fit into a standard biosafety cabinet.

7.2.2.1.5 BIOFACTORY AND 3D DISCOVERY®

Biofactory is a highly versatile 3D bioprinter manufactured by Delta-Robotics, which is currently known as regenHU from Switzerland (regenHU biosystems architects n.d.). Biofactory bioprinters entail EBB and DBB modalities in a single platform. Therefore, Biofactory allows working with a wide range of biomaterials including photo-crosslinkable hydrogels (wavelength of 355 nm), proteins, and high viscosity biomaterials (regenHU biosystems architects n.d.). Biofactory is a built-in system in a laminar flow hood maintaining a sterile environment and a controlled temperature, humidity, and gas composition. Researchers have recently used Biofactory bioprinters in different applications, such as skin tissue regeneration (Ng et al., 2016), in vitro models (Horváth et al., 2015), and 3D tubular construct (Tan and Yeong, 2015). 3D Discovery® bioprinter is capable of dispensing up to four different materials in 2D or 3D using

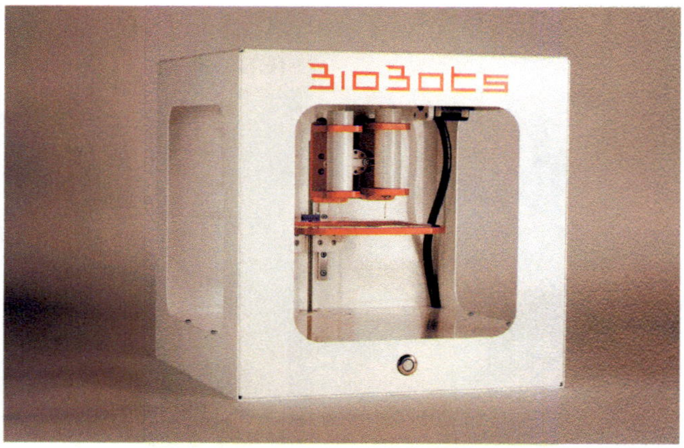

FIGURE 7.4 Biobot 1 *(Courtesy of Biobots).*

multiple fluid dispenser heads (droplet-based) or printerheads (extrusion-based) (Root Analysis, 2014). The fluid dispenser head has a resolution down to a picoliter enabling fabrication of high-throughput arrays on well plates of various dimensions for chemotaxis assays. The bioprinter has heating (up to 80°C) and cooling chambers allowing bioprinting of biomaterials within a wider range of viscosity.

7.2.2.1.6 BIO3D SYN^ AND BIO3D EXPLORER

Bio3D Technologies from Singapore has developed two different 3D bioprinting platforms including "Bio3D SYN^" and "Bio3D Explorer" (Bio3D Technologies n.d.). Bio3D SYN^ was designed with a high resolution (around 1 μm) on each axes. Bio3D SYN^ does not only facilitate EBB but also jetting and photopolymerization. This bioprinter has brought a new concept into the bioprinter market as it entails multiple configurations for different bioprinting modalities. Bio3D SYN^ has an antivibration levitation build platform, which enables precise control on the distance between the nozzle tip and the platform (Bio3D Technologies n.d.). In addition, Bio3D SYN^ enables real-time monitoring of the process as it possesses an advanced control mechanism. Bio3D SYN^ is capable of bioprinting multiple types of biomaterials, including but not limited to hydrogels, proteins, and cells, for the fabrication of living tissue substitutes for tissue engineering and regenerative medicine. Designed for educational or training purposes, Bio3D Explorer was developed in a less sophisticated manner than Bio3D SYN^ with a motion resolution five times less than that of Bio3D SYN^. One of the major advantages of this bioprinter is that it ensures a portable system which can operate up to four printheads.

7.2.2.1.7 FAB@HOME

Fab@Home was one of the first open-source 3D printer available to the public. Up until 2005, all 3D printers were industrial scale, expensive, and proprietary. The high cost and closed nature of the 3D printing industry at the time limited the accessibility of the technology to the masses, the range of materials that could be used, and the level of exploration that could be done by users. The goal of the Fab@Home project was to change this situation by creating a versatile, low-cost, open-source printer to accelerate technology innovation and its migration into the consumer and maker space (Malone and Lipson, 2007). Since its open-source release in 2006, hundreds of Fab@Home 3D printers were built across the world and its design elements could be found in many recent printers, most notably the Makerbot Replicator. The printer's multiple syringe-based deposition mechanism allowed for some of the first multimaterial prints, including food and cell printing. Fab@Home bioprinters are currently commercialized by Seraph Robotics in the United States, and the bioprinters have been utilized by various research and academic institutions (Seraph Robotics n.d.). Fab@Home bioprinters, including Fab@Home M3, Scientist, and Fab@Home M4 models, have been utilized to bioprint tissue constructs including but not limited to cartilage (Cohen et al., 2010b), bone (Cohen et al., 2010a), and heart valve (Duan et al., 2014).

7.2.2.1.8 INKREDIBLE

Cellink is a recently established company in the United States commercializing their first bioprinter "Inkredible."(Cellink n.d.) The Inkredible has a printhead with a dual extruder for bioprinting hydrogel solutions and can easily fit under a standard biosafety cabinet allowing the operator to run it under sterile conditions. The Inkredible was launched to facilitate bioprinting of various tissue substitutes for academic and research institutes within an affordable price range.

7.2.2.1.9 NOVOGEN MMX™

NovoGen MMX™ bioprinter was commercialized by Organovo when the company was first launched. Although it is currently not commercially available, it has been extensively used by the company to bioprint various tissue types such as liver model and the breast tissue model for cancer screening (King et al., 2014; Roskos et al., 2015). With its multihead dispensers, NovoGen MMX™ during its early years was used to bioprint tissue spheroids along with a support structure made of agarose hydrogel. After the bioprinting process, tissue spheroids fused together and further matured into a tissue-like organization. As this occurred, the agarose supporting mold was dissolved away or removed, thereby leaving a final bioprinted tissue (Norotte et al., 2009). This point powerfully illustrated the fact that the cells contained in tissue spheroids were capable of rearranging themselves postbioprinting and facilitating the rapid maturation of tissues. For example, blood vessels were bioprinted using tissue spheroids comprised of a mix of endothelial, smooth muscle, and fibroblast cells. Once placed in position by the printhead, and with no technological intervention, endothelial cells migrated toward the luminal surface of the blood vessel and fibroblasts migrated toward the outer surface. As loading tissue spheroids is an extremely challenging task (Ozbolat, 2015b), the company has recently proceeded with bioprinting preaggregates into a designed shape for engineering of tissues for drug testing and cancer modeling using a new model of their bioprinter (see Fig. 7.5).

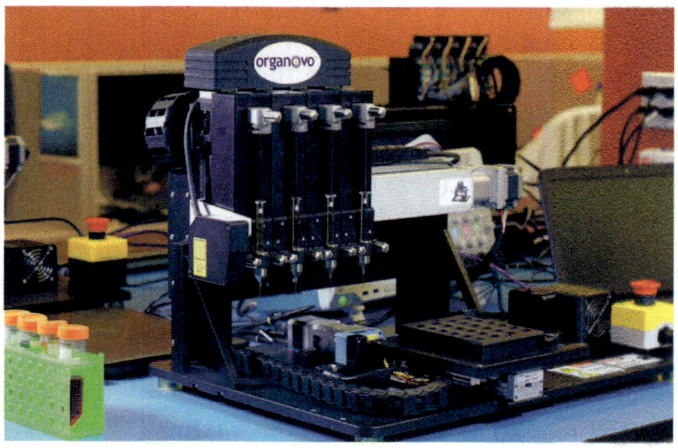

FIGURE 7.5 NovoGen MMX™ bioprinter *(Image courtesy of Organovo Holdings, Inc.).*

7.2.2.1.10 REGEMAT 3D

REGEMAT 3D company, founded in Spain, focuses on 3D bioprinting technologies to find new solutions to tissue engineering and regenerative medicine problems (Regemat3D n.d.). The company has produced their first commercially available 3D bioprinter system called REGEMAT 3D V1 (see Fig. 7.6), a multihead system, which allows bioprinting of multiple types of biomaterials. REGEMAT 3D V1 enables pore filling (IPF), injection filling (IF), or fused deposition modeling (FDM) processes using REGEMATs printhead technologies. Additionally, REGEMAT 3D V1 bioprinter and its components can be customized based on custom tissue bioprinting requirements.

7.2.2.1.11 REGENOVO

In another spot on the world, researchers from Hangzhou Dianzi University in China announced the invention of the first 3D bioprinter with independent intellectual property rights in China in 2013 (Regenovo Biotechnology Co., Ltd. n.d.). The bioprinter, named Regenovo Bio-printer^{TM} (with models including Bio-Printer^{TM}—Lite, Bio-Printer^{TM}—Pro, Bio-Printer^{TM}—WS), has already been used in bioprinting multiple tissue types, including liver and human ear cartilage constructs (Regenovo Biotechnology Co., Ltd. n.d.). Regenovo bioprinters do not only realize bioprinting in aseptic conditions, but also have temperature-controlled cartridges supporting bioprinting of various bioink solutions within the temperature range from −5 to 260°C.

7.2.2.1.12 nScrypt

nScrypt from the United States previously manufactured a bioprinter for precise deposition of bioink materials comprised of three essential elements including a robotic precision position system (with a movable x—y stage and three z-directional printheads), automated biomaterial dispensers, and a computer-based software enabled operational

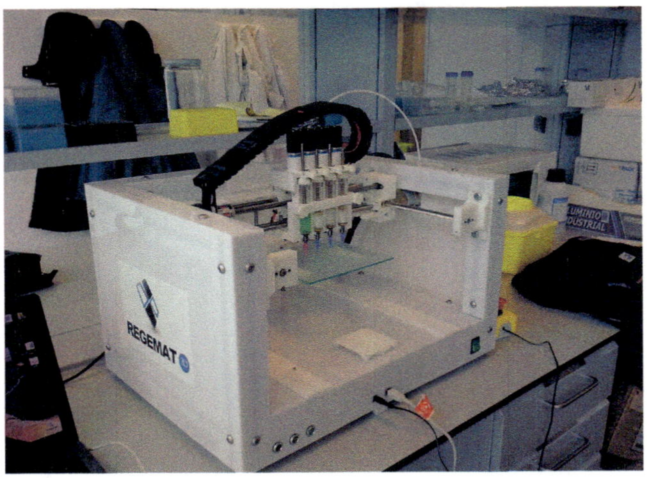

FIGURE 7.6 Regemat 3D V1 bioprinter *(Image courtesy of REGEMAT 3D).*

control (Dababneh and Ozbolat, 2014). The first two printheads were used to bioprint the bioink, where the biopaper substrate was printed by the third head. The company currently offers the nScrypt 3Dn model (see Fig. 7.7) for cell bioprinting, which can hold four different bioink solutions at a time and facilitate high cell viability using the SmartPump™ dispenser (nScript, 2016). The dispenser can bioprint a variety of ECM components such as collagen and hyaluronic acid in a heated or cooled condition. In addition, nScrypt 3Dn can also be mounted with a high-precision nFD™ printhead for deposition of a wide range of thermoplastic-based biopolymers.

Table 7.2 presents a detailed list of commercially available extrusion-based bioprinters along with their use and features.

7.2.2.2 Droplet-Based Bioprinters

Engineering tissues with native-like characteristics are not trivial (Xu et al., 2013b). DBB, among all of the available bioprinting modalities, fabricates tissues with comparable native-like characteristics because of its ability to bioprint various cell types accurately and simultaneously (Gao et al., 2014).

Commercially available multinozzle inkjet printheads such as EPSON SEA-Jet™ (electrostatic DOD), Fuji Dimatix™ (piezoelectric DOD), and Xaar-126 (piezoelectric DOD) have since been used for bioprinting various cell types and several other biologics (Choi et al., 2011; Ferris et al., 2013; Nishiyama et al., 2008). The printheads generate droplets of 1–100 picoliters in volume (droplet diameters of 10–60 μm), indicating very

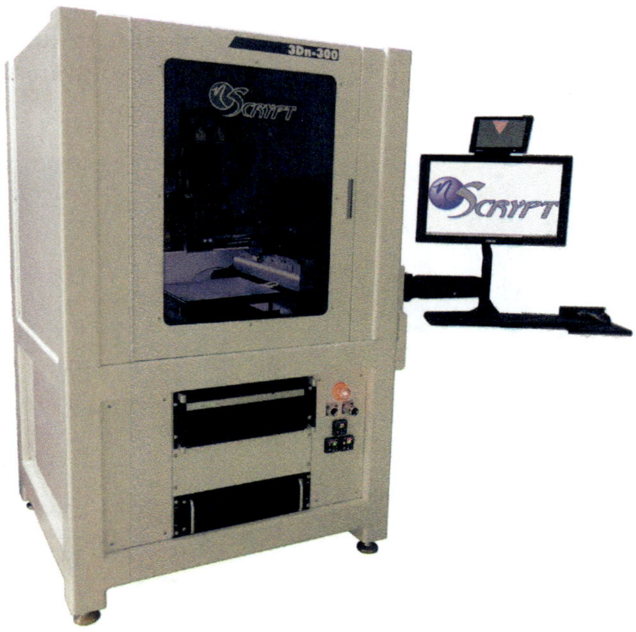

FIGURE 7.7 3Dn-300 TE bioprinter *(Image courtesy of nScrypt, Inc.).*

Table 7.2 Commercially Available Extrusion-Based Bioprinters

	Bioprinter Name	Country	Bioprinting Mechanism	Company	Use	Dual Bioink Printability	Features
Extrusion-based bioprinters	Novogen MMX™	USA	Mechanical microextrusion	Organovo	Bone (Edwin et al. n.d.), liver (Robbins et al., 2013), breast cancer (King et al., 2013), vascularization (Bertassoni et al., 2014)	+	Precision: 20 μm (Root Analysis, 2014)
	BioScaffolder	Germany	Pneumatic microextrusion	SYS + ENG	Encapsulated proteins (Poldervaart et al., 2013), cartilage (Visser et al., 2013), vascularization (Fedorovich et al., 2011), bone (Seyednejad et al., 2011)	+	Stepper motor with 5 μm/step (SYS + ENG n.d.)
	3D BioPlotter	Germany	Pneumatic microextrusion	EnvisionTec	Bone (Fedorovich et al., 2008), acellular scaffolds (Chien et al., 2012)	+	Axis resolution: 1 μm (x–y–z axis) (EnvisionTEC) Speed: 0.1–150 mm/s (EnvisionTEC), price > $145,000§
	Regenovo	China	Extrusion	Regonovo Biotechnology Co., Ltd	β-TCP bone scaffold (Zou et al., 2016), 3D gelatin/alginate scaffolds (Wang et al., 2016)	+	Resolution 20 μm (Bodrum et al., 2015)
	BioAssembly tool (BAT)	USA	Pneumatic microextrusion	Sciperio/ nScrypt	Vascularization and skin (Smith et al., 2004)	+	Price range: $200,000–$400,000 (Root Analysis, 2014)
	3D Discovery	Switzerland	Pneumatic microextrusion	RegenHU	Cartilage (Markstedt et al., 2015)	+	Printing materials up to viscosity 10,000 mPa (Root Analysis, 2014)
	BioFactory	Switzerland	Pneumatic microextrusion	RegenHU	Air-blood tissue barrier (Horváth et al., 2015)	+	Printing resolution: < 5 μm (Horváth et al., 2015)
	BioBot 1	USA	Pneumatic micro-extrusion	BioBots	GelMA hydrogel extrusion optimization (Ersumo and Spiller, 2015)	+	Printing resolution: 100 μm (BioBots, n.d.) Position precision: 5.5 μm (x–y axis)¥ 5 μm(z axes)¥ Price: $10,000 (BioBots, n.d.)
	Bioassembly Bot	USA	Pneumatic microextrusion	Advanced solutions	Human heart (Root Analysis, 2014)	+	Repeatedly up to 20 μm (Advanced Solutions n.d.) Price > $159,995 (Advanced Solutions n.d.)
	Fab@Home	USA	Mechanical microextrusion	Seraph Robotics	Aortic valves (Duan et al., 2013), filling chondral and osteochondral defects (Cohen et al., 2010a), and ear (Mannoor et al., 2013)	+	Positioning resolution: 15.8 μm per full step, a nominal top speed of 25 mm/s (x–y–z axes) (Malone and Lipson, 2007)

Continued

Table 7.2 Commercially Available Extrusion-Based Bioprinters—cont'd

Bioprinter Name	Country	Bioprinting Mechanism	Company	Use	Dual Bioink Printability	Features
The Alpha Bioprinter	UK	Pneumatic extrusion	3Dynamic Systems (3DS)	NI	−	Accuracy: ± 75 μm (3Dynamic Systems n.d.) Price: £9,480[§]
The Omega Bioprinter	UK	Pneumatic extrusion	3Dynamic Systems (3DS)	NI	+	Accuracy: ±50 μm (3Dynamic Systems n.d.) Price: £14,480[§]
Regemat 3D V1	Spain	Pneumatic extrusion	Regemat 3D	NI	+	Axis resolution: 150 μm (x–y axis), 400 nm (z-axis) (Regemat3D n.d.) Price > 11,700 euros[§]
Fab@Home MD4	USA	Pneumatic extrusion	Seraph Robotics	NI	+	50 μm Gantry (Seraph Robotics n.d.)
Scientist 3D printer	USA	Pneumatic extrusion	Seraph Robotics	NI	+	5–10 μm Gantry (Seraph Robotics n.d.)
Bio3D SYN˙	Singapore	Microextrusion	Bio3D Technologies	NI	+	1 μm (x–y–z resolution) (Bio3D technologies n.d.) Speed: 10–300,000 μm/min (Bio3D technologies n.d.)
Bio3D Explorer	Singapore	Microextrusion	Bio3D technologies	NI	+	5 μm (x–y–z resolution) (Bio3D technologies n.d.)
Inkredible	USA	Microextrusion	Cellink	NI	+	x–y resolution per microstep: 10 μm z resolution per microstep: 2.5 μm **Layer resolution: 50–100 μm (Cellink n.d.)**

NI, No published research article has been identified; +, capable of bioprinting one or more bioink at a time; −, capable of bioprinting only one bioink at a time.
[§]Pricing information has been obtained from the company.
[¥]Information has been obtained from the company.

small nozzle orifice diameters. Thus the printheads are prone to clogging when bioprinting viscous or fibrous bioink such as cell-laden collagen (Yamaguchi et al., 2012). Consequently, a very limited number of cell types and biologics are bioprintable using these printheads. At the same time, single-nozzle piezoelectric dispensers, including but not limited to, Microfab Technologies MJ series, Microdrop Technologies MD series, and Nordson Pico® series are versatile and offer greater control over droplet generation and placement. Hence, the dispensers have been extensively used for high-throughput and high-resolution bioprinting applications (Suntivich et al., 2014; Xu et al., 2012; Christensen et al., 2015). However, small secondary droplets known as satellite droplets often accompany the primary droplets (Morrison and Harlen, 2010) and can reduce the bioprinting accuracy and precision (Christensen et al., 2015). Similar to multinozzle inkjet printheads, the single-nozzle dispensers are prone to clogging when bioprinting viscous bioink solutions.

Microvalve bioprinters, in contrast, have not been reported to generate satellite droplets to date in the literature. Commercially available microvalve dispensers such as TechElan G100-150300NJ, Fritz Gyger SMLD, Offshore Solutions microvalve nozzle, and Lee Products VHS nanoliter dispense valve have been used for bioprinting a myriad of living cells and other biologics (Xu et al., 2010, 2011; Moon et al., 2010; Gurkan et al., 2014; Lee et al., 2009a; Lee et al., 2010b; Faulkner-Jones et al., 2013; Faulkner-Jones et al. 2015; Li et al., 2015a,b; Lee et al., 2014; Xu et al., 2013b). However, the dispensers generate larger droplets compare to other DBB modalities under identical conditions (Tasoglu and Demirci, 2013). Hence, they are not suitable for high-resolution bioprinting applications. In contrast, electrohydrodynamic (EHD) jet bioprinters are capable of generating droplets that are smaller than the nozzle orifice opening (diameter) (Jayasinghe et al., 2006; Jayasinghe and Edirisinghe, 2004). Thus, these bioprinters are suitable for propelling highly concentrated bioink solutions (up to 20% weight by volume) through extremely small nozzles (orifice diameters $\leq 100\ \mu m$) (Jayasinghe et al., 2006). Several in-house built EHD bioprinters, assembled from commercially available components, have been used to bioprint various biologics such as living cells and proteins (Eagles et al., 2006; Workman et al., 2014; Xie and Wang, 2007; Kim et al., 2007; Poellmann et al., 2011). But, these bioprinters eject a continuous jet or a stream of multiple droplets at a time (Onses et al., 2015; Sutanto et al., 2012; Gasperini et al., 2015), and they are not ideal for high-precision (precise placement of droplets) bioprinting applications.

On the other hand, acoustic bioprinters employ a gentle acoustic field to eject droplets from an open pool of bioink solution unlike inkjet, EHD, or microvalve bioprinters, which eject droplets through a nozzle (Demirci and Montesano, 2007). Constituent living cells of the bioink are consequently not subjected to detrimental stressors such as heat, high pressure, large voltage, and shear stress during droplet ejection. However, 3D construct fabrication requires printhead and/or substrate movement which can introduce undesirable disturbances. As a result, the disturbances can diminish the control over the droplet generation and placement in acoustic bioprinting. In addition, the bioprinters may not be suitable for bioprinting viscous bioink materials such as cell-laden collagen as the gentle acoustic waves may not be sufficient to generate droplets. Thus, the bioprinters have been employed limitedly for bioprinting a very few biologics (Fang et al., 2012; Demirci and Montesano, 2007).

Overall, in-house assembled bioprinters using commercially available components are economical and offer greater freedom; however, their design is time-consuming at times and requires specialized skills and knowledge in the areas of electrical and computer engineering, pertaining to system integration. A typical 3D bioprinter, for instance, requires coordinated movement of printhead and substrate along the three axes and a software program to control the movement as well as the droplet jetting mechanism, according to print job file or the operator's input. On the other hand, commercially available complete bioprinting systems (bioprinters) save the development time and the subsystems are often well integrated. However, they are expensive and may limit the level of customization. Table 7.3 presents the commercially available and noncommercial droplet-based bioprinters along with their application areas. A limited number of complete bioprinting systems are commercially available, which are discussed herein.

7.2.2.2.1 AUTODROP COMPACT AND AD-P-8000

Autodrop Compact bioprinters by Microdrop Technologies (Germany) rely on piezoelectric drop-on-demand inkjet (PIJ) mechanism to generate droplets (Microdrop Technologies, 2016). Bioink solution in PIJ bioprinters is stored in a fluid reservoir and is held in place at the nozzle orifice because of the surface tension (Derby, 2010). A voltage pulse is applied to deform the piezoelectric actuator of the bioprinter which in turn deforms the fluid reservoir (Wijshoff, 2010). The sudden change in the volume of the fluid reservoir causes a pressure wave when the surface tension at the nozzle orifice is overcome. Consequently, a droplet of the bioink is ejected (Singh et al., 2010). Some PIJ bioprinters also require pneumatic pressure (static pressure through means of pressurized-air) commonly referred to as the back pressure to supplement the pressure pulses to overcome the surface tension at the nozzle orifice. Autodrop Compact bioprinters, as their name indicates, are compact PIJ bioprinters. Their substrate dimensions are 200 × 200 mm. At the same time, the bioprinters position accuracy (x–y–z axis) is ± 25 μm and the travel velocity is 75 mm/s (acceleration 500 mm/s^2). Further, the payload capacity of the bioprinters is 5 kg for y-axis and 1 kg for x- and z-axis. An electronic controller is provided to regulate the voltage pulse characteristics and the simultaneous operation of up to two piezoelectric dispensers. Similarly, a graphical editor is provided for defining custom design patterns and it also supports the import of vector-based graphic files. Autodrop AD-P-8000 bioprinters have better accuracy, greater travel velocity and higher payload capacity than Autodrop Compact bioprinters. The position accuracy (x–y) of the bioprinters is ± 5 μm and the travel–velocity is 125 mm/s (acceleration 1000 mm/s^2). Further, the payload capacity of the bioprinters is 10 kg for y-axis and 1.5 kg for x- and z-axis. The included electronic controller simultaneously

Table 7.3 Droplet-based Bioprinters

	Availability	Bioprinter Name	Country	Bioprinting Mechanism	University/Company	Use	Dual Bioink Printability
Droplet-based bioprinters	Commercial	Fujifilm Dimatrix Printer	USA	Piezoelectric drop-on-demand	Fujifilm Dimatix, Inc.	Study of cell-to-cell communications among bioprinted bacterial cells (Choi et al., 2011)	–
		MicroFab JetLab II	USA	Piezoelectric drop-on-demand	MicroFAB Technologies, Inc.	Cell and biologics 3D bioprinting including silk nest arrays for hosting cells (*Escherichia coli*) for biosensing (Suntivich et al., 2014)	+
		MicroFab JetLab 4	USA	Piezoelectric drop-on-demand	MicroFAB Technologies, Inc.	Bioprinting	+
		Autodrop Compact	Germany	Piezoelectric drop-on-demand	Microdrop Technologies	Bioprinting	+
		Autodrop AD-P-8000	Germany	Piezoelectric drop-on-demand	Microdrop Technologies	Bioprinting	+
		Cluster Technology DeskViewer	Japan	Piezoelectric drop-on-demand	Cluster Technology Co., Ltd.	Human liver tissue chips comprising of hepatocytes (HepG2) and human umbilical vein endothelial cells (HUVECs) (Matsusaki et al., 2013)	+
		Cell Jet Cell Printer	USA	synQUAD drop-by-drop technology (micro-valve and syringe pump)	Digilab, Inc.	Cell printing	–
	Noncommercial	Custom printer with MicroJet™ piezoelectric actuator with MicroFab Technologies nozzle	USA	Piezoelectric drop-on-demand	Carnegie Mellon University and University of Pittsburgh Medical Center (UPMC)	FGF-2 dose impact on human MG-63 osteosarcoma cell response (Campbell et al., 2005; Miller et al., 2006), BMP-2 to evaluate spatially controlled differentiation of MDSCs (Phillippi et al., 2008)	–
		Custom printer with MicroFab MJ-ABP-01 piezoelectric nozzle	Canada	Piezoelectric drop-on-demand	University of British Columbia	MCF-7 movement within in the nozzle during the printing process (Cheng et al., 2014)	–

Continued

Table 7.3 Droplet-based Bioprinters—cont'd

Availability	Bioprinter Name	Country	Bioprinting Mechanism	University/Company	Use	Dual Bioink Printability
	Custom printer with MicroFab MJ-ABL-01-120-6MX piezoelectric nozzle	USA	Piezoelectric drop-on-demand	Clemson University and University of Florida	Complex tubular tissue (NIH 3T3 cells and alginate) constructs with bifurcations (Xu et al., 2012; Christensen et al., 2015)	–
	Modified Canon Bubble Jet printer (BJC-2100) and modified Hewlett–Packard Deskjet printers (HP 550C, HP 500, and HP 340)	USA	Thermal drop-on-demand	Clemson University and the University of Texas at El Paso	Collagen scaffolding patterns (Roth et al., 2004), mammalian cell (CHO cells and rat primary embryonic motoneural cells) constructs (Xu et al., 2005), neural cell (rat hippocampal and cortical cell) constructs (Xu et al., 2006), alginate 3D constructs (Boland et al., 2007), cardiac 3D constructs (feline and H1 cardiomyocytes with alginate), vascular (HMVECs and fibrin) constructs (Cui and Boland, 2009), skin transplants (NHDF and NHEK) with built-in vascular networks (HMVECs) for in vivo wound healing studies (Yanez et al., 2014)	+
	Modified Hewlett–Packard Deskjet printer (HP 550C)	USA	Thermal drop-on-demand	Wake Forest University	Alginate microspheres with single-encapsulated cells (beta-TC6) (Xu et al., 2008), complex heterogeneous 3D tissue models with hAFCS, dSMCs, and bECs (Xu et al., 2013a)	+
	Modified Hewlett–Packard Deskjet printer (HP 500)	USA	Thermal drop-on-demand	The Scripps Research Institute	In situ bioprinting of chondrocytes and PEGDMA hydrogel for direct cartilage repair (Cui et al., 2012a), cartilage constructs (human articular chondrocytes) to study FGF-2 and TGF-β1 growth factors impact on printed cartilage formation (Cui et al., 2012b)	+
	Modified Hewlett–Packard ink-jet printer	USA	Thermal drop-on-demand	TeVido BioDevices	Breast tissue	+

Modified Hewlett–Packard deskjet printer	USA, Germany, Japan, and China	Thermal drop-on-demand	Stemorgan Therapeutics, Technical University Munich, The Scripps Research Institute, Tokyo University of Science, Rensselaer Polytechnic Institute, Wuhan University of Technology	Stem cell tissue constructs (hMSCs with PEG) and their directed differentiation into bone and cartilage (Gao et al., 2014; Gao et al. 2015)	+
Modified Hewlett–Packard 5360 printer	USA and China	Thermal drop-on-demand	University of Texas at El Paso, Shanghai Jiao Tong University, Sun Yat-sen University, and Texas Tech University Health Sciences	High-throughput miniature drug-screening platform employing bioprinted *E. coli*-laden alginate and three different antibiotics (penicillin/streptomycin, antimycotic, and kanamycin sulfate) (Rodríguez-Dévora et al., 2012)	+
Lab-on-a-printer	Canada	Microchannel-based thermal inkjet	Aspect Biosystems	3D tissue fabrication, drug testing, toxicity testing	+
Modified Hewlett–Packard (HP 660C) printer with add-on piezoelectric pump	USA	Piezoelectric drop-on-demand	Clemson University	Protein (bovine serum albumin and streptavidin) and cell (bovine aortal endothelial cell) 2D constructs (Wilson and Boland, 2003)	N/A
Custom printer with Epson SEA-Jet printhead	Japan	Electrostatic drop-on-demand	University of Toyama and Kanagawa Academy of Science and Technology	3D tissue (HeLa cells) constructs (hollow tubes) (Nishiyama et al., 2008)	–
Custom printer	Ireland and Germany	Piezoelectric drop-on-demand	University of Freiburg, Trinity College and Women and Infants University Hospital	Microspheres with single-encapsulated cells (HeLa cells) (Yusof et al., 2011)	–
Custom printer with Xaar-126 piezoelectric printhead	Australia	Piezoelectric drop-on-demand	University of Wollongong	2D tissue (C2C12 and PC12 cells) constructs (Ferris et al., 2013)	+
Custom EHD printer using commercially available subsystems	UK	Electrohydrodynamic (EHD) jetting	University of London	EHD as a viable bioprinting strategy using Jurkat cells (Jayasinghe et al., 2006), CAD (Cath.-a-differentiated) mouse neural cells (Eagles et al., 2006), human astrocytoma cells (Jayasinghe and Townsend-Nicholson, 2006), white blood cells, erythrocytes (Mongkoldhumrongkul et al., 2009), and THP-1 cells with alginate and collagen (Workman et al., 2014)	–

Continued

Table 7.3 Droplet-based Bioprinters—cont'd

Availability	Bioprinter Name	Country	Bioprinting Mechanism	University/Company	Use	Dual Bioink Printability
	Custom EHD printer using commercially available subsystems	Singapore	EHD jetting	National University of Singapore and Molecular Engineering of Biological and Chemical Systems	Microencapsulation of cells (hepatocytes G2 cells) with alginate (Xie and Wang, 2007)	–
	Custom EHD printer using commercially available subsystems	South Korea	EHD jetting	Yonsei University	Collagen scaffold patterns (Kim et al., 2007)	–
	Custom EHD printer using commercially available subsystems	USA	EHD jetting	University of Illinois at Urbana—Champaign, University of Michigan, and Rensselaer Polytechnic Institute	Rabbit Immunoglobulin-G and fibronectin scaffold patterns (Poellmann et al., 2011)	–
	Custom EHD printer using commercially available subsystems	Italy	EHD jetting	University of Trento	Microencapsulation of cells (B50 rat neural cells) with alginate (Gasperini et al., 2013), 3T3 fibroblasts and alginate constructs (Gasperini et al., 2015)	–
	Custom acoustic picoliter droplet ejection system	USA	Acoustic droplet ejection	Harvard University	Encapsulation of a single to multiple cells (mESC, RAJI, HL-1, 3T3, and AML-12) (Demirci and Montesano, 2007)	+
	Custom acoustic droplet ejection system	USA	Acoustic droplet ejection	University of Michigan	2D heterogeneous tissue (MDA MB 231 breast cancer cells and HEK 239 cells with dextran) constructs (Fang et al., 2012)	–
	Custom printer with TechElan solenoid valve ejector (G100-150300nj)	USA and Finland	Microvalve (Solenoid)	Harvard University, Massachusetts Institute of Technology, Clemson University, and University of Helsinki	Cells (mESC, RAJI, HL-1, 3T3, and AML-12) encapsulation, cell encapsulation (rat bladder smooth muscle cells with collagen) (Xu et al., 2010), 3D tissue constructs (rat bladder smooth muscle cells and collagen) fabrication (Moon et al., 2010), heterogeneous tissue (NIH: OVCAR-5 human ovarian cancer cells and MRC-5 normal human fibroblasts) constructs (Xu et al., 2011), 3D fibrocartilage tissue models by bioprinting mesenchymal stem cells with GelMA precursor solution and photointiator (Gurkan et al., 2014)	+

Custom printer with Fritz Gyger SMLD solenoid valve ejector	USA and South Korea	Microvalve (Solenoid)	Harvard Medical School, Rensselaer Polytechnic Institute, Albany Medical College, and Korea Advanced Institute of Science and Technology (KAIST)	3D skin tissue (human dermal fibroblasts, human epidermal keratinocytes, and collagen) constructs (Lee et al., 2009a), 2D neural tissue (rat astrocytes, neurons, and collagen) constructs (Lee et al., 2009b), VEGF-releasing fibrin gel scaffolds for neural stem cell (murine NSC) culture (Lee et al., 2010b), Angiogenic sprouting of vascular networks at cellular level through bioprinted HUVECs and NHLFs (Lee et al., 2014)	+
Custom printer with Offshore Solutions solenoid inkjet valve	USA	Microvalve (Solenoid)	Wake Forest University	Cartilage tissue constructs (chondrocytes, fibrinogen, and collagen) (Xu et al., 2013b)	−
Custom printer with Lee Products VHS Nanoliter dispense valve with Lee Products Minstac Nozzle	UK	Microvalve (Solenoid)	Heriot-Watt University and Roslin Biocentre	Tissue (HEK293 and hESC cells) spheroids (Faulkner-Jones et al., 2013), 3D hepatocyte constructs (HLCs differentiated from hESCs and hiPSCs with alginate) (Faulkner-Jones et al., 2015), DNA based hydrogel bioprinting (Li et al., 2015a,b)	+
Custom printer	Australia	Microvalve (Solenoid)	University of Wollongong	2D tissue (C2C12 cells) constructs (Ferris et al., 2013)	−

N/A, Information not available; +, capable of bioprinting one or more bioink at a time; −, capable of bioprinting only one bioink at a time.

supports up to eight piezoelectric dispensers. The bioprinter is comparable to the Autodrop Compact in other aspects.

7.2.2.2.2 MICROFAB JETLAB®

MicroFab jetlab® bioprinters from MicroFab Solutions Inc. from the United States employ PIJ mechanism to generate droplets and are available in two configurations, jetlab® II (see Fig. 7.8A) and jetlab® 4 (see Fig. 7.8B) (MicroFab Technologies Inc. n.d.). The jetlab® 4 is compact and relatively inexpensive compared to jetlab® II. The substrate size of jetlab® 4 is 160 × 120 mm as compared to 200 × 200 mm of jetlab® II. However, jetlab® II has higher positioning (x–y axis) accuracy of ± 15 μm than jetlab® 4, which is ± 30 μm. In addition, jetlab® II is faster (100 mm/s velocity and 400 mm/s^2 acceleration) than jetlab® 4 (50 mm/s velocity and 1500 mm/s^2 acceleration). Furthermore, jetlab® II has greater payload capacity (x and y stage maximum payload is 10 kg and z stage maximum payload is 3 kg) than jetlab® 4 (x and y stage maximum payload is 20 kg and z stage maximum payload is 5 kg). The two configurations are available with various integrated control mechanisms (controllers) for regulating motion, pneumatic pressure, voltage pulse generation and pulse characteristics, temperature, and alignment. In addition, a software graphical user interface is provided to define the process parameters. Hence, very little training is necessary for the bioprinters operation and familiarization.

7.2.2.3 Laser-Based Bioprinters

LBB relies on two different mechanisms including processes based on cell transfer and processes involving photopolymerization. Processes involving photopolymerization (i.e., stereolithography and its modifications) utilize modified commercial 3D printers or custom-made platforms. The author excludes the discussion on such content here but refers the reader to Chapter 6 for more details of modified configurations. Processes based on cell transfer are laser-guided direct writing (LGDW) (Odde and Renn 1999, 2000), matrix-assisted pulsed-laser evaporation-direct write (MAPLE-DW)

(A) (B)

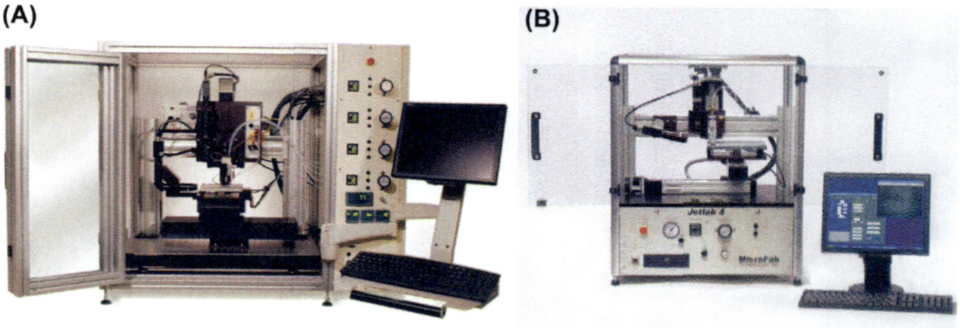

FIGURE 7.8 Commercially available droplet-based bioprinters: (A) jetlab® II and (B) jetlab® 4 bioprinter *(Image courtesy of MicroFab Solutions Inc.)*.

(Lin et al., 2009; Doraiswamy et al., 2006; Ringeisen et al., 2002), and laser-induced forward transfer (LIFT) (Ringeisen et al., 2002, 2004) to deposit bioink droplets.

LGDW employs optical trapping forces of a weakly focused laser beam for guided disposition of individual biologics such as living cells with micrometer-scale accuracy (Renn et al., 1999; Xu et al., 2003; Nahmias et al., 2005; Ringeisen et al., 2006). However, the refractive index of the individual biologics significantly impacts the magnitude of the optical forces (a 4% decrease in refractive index decreases the trapping force by four times and the pushing force by 25 times) (Nahmias et al., 2005). Consequently, a very few cell types and other biologics are bioprintable and hence LGDW bioprinters, in-house built from commercially available subsystems, have been used in a very few studies (Odde and Renn, 2000; Xu et al., 2003; Nahmias et al., 2005; Odde and Renn, 1999).

MAPLE-DW- or LIFT-based bioprinters, in contrast, are suitable for bioprinting a myriad of biologics as they are nozzle free and are not constrained by the viscosity of bioink solutions (Lin and Huang, 2011). In addition, the bioprinters are suitable for fabricating 3D tissue constructs, including hollow tubular tissue constructs, as they are not limited by the bioink viscosity (Yan et al., 2013; Xiong et al., 2015a). The difference between MAPLE-DW and LIFT is that an energy-absorbing IR-transparent inter layer of thin film is present above the bioink coating in LIFT. Bioprinters based on LIFT and its variations are known by various names such as biological laser printing (BioLP) (Barron et al., 2004a,b,c; Barron et al., 2004c), absorbing film assisted-LIFT (AFA-LIFT) (Hopp et al., 2005), and laser-assisted bioprinting (LaBP) (Gruene et al., 2011a,b). However, their principal working mechanism is the same (Ringeisen et al., 2006). That is, the bioprinters use focused laser pulses to generate bioink droplets by locally heating the bioink directly (MAPLE-DW) or alternatively the sacrificial absorbing inter layer (BioLP, LaBP, and AFA-LIFT), which are applied as layers on a quartz ribbon support. The localized heating causes a vapor bubble, which rapidly expands and collapses (bursts), generating a pressure wave. The pressure wave consequently propels bioink droplets (or jets depending on the process parameters such as the bioink viscosity and laser energy) on to a receiving substrate (Lin et al., 2010; Koch et al., 2012; Barron et al., 2004c). Modified LIFT-based bioprinters have been used for bioprinting applications involving living cells such as stem cells (Koch et al., 2010; Gruene et al., 2011a,b) and other biologics such as proteins (Ringeisen et al., 2002). Although, the bioprinters are not constrained by the bioink viscosity, their bioprinting speed is limited by the ribbon preparation time at present (Skardal and Atala, 2015) and is often slower than other bioprinting modalities. Nearly all of laser-based bioprinters (see Table 7.4), reported to date, rely on neodymium-doped yttrium aluminum garnet (Nd:YAG) or excimer [argon fluoride (ArF) or krypton fluoride (KrF)] lasers for pulse generation and have been assembled from commercially available subsystems. In-house built bioprinters are generally expensive as compared to EBB and DBB bioprinters. Currently, there is no commercially available laser-based bioprinters in the market.

Table 7.4 Laser-Based Bioprinters*

	Availability	Bioprinter Name	Country	Bioprinting Mechanism	University/Institution	Use	Dual Bioink Printability
Laser-based bioprinters	Noncommercial	Custom-built laser-based bioprinter	USA	LGDW	University of Minnesota and Michigan Technological University	Embryonic chick spinal cord cells to demonstrate LGDW capabilities (Odde and Renn, 2000), 2D and 3D HUVEC patterns on Matrigel (Nahmias et al., 2005)	–
		Custom-built laser-based bioprinter	USA	LGDW	Michigan Technological University and University of Missouri—Columbia	Evaluation of laser-induced damage on bioprinted avidin biomolecules (proteins) (Xu et al., 2003)	–
		Custom-built laser-based bioprinter based on ArF excimer laser	USA	LIFT and MAPLE-DW	US Naval Research Laboratory	Biotinylated bovine serum albumin (BSA) protein microarray fabrication by using MAPLE-DW (Ringeisen et al., 2002), 2D patterning of human osteosarcoma and rat cardiac cells by using MAPLE-DW (Barron et al., 2004c), 3D patterning of human osteosarcoma cells by using BioLP (Barron et al., 2004c), single cell patterns of human osteosarcoma cells by using BioLP (Barron et al., 2005)	–
		Custom-built laser-based bioprinter based on ArF excimer laser		MAPLE-DW	US Naval Research Laboratory, University of North Carolina at Chapel Hill, Georgia Institute of Technology, Paul Scherrer Institute, Laboratory for Functional Polymers EMPA Swiss Federal Laboratories for Materials Testing and Research Uberlandstrasse, Hungarian Academy of Sciences and University of Szeged, National Institute for Laser and Plasma and Radiation Physics (Romania)	Patterning of viable B35 neuroblasts by using triazene polymer intermediate absorbing layer (Doraiswamy et al., 2006)	–

Custom-built laser-based bioprinter based on ArF excimer laser	USA	MAPLE-DW	US Naval Research Laboratory and University of North Carolina at Chapel Hill	Codeposition of hydroxyapatite and viable MG 63 osteoblast-like cells (Doraiswamy et al., 2007)	–
Custom-built laser-based bioprinter based on ArF excimer laser	USA	MAPLE-DW	Clemson University, University of Florida, Rensselaer Polytechnic Institute, and Tulane University	Laser fluence (energy) impact on yeast (Lin et al., 2009) and human colon cancer cells viability (Lin et al., 2010), alginate long tubes and annular constructs fabrication (Yan et al., 2013), alginate gelation impact on bioprinted NIH 3T3 cell viability (Gudapati et al., 2014) and bifurcated hollow tubular tissue (NIH 3T3 cells and alginate) constructs (Xiong et al., 2015a)	–
Custom-built laser-based bioprinter based on Nd:YAG laser	Germany	LIFT	Laser Zentrum Hannover e.V., Hannover Medical School, and Helmholtz Institute of the RWTH Aachen University	3D cell arrays comprising endothelial colony forming cells (ECFCs) and adipose-derived stem cells (ASCs) to study cell-to-cell interactions in 3D environments (Gruene et al., 2011a,b), skin tissue consisting of NIH-3T3 fibroblasts, human keratinocyte cells and collagen (Koch et al., 2012), and LaBP process impact on adipogenic stem cell proliferation and differentiation (Gruene et al., 2011a,b)	–
Custom-built laser-based bioprinter based on KrF excimer laser	USA and Hungary	LIFT	Hungarian Academy of Sciences and University of Szeged, University of Szeged, and US Naval Research Laboratory	AFA–LIFT impact on viability and proliferation of bioprinted rat Schwann and astroglial cells and pig lens epithelial cells (Hopp et al., 2005)	–

N/A, Information not available; –, capable of bioprinting only one bioink at a time; *ArF*, argon fluoride; *BioLP*, biological laser printing; *LGDW*, laser-guided direct writing; *HUVEC*, human umbilical vein endothelial cell; *LIFT*, laser-induced forward transfer; *MAPLE-DW*, matrix-assisted pulsed-laser evaporation-direct writes.

*Modified or custom-built 3D printers used in photopolymerization-involved processes are excluded in this table.

7.3 Limitations

Despite the great progress in bioprinting processes and the latest advancements in bioprinter technologies along with a number of bioprinters recently introduced into the market, bioprinter technologies still exhibit a myriad of weaknesses, as outlined below, that are vital to make the technology highly robust and affordable for functional tissue fabrication, and available for clinical use (Ozbolat and Hospodiuk, 2016).

7.3.1 Limited Variety of the Commercially Available Bioprinters

Despite the great progress in commercialization of bioprinter technologies, a vast majority of the efforts is limited to extrusion-based bioprinters and a very small attention has been paid to other bioprinting technologies such as LBB and DBB. Currently available extrusion-based bioprinters, on the other hand, are similar to each other with small variations in their functionality such as advanced automation in cartridge replacement, automated loading and unloading capability of the bioink solution, and different software capabilities in terms of the motion system. Although there is a wide variety of inkjet-based printers in the market, the majority of the inkjet printers are equipped with a highly small nozzle orifice opening, which is not convenient for bioprinting mammalian cells with an average diameter of 20–25 μm. In addition to commercially available bioprinters, commercial 3D printers with open-source architecture is also highly helpful for researchers as some research groups prefer to customize their own bioprinters based on the final use. For example, Fig. 7.9A shows a bioprinter modified from a Solidoodle Workbench Apprentice, which is an open-source 3D printer. After modifying its FDM extruders into a pneumatically driven EBB mechanism (Fig. 7.9B), Pluronic F-127 hydrogel was printed on a thermally controlled table in the form of concentric cylinders (Fig. 7.9C).

7.3.2 Cartridge and Nozzle Design

Current technologies have major issues with the cartridge and nozzle design as loading and unloading a bioink solution, as well as bioprinting of it, is highly vital for the success of a bioprinting process. Majority of the cartridge technologies allow an operator to load the bioink before starting the bioprinting process. In general, keeping cells in a precursor hydrogel solution during a prolonged bioprinting period can be harmful for cells. NovoGen MMX™ bioprinter overcame that issue by using a dispensing system with aspiration ability that allows operator to load the solution into the pipette automatically using a back pressure mechanism. Although, this provides a great ability for thermally reversible materials (i.e., agarose) and some flexibility to the operator, if there is any clogging occurs, the system is limited to lower viscosity biomaterials particularly during the aspiration process (Kucukgul et al., 2015).

One of the other important aspects of bioprinting is the nozzle selection as the coefficient of friction on the wall of the nozzle tip mediates the shear stress, which might be

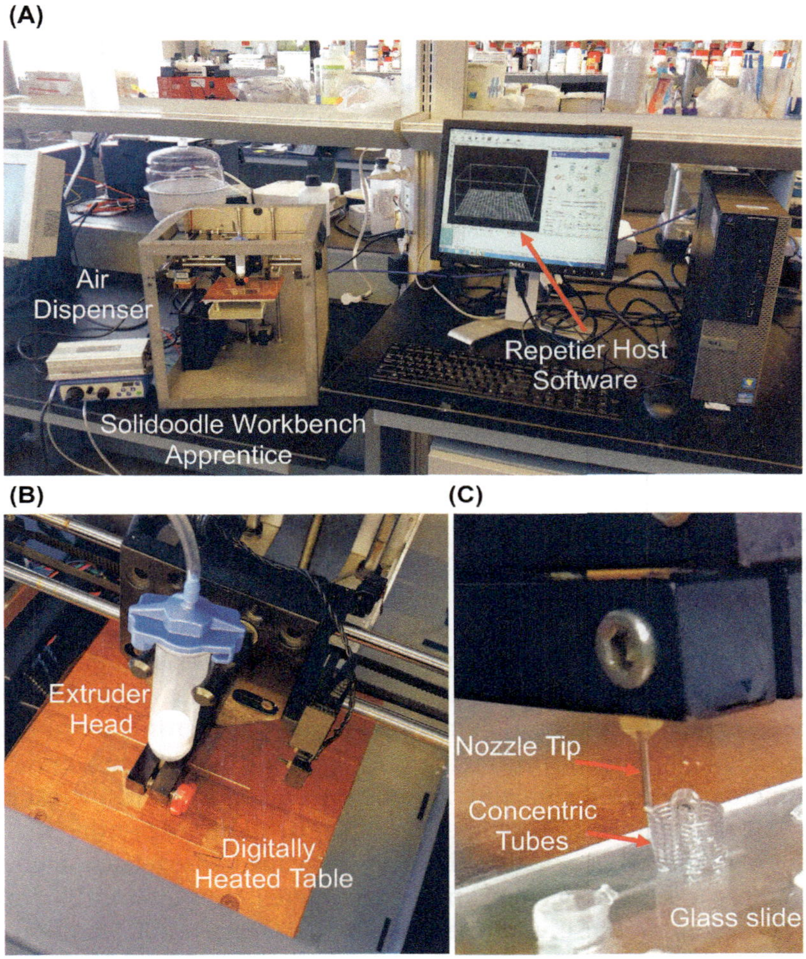

FIGURE 7.9 A Modified low-cost bioprinter. (A) The Solidoodle Workbench Apprentice was modified into an extrusion-based bioprinter (B) with a pneumatic-driven dispensing mechanism and (C) used to bioprint concentric tubes of Pluronic F-127 hydrogel at the Pennsylvania State University, USA.

detrimental for cells. Thus, a surface with a small coefficient of friction and one that is easy to sterilize would be ideal for bioprinting cells, e.g., glass pipettes or ceramic-coated nozzles (Bruzewicz et al., 2012). In addition, new nozzle designs can be considered to decrease the shear stress on cells as well as improve the resolution of bioprinting. In this regards, a cone-shaped nozzle (i.e., Taylor cone or regular cone) might be helpful to alleviate the applied shear stress, which reaches its maximum at the end of the nozzle tip and affects cells at a minimum duration (Franco et al., 2011). In addition to these approaches, a highly innovative approach might be using a nozzle-free extrusion system that enables the bioink to overcome surface tension–induced droplet formation. Only laser- (Xiong et al., 2015b) and acoustic-based (Demirci and Montesano, 2007) bioprinting technologies have nozzle-free configurations, which facilitates the delivery of cells without exposing them to the shear stress.

7.3.3 Size and Speed of Bioprinters

The other limitation in bioprinter technologies is the size of bioprinters. In general, all bioprinters are designed to enable fabrication of small parts in the range of sub centimeter scale and the majority of them are built in very large working envelopes, which bring a major issue during tissue bioprinting mission, such as fitting them into a standard biosafety cabinet. In the mean time, there are bioprinters that are highly compact that do not allow operators to intervene whenever needed. This makes the learning curve of the bioprinter steeper as the operator should interact with the bioprinter head substantially. When the technology transition into a more robust and automated state, bioprinters can be built in a highly compact size in such a way that envisioned tissue fabrication lines can be built within bioreactor chambers under physiologically relevant conditions (Ozbolat and Yu, 2013).

The speed of bioprinting is another concern as the majority of EBB technologies try to cover a large area using a relatively small resolution, which takes significant time when considering several layers in 3D. This becomes even a more serious issue when using other bioprinting modalities, particularly LBB and DBB. DBB can circumvent that situation using multiple nozzles spontaneously; however, smaller resolution contributes to the low speed of bioprinting considerably. Laser-based bioprinters are highly slow as there is only a single laser beam tracing the region of interest; however, the recently developed microarray-based stereolithography systems provide highly fast platforms for bioprinting (Hribar et al., 2014; Zhang et al., 2012). In addition, printing in 3D using soft materials such as hydrogels is highly challenging, while hydrogel shape does not retain itself and changes (i.e., swelling, buckling, bending, etc.), thus bioprinting time should be minimized to overcome these unforeseeable issues. One possible solution to this is to increase the number of printing arms using MABP concept (Ozbolat et al., 2014). An alternative solution is to have an array of nozzles [attached on single arm (Horváth et al., 2015)] separated from each other by a distance close to the desired porosity, which has the ability to rotate along the z-axis to bioprint in x- and y-axis interchangeably.

7.3.4 Limited Motion Capabilities

Although modification of commercially available inkjet printers has been performed for bioprinting of biologics such as cells, DNA, and growth factors, the motion system is limited to 1D or 2D depending on the technology. Therefore, further motion stages are required to expand the motion in 3D such as integrating a motorized table for the movement in z-axis. This can be sometimes highly expensive and difficult to make as it involves cross talk between the existing motion system and the newly integrated one. The vast majority of the bioprinter technologies are limited to 3-axis motion, which is hard to operate when the technology translates into operating rooms for in situ bioprinting purposes (Ozbolat, 2015a). Naturally forming defects are highly complicated in shape and bioprinting for concave cavities or nonplanar defect surfaces may necessitate omnidirectional motion (Ozbolat, 2015a). Thus, additional axes should be integrated to create more freedom, which has a great potential for in situ bioprinting. BioAssemblyBot technology has the potential to overcome the current challenges associated with 3-axis bioprinters.

7.3.5 Lack of Full Automation

Another limitation of bioprinting technologies is the lack of full automation compared to conventional 3D printing processes such as FDM, selective laser sintering, stereolithography, and powder-bed printing. One of the most important facts contributing to this drawback is the raw materials used in 3D printing technologies. For example, materials used in 3D printing processes including plastics, ceramics, or metals are in general in solid form before or after the 3D printing process, which are highly stable. In contrast, biomaterials used in bioprinting processes are in gel or sol—gel form, which cannot be easily formed in high resolution and cannot preserve the given original shape. During the bioprinting process, the shape of the gel can easily change such as it can collapse, swell, or sometimes dehydrate. When the original path-plan is applied, several issues are encountered such as printing level might be higher than the top surface of the printed construct or sometimes the nozzle can hit to the bioprinted construct and drag it. In this case, bioprinting process needs to be restarted from scratch. This issue becomes even more problematic when bioprinting multiple bioink solutions, which can easily mass up the bioprinted constructs. Thus, vision-based process monitoring technologies have been used to detect the bioprinted construct height and inform the bioprinter in real time. Despite these technologies, errors are anticipated and build up gradually, which can affect the overall quality of the bioprinted constructs.

Existing widely used bioink materials, which have greater bioprintability properties such as alginate and Pluronic F-127, do not favor cell growth and proliferation compared to ECM-based bioink materials (Ozbolat and Hospodiuk, 2016). Therefore, researchers acquiring commercially available bioprinters do not employ those bioink materials, rather, most of the bioprinting efforts are embodied to the extent that new biomaterials are investigated and evaluated. Researchers devote a significant effort in understanding the behaviors of these biomaterials. Thus, there is no standardization in bioprinting processes and nearly all bioprinters necessitates a substantial time for the user to ramp up in learning the process.

7.3.6 High Cost of Bioprinting and Bioprinters

One of the other limitations in bioprinting is the high cost of bioprinting and bioprinters. First of all, bioprinting living cells and following in vitro culture is expensive. Particularly, scaffold-free bioprinting approach requires significantly high number of cells in the order of 50–100 million cells to be able to obtain a printable range of sample. Expanding this many cells requires a few months as well as considerable consumption of reagents (Ozbolat, 2015a,b). In addition, the obtained bioink will be highly small in size; thus, the operator does not have much chance to practice the bioprinting process. Therefore, setting up experiments and running them is a challenge and expensive.

The cost of bioprinters is also another concern as the technology is still in its infancy (Ozbolat and Yu, 2013); however, we expect a decrease in the cost of bioprinters as what has been experienced with 3D printers. Currently, the majority of the high-quality and high-resolution bioprinters that are highly automated, lie in the price range of \$150–\$200k. Laser-based bioprinters are not commercially available but the system can be gathered for more than a few hundred thousand dollars in price depending on its capabilities. Inkjet bioprinters can be highly cheap if a commercially available inkjet printer is modified to a bioprinter, but these bioprinters do not support cell printing easily in a highly repeatable form and most of them lack 3D motion capabilities (Xu et al., 2005). More expensive systems are commercially available for biological applications around \$20–70k depending on the number of printhead and the resolution and automation of the system. A great number of start-up companies have been emerging to provide cost-effective and affordable bioprinters for researchers as well as for industry use. For example, affordable dual head bioprinters with thermal and photocrosslinking capabilities range from \$5000 to 10,000; however, the quality, resolution, and operability of these cost-effective bioprinters are not at high standard. Nonetheless, these bioprinters provide unique opportunities as a training tool for researchers. The cost of a basic modified bioprinter, such as the Solidoodle Workbench Apprentice in Fig. 7.9, can even cost less than \$500 excluding the fluid-dispensing system.

7.3.7 Low Process Resolution

The resolution of the bioprinting technology is currently a big impediment in bioprinting high-definition constructs. Here, the author discusses the resolution in the context of the smallest feature size that can be bioprinted rather than the resolution of the motion system. As already discussed before, the resolution of the motion system is considerably higher than that of the bioprinting process itself. Although highly accurate motion stages can be made, a high resolution cannot be achieved on the bioprinted constructs due to several reasons such as instability of hydrogels, swelling and dehydration behavior of hydrogel-based bioink solutions, and the limitations with the nozzle size such as clogging. In general, LBB and DBB processes have high resolution (Dababneh and Ozbolat, 2014); however, the most commonly used bioprinting modality, EBB, suffers tremendously from the resolution perspective. In general, roughly 100 μm is the highest resolution ranges achieved in EBB (Ozbolat and Hospodiuk, 2016). Recent technology using bioplotting (Hinton et al., 2015), on the other hand, facilitates higher resolution, where a plotting medium with microparticles acts line a Bingham plastic possessing solid-like behavior in static condition at low shear stresses (when there is no plotting) and viscous fluid-like behavior at higher shear stresses (when there is plotting). Such system enables retention of the original shape of extruded filaments without spreading and swelling. With this capability, structurally integrated well-defined scaffolds have recently been bioprinted for developing branched vascular constructs and highly complex heart constructs, where the resolution can be further improved using smaller microparticles.

7.3.8 Lack of Compatible Bioink Materials

Bioprintable biomaterials constitute a very small percentage of the biomaterials used in tissue engineering (Ozbolat and Hospodiuk, 2016). When designing and processing new biomaterials, the majority of researchers in the biomaterials field do not consider bioprinting as an end application. Despite the great progress in the last decade, bioprintable biomaterials or bioink materials have several limitations associated with their biological, immunological, microstructural, mechanical, rheological, and chemical properties.

Most of the hydrogel-based bioink materials lack the native-like environment for promoting differentiation and growth of cells into multiple lineages (Ker et al., 2011). While tissues and organs comprise multiple cell types organized spatially, a bioink that supports organization of the heterocellular nature of the tissue microstructure should be developed. As each cell type entails the requirement of using different bioink materials, standardization of bioink materials is of a challenge. In addition, the bioprintability of hydrogels depends on their shear-thinning property, which increases when the viscosity of hydrogels increases. This also favors mechanical and structural properties as well as the formability of complex shapes; however, higher concentration of hydrogels does not favor cell viability and proliferation. In addition, hydrogels do not facilitate close cell-to-cell contact while cells are immobilized and isolated from each other. Thus, scaffold-free bioink materials are highly appealing in that sense as physiologically relevant tissues can be bioprinted but bioprinting of scaffold-free bioink materials is highly challenging as well as their preparation, handling, and cultivation are labor-intensive and expensive (Ozbolat, 2015a,b).

7.3.9 Progress in Bioprinting and Tissue Engineering Research

Advances in bioprinter technologies vitally depend on the progress in various areas including bioprinting, biomaterials, and tissue engineering. More advanced bioprinting processes, which are highly practical for functional tissue fabrication, will support commercialization of these technologies. Although there is a wide spectrum of work has been done in the context of bioprinting, most of them did not aim to generate functional tissues, rather viability and short-term functionality of cells have been evaluated. To translate bioprinter technologies from bench to bedside, new bioprinting and tissue engineering approaches need to be explored and discovered. Most of the work in bioprinting is limited to scaffold-based approach and there is very a few work demonstrated the use of scaffold-free approach facilitating better tissue biomimicry; however, scaffold-free approach lacks mechanical integrity and rigidity (Ozbolat, 2015a,b). Therefore, hybrid technologies are needed to generate mechanically supporting scaffold-based structures along with physiologically relevant scaffold-free tissue modules.

7.3.10 Limited Clinical Translation

The vast majority of the efforts in bioprinting research has taken place in the area of basic science and a limited number of animal trials has been performed for the bioprinted tissues, which is highly critical for translation of the technology into clinics (Ozbolat and Hospodiuk, 2016). This will ultimately necessitate bioprinter technologies and bioprinted tissues and organs to be regulated by Food and Drug Administration (FDA) through a long pathway. FDA currently does not have a classification for bioprinters and bioprinted tissues yet (King et al., 2014). Because of this issue, the emerging bioprinting businesses prefer to stay on the safe side and deliver products that are close to commercialization such as tissues for drug testing and high-throughput screening. One of the other issues slowing down that process is the lack of scale-up tissues at the clinically relevant sizes (Ozbolat, 2015a). Current approaches entail highly small tissue and organ models due to lack of vascularization from arteries and veins down to capillaries. In addition, there are other impediments that should be circumvented such as ethical concerns with the transplantation of bioprinted tissues and organs, consent of the patients regarding use of their cells going through several processes to be used as bioink, mechanical strength and stability of the tissues, long-term in vivo functionality, immune rejection issues as well as other issues related to the engraftment, and innervation of the tissues and organs.

7.4 Future Directions

Despite the great progress in bioprinting technologies, there exists a plethora of room for improvement as well as new directions for investigations. Although several commercial technologies are currently available for EBB, very limited products are available in LBB and DBB. Only a few companies commercialize the inkjet bioprinting technology, therefore more investment can be considered in these areas to utilize the unique strengths of these technologies. Although extrusion-based technologies have been widely preferred for commercialization due to their flexibility and ability to create porous structures (Khoda et al., 2013), further consideration and technological translational effort should be made for other bioprinting modalities.

Although a great progress has been made with novel biomaterials and biomaterial processing techniques, the development of bioink materials that are well suited for bioprinting and allow one to bioprint mechanically and biologically enhanced tissue constructs is still a great need. Particularly, new biomaterials with very quick gelation or solidification capabilities providing a mild environment for cells would be highly desirable. Despite the great success in developing new hydrogels for tissue engineering, not all of them have been adopted to bioprinting. Thus, a new field of study such as "bioprintable biomaterials" under the biomaterials and biofabrication fields could be a great leap to promote research in this direction. In general, highly novel hydrogels should be developed to do the following: promote cell adhesion, proliferation, aggregation, and differentiation toward multiple lineages; exhibit high mechanical integrity and structural stability without dissolving after bioprinting; facilitate engraftment with the endogenous tissue without generating immune response; demonstrate bioprintability with ease of shear thinning, rapid solidification and formability; and be affordable, abundant, and commercially available with appropriate regulatory guidelines for clinical use.

As more standardized bioink materials are introduced for different bioprinting modalities, it will be highly easier for bioprinter builders to standardize and automate their bioprinters and bioprinting processes according to standard properties, which can enable rapid adoption of bioprinter technologies into nonbioprinting communities such as pharmaceutics, clinics, and cancer research. As currently available, LBB is highly challenging to operate and extrusion-based bioprinters need significant learning curve, it is not trivial for someone out of the field to practice these modalities. As inkjet bioprinters are highly automated, its translation into other fields such as pharmaceutics can take place sooner as some pharmaceutical companies have already started experimenting such platforms (Root Analysis, 2014).

For bioprinting scale-up tissues and organs, hybrid bioprinting technologies are desirable in a sense that vascularization can be easily integrated. Current modalities alone do not enable fabrication of blood vessels and the rest of the organs at the same time but integrating multiple modalities, such as EBB for vascular network bioprinting using indirect bioprinting, are extensively explained in our recent work (Ozbolat and Hospodiuk, 2016), and inkjet bioprinting for the rest of the parenchymal tissue. As scale-up tissues and organs necessitate prolonged bioprinting times, faster bioprinters are highly desirable. Alternatively, bioprinters with independent arms running in tandem can be another solution to increase the speed of bioprinting process. Such arms can also be further enhanced by adding extra motion capabilities such as expanding motion capabilities from three axes to five to six axes to bioprint on nonhorizontal or nonplanar surfaces. This is particularly highly vital for in situ bioprinting when the technology translate into clinics (Ozbolat, 2015a).

In addition, online monitoring and inspection capabilities should be integrated into the bioprinter technologies as the quality of bioprinted tissue construct is highly vital as the technology has recently translated into pharmaceutical market for tissue fabrication. In this regard, in situ monitoring capabilities will be quite beneficial such as monitoring the structural integrity and geometric morphology of bioprinted tissue constructs using a machine vision system and the biological quality of the constructs by monitoring the cellular activity through permittivity spectra of cells using a real-time nondestructive metrology tools (Pavillon et al., 2013).

7.5 Summary

With the recently growing demand in bioprinters, bioprinting technology has been further adopted by a broad spectrum of application areas including but not limited to transplantation and clinics, pharmaceutics, high-throughput screening, cancer research, and cosmetology. This chapter discussed the bioprinter technologies and their components along with their working mechanisms and presented an evaluation of commercially existing bioprinters under three different modalities including EBB, DBB, and LBB. Bioprinters currently suffer from several limitations such as low resolution, high cost and size, limited motion freedom and capacity, narrow range of compatible bioink materials, low level of diversity in bioprinter modalities, and nonfunctional end products; however, the author envisions greater progress in bioprinting field in the next decade as well as more emerging businesses that will further advance the state of the art in bioprinter technologies.

References

3Dynamic Systems. Available at: <http://bioprintingsystems.com> (12.03.16.).

Advanced Solutions. BioAssemblyBot—Life Sciences—Advanced Solutions. Available at: <http://www.bioassemblybot.com> (12.03.16.).

Barron, J.A., et al., 2004a. Application of laser printing to mammalian cells. Thin Solid Films 383–387, 453–454.

Barron, J.A., et al., 2004b. Biological laser printing: a novel technique for creating heterogeneous 3-dimensional cell patterns. Biomedical Microdevices 6 (2), 139–147.

Barron, J.A., Krizman, D.B., Ringeisen, B.R., 2005. Laser printing of single cells: statistical analysis, cell viability, and stress. Annals of Biomedical Engineering 33 (2), 121–130.

Barron, J.A., Spargo, B.J., Ringeisen, B.R., 2004c. Biological laser printing of three dimensional cellular structures. Applied Physics A 79 (4–6), 1027–1030.

Bertassoni, L.E., et al., 2014. Hydrogel bioprinted microchannel networks for vascularization of tissue engineering constructs. Lab on a Chip 14 (13), 2202–2211.

Bio3D Technologies. Available at: <http://bio3d.tech/index.html> (12.03.16.).

BioBots. Available at: <https://www.biobots.io> (27.03.16.).

Bodrum, V.H., et al., 2015. Design and construction of a 3D bioprinter for bioprinting of tissues and organs. In: Proceedings of the National Medical Technologies Congress, Mugla, Turkey, pp. 153–157.

Boland, T., et al., 2007. Drop-on-demand printing of cells and materials for designer tissue constructs. Materials Science and Engineering: C 27 (3), 372–376.

Bruzewicz, D.A., Reches, M., Whitesides, G.M., 2012. Low-cost printing of PDMS barriers to define microchannels in paper. Changes 29 (9), 997–1003.

Campbell, P.G., et al., 2005. Engineered spatial patterns of FGF-2 immobilized on fibrin direct cell organization. Biomaterials 26 (33), 6762–6770.

Cellink. No Title. Available at: <http://www.cellink3d.com/>(accessed 27.02.16.).

Cheng, E., Ahmadi, A., Cheung, K.C., 2014. Investigation of the hydrodynamics of suspended cells for reliable inkjet cell printing. In: Processings of the 12th International Conference on Nanochannels, Microchannels and Minichannels, August 3–7.

Chien, K.B., Makridakis, E., Shah, R.N., 2012. Three dimensional printing of soy protein scaffolds for tissue regeneration. Tissue Engineering Part C: Methods 19 (6), 417–426.

Choi, W.S., et al., 2011. Synthetic multicellular cell-to-cell communication in inkjet printed bacterial cell systems. Biomaterials 32 (10), 2500–2507.

Christensen, K., et al., 2015. Freeform inkjet printing of cellular structures with bifurcations. Biotechnology and Bioengineering 112 (5), 1047–1055.

Coatnye, S., et al., 2013. 3D Bio-Printing. Technical Report No. 2013.04.07.

Cohen, D.L., et al., 2010a. Additive manufacturing for in situ repair of osteochondral defects. Biofabrication 2 (3), 035004.

Cohen, D.L., et al., 2010b. Increased mixing improves hydrogel homogeneity and quality of three-dimensional printed constructs. Tissue Engineering Part C: Methods 17 (2), 239–248.

Cui, X., et al., 2012a. Direct human cartilage repair using three-dimensional bioprinting technology. Tissue Engineering Part A 18 (11–12), 1304–1312.

Cui, X., et al., 2012b. Synergistic action of fibroblast growth factor-2 and transforming growth factor-beta1 enhances bioprinted human neocartilage formation. Biotechnology and Bioengineering 109 (9), 2357–2368.

Cui, X., Boland, T., 2009. Human microvasculature fabrication using thermal inkjet printing technology. Biomaterials 30 (31), 6221–6227.

Dababneh, A.B., Ozbolat, I.T., 2014. Bioprinting technology: a current state-of-the-art review. Journal of Manufacturing Science and Engineering 136 (6), 061016.

Demirci, U., Montesano, G., 2007. Single cell epitaxy by acoustic picolitre droplets. Lab on a Chip 7 (9), 1139–1145.

Derby, B., 2010. Inkjet printing of functional and structural materials: fluid property requirements, feature stability, and resolution. Annual Review of Materials Research 40 (1), 395–414.

Doraiswamy, A., et al., 2006. Excimer laser forward transfer of mammalian cells using a novel triazene absorbing layer. Applied Surface Science 252 (13), 4743–4747.

Doraiswamy, A., et al., 2007. Laser microfabrication of hydroxyapatite-osteoblast-like cell composites. Journal of Biomedical Materials Research. Part A 80 (3), 635–643.

Duan, B., et al., 2013. 3D bioprinting of heterogeneous aortic valve conduits with alginate/gelatin hydrogels. Journal of Biomedical Materials Research Part A 101A (5), 1255–1264.

Duan, B., et al., 2014. Three-dimensional printed trileaflet valve conduits using biological hydrogels and human valve interstitial cells. Acta Biomaterialia 10 (5), 1836–1846.

Eagles, P.A., Qureshi, A.N., Jayasinghe, S.N., 2006. Electrohydrodynamic jetting of mouse neuronal cells. The Biochemical Journal 394 (Pt 2), 375–378.

Edwin, G., et al., Three-dimensional (3D) bone tissues derived from stem cells as a novel model for mineralization, p. Poster no. 23.

EnvisionTEC. Available at: <http://envisiontec.com> (27.02.16.).

Ersumo, N.T., Spiller, K.L., 2015. Effects of hydrogel properties and extrusion parameters on 3D bio-printing. IEEE 25–26.

Fang, Y., et al., 2012. Rapid generation of multiplexed cell cocultures using acoustic droplet ejection followed by aqueous two-phase exclusion patterning. Tissue Engineering Part C: Methods 18 (9), 647–657.

Faulkner-Jones, A., et al., 2015. Bioprinting of human pluripotent stem cells and their directed differentiation into hepatocyte-like cells for the generation of mini-livers in 3D. Biofabrication 7 (4), 044102.

Faulkner-Jones, A., et al., 2013. Development of a valve-based cell printer for the formation of human embryonic stem cell spheroid aggregates. Biofabrication 5 (1), 015013.

Fedorovich, N.E., et al., 2011. Distinct tissue formation by heterogeneous printing of osteo- and endothelial progenitor cells. Tissue Engineering Part A 17, 2113–2121.

Fedorovich, N.E., et al., 2008. Three-dimensional fiber deposition of cell-laden, viable, patterned constructs for bone tissue printing. Tissue Engineering Part A 14 (1), 127–133.

Ferris, C.J., et al., 2013. Bio-ink for on-demand printing of living cells. Biomaterials Science 1 (2), 224–230.

Franco, J., Hunger, P., Launey, M.E., Tomsia, A.P., Saiz, E., 2011. Direct-write assembly of calcium phosphate scaffolds using a water-based hydrogel. Acta Biomaterialia 6 (1), 218–228.

Gao, G., et al., 2014. Bioactive nanoparticles stimulate bone tissue formation in bioprinted three-dimensional scaffold and human mesenchymal stem cells. Biotechnology Journal 9 (10), 1304–1311.

Gao, G., et al., 2015. Inkjet-bioprinted acrylated peptides and PEG hydrogel with human mesenchymal stem cells promote robust bone and cartilage formation with minimal printhead clogging. Biotechnology Journal 10 (10), 1568–1577.

Gasperini, L., et al., 2015. An electrohydrodynamic bioprinter for alginate hydrogels containing living cells. Tissue Engineering Part C: Methods 21 (2), 123–132.

Gasperini, L., Maniglio, D., Migliaresi, C., 2013. Microencapsulation of cells in alginate through an electrohydrodynamic process. Journal of Bioactive and Compatible Polymers 28, 413–425.

Gruene, M., et al., 2011a. Adipogenic differentiation of laser-printed 3D tissue grafts consisting of human adipose-derived stem cells. Biofabrication 3 (1), 015005.

Gruene, M., et al., 2011b. Laser printing of three-dimensional multicellular arrays for studies of cell–cell and cell–environment interactions. Tissue Engineering Part C: Methods 17 (10), 973–982.

Gudapati, H., et al., 2014. Alginate gelation-induced cell death during laser-assisted cell printing. Biofabrication 6 (3), 035022.

Gurkan, U.A., et al., 2014. Engineering anisotropic biomimetic fibrocartilage microenvironment by bioprinting mesenchymal stem cells in nanoliter gel droplets. Molecular Pharmaceutics 11 (7), 2151–2159.

Hinton, T.J., et al., 2015. Three-dimensional printing of complex biological structures by freeform reversible embedding of suspended hydrogels. Science Advances 1 (9).

Hong, S., et al., 2013. Cellular behavior in micropatterned hydrogels by bioprinting system depended on the cell types and cellular interaction. Journal of Bioscience and Bioengineering 116 (2), 224–230.

Hopp, B., et al., 2005. Survival and proliferative ability of various living cell types after laser-induced forward transfer. Tissue Engineering 11 (11–12), 1817–1823.

Horváth, L., et al., 2015. Engineering an in vitro air-blood barrier by 3D bioprinting. Scientific Reports 5, 7974.

Hribar, K.C., et al., 2014. Light-assisted direct-write of 3D functional biomaterials. Lab on a Chip 14 (2), 268–275.

Jayasinghe, S.N., Edirisinghe, M.J., 2004. Electrostatic atomisation of a ceramic suspension. Journal of the European Ceramic Society 24 (8), 2203–2213.

Jayasinghe, S.N., Qureshi, A.N., Eagles, P.A.M., 2006. Electrohydrodynamic jet processing: an advanced electric-field-driven jetting phenomenon for processing living cells. Small (Weinheim an der Bergstrasse, Germany) 2 (2), 216–219.

Jayasinghe, S.N., Townsend-Nicholson, A., 2006. Stable electric-field driven cone-jetting of concentrated biosuspensions. Lab on a Chip 6 (8), 1086–1090.

Jia, J., et al., 2014. Engineering alginate as bioink for bioprinting. Acta Biomaterialia 10 (10), 4323–4331.

Ker, E.D.F., et al., 2011. Engineering spatial control of multiple differentiation fates within a stem cell population. Biomaterials 32 (13), 3413–3422.

Khalil, S., Nam, J., Sun, W., 2005. Multi-nozzle deposition for construction of 3-D biopolymer tissue scaffolds. Rapid Prototyping Journal 11, 9–17.

Khoda, A.K.M., Ozbolat, I.T., Koc, B., 2013. Designing heterogeneous porous tissue scaffolds for additive manufacturing processes. Computer Aided Design 45 (12), 1507–1523.

Khoda, A.K.M., Ozbolat, I.T., Koc, B., 2011. Engineered tissue scaffolds with variational porous architecture. Journal of Biomechanical Engineering 133 (1), 011001.

Kim, H.S., et al., 2007. Optimization of electrohydrodynamic writing technique to print collagen. Experimental Techniques 31 (4), 15–19.

King, S.M., et al., 2013. Development of 3D bioprinted human breast cancer for in vitro screening of therapeutics targeted against cancer progression. In: Poster Presented to American Society of Cell Biology Annual Meeting, New Orleans, 14–18 December.

King, S.M., Presnell, S.C., Nguyen, D.G., 2014. Development of 3D bioprinted human breast cancer for in vitro drug screening. Cancer Research 74 (19), 2034.

Klebe, R.J., 1988. Cytoscribing: a method for micropositioning cells and the construction of two- and three-dimensional synthetic tissues. Experimental Cell Research 179 (2), 362–373.

Koch, L., et al., 2010. Laser printing of skin cells and human stem cells. Tissue Engineering Part C Methods 16 (5), 847–854.

Koch, L., et al., 2012. Skin tissue generation by laser cell printing. Biotechnology and Bioengineering 109 (7), 1855–1863.

Kolesky, D., et al., 2014. Bioprinting: 3D bioprinting of vascularized, heterogeneous cell-laden tissue constructs. Advanced Materials 26 (19), 2966.

Kucukgul, C., et al., 2015. 3D bioprinting of biomimetic aortic vascular constructs with self-supporting cells. Biotechnology and Bioengineering 112 (4), 811–821.

Landers, R., et al., 2002. Rapid prototyping of scaffolds derived from thermoreversible hydrogels and tailored for applications in tissue engineering. Biomaterials 23 (23), 4437–4447.

Lee, V., et al., 2014. Generation of multi-scale vascular network system within 3D hydrogel using 3D bioprinting technology. Cellular and Molecular Bioengineering 7 (3), 460–472.

Lee, W., et al., 2009a. Multi-layered culture of human skin fibroblasts and keratinocytes through three-dimensional freeform fabrication. Biomaterials 30 (8), 1587–1595.

Lee, W., et al., 2010a. On-demand three-dimensional freeform fabrication of multi-layered hydrogel scaffold with fluidic channels. Biotechnology and Bioengineering 105 (6), 1178–1186.

Lee, W., et al., 2009b. Three-dimensional bioprinting of rat embryonic neural cells. NeuroReport 20 (8), 798–803.

Lee, Y.-B., et al., 2010b. Bio-printing of collagen and VEGF-releasing fibrin gel scaffolds for neural stem cell culture. Experimental Neurology 223 (2), 645–652.

Li, C., et al., 2015a. Rapid formation of a supramolecular polypeptide-DNA hydrogel for in situ three-dimensional multilayer bioprinting. Angewandte Chemie (International ed. in English) 54 (13), 3957–3961.

Li, Y., et al., 2015b. Current status of additive manufacturing for tissue engineering scaffold. Rapid Prototyping Journal 21 (6), 747–762.

Lin, Y., et al., 2010. Effect of laser fluence in laser-assisted direct writing of human colon cancer cell. Rapid Prototyping Journal 16 (3), 202–208.

Lin, Y., et al., 2009. Effect of laser fluence on yeast cell viability in laser-assisted cell transfer. Journal of Applied Physics 106 (4), 043106.

Lin, Y., Huang, Y., 2011. Laser-assisted fabrication of highly viscous alginate microsphere. Journal of Applied Physics 109 (8), 083107.

Malone, E., Lipson, H., 2007. Fab@Home: the personal desktop fabricator kitnull. Rapid Prototyping Journal 13 (4), 245–255.

Mannoor, M.S., et al., 2013. 3D printed bionic ears. Nano Letters 13 (6), 2634–2639.

Markstedt, K., et al., 2015. 3D bioprinting human chondrocytes with nanocellulose–alginate bioink for cartilage tissue engineering applications. Biomacromolecules 16 (5), 1489–1496.

Matsusaki, M., et al., 2013. Three-dimensional human tissue chips fabricated by rapid and automatic inkjet cell printing. Advanced Healthcare Materials 2 (4), 534–539.

Microdrop Technologies. Available at: <http://microdrop.com> (3.03.16.).

Miller, E.D., et al., 2006. Dose-dependent cell growth in response to concentration modulated patterns of FGF-2 printed on fibrin. Biomaterials 27 (10), 2213–2221.

Mongkoldhumrongkul, N., et al., 2009. Bio-electrospraying whole human blood: analysing cellular viability at a molecular level. Journal of Tissue Engineering and Regenerative Medicine 3 (7), 562–566.

Moon, S., et al., 2010. Layer by layer three-dimensional tissue epitaxy by cell-laden hydrogel droplets. Tissue engineering Part C, Methods 16 (1), 157–166.

Morrison, N.F., Harlen, O.G., 2010. Viscoelasticity in inkjet printing. Rheologica Acta 49 (6), 619–632.

Murphy, S.V., Skardal, A., Atala, A., 2013. Evaluation of hydrogels for bio-printing applications. Journal of Biomedical Materials Research - Part A 101 A (1), 272–284.

Nahmias, Y., et al., 2005. Laser-guided direct writing for three-dimensional tissue engineering. Biotechnology and Bioengineering 92 (2), 129–136.

Ng, W.L., Yeong, W.Y., Naing, M.W., 2016. Polyelectrolyte gelatin-chitosan hydrogel optimized for 3D bioprinting in skin tissue engineering. International Journal of Bioprinting 2 (1), 53–62.

Nishiyama, Y., et al., 2008. Development of a three-dimensional bioprinter: construction of cell supporting structures using hydrogel and state-of-the-art inkjet technology. Journal of Biomechanical Engineering 131 (3), 35001.

Norotte, C., et al., 2009. Scaffold-free vascular tissue engineering using bioprinting. Biomaterials 30 (30), 5910–5917.

nScript. Available at: <http://nscrypt.com> (27.02.16.).

Odde, D.J., Renn, M.J., 1999. Laser-guided direct writing for applications in biotechnology. Trends in Biotechnology 17 (10), 385–389.

Odde, D.J., Renn, M.J., 2000. Laser-guided direct writing of living cells. Biotechnology and bioengineering 67 (3), 312–318.

Onses, M.S., et al., 2015. Mechanisms, capabilities, and applications of high-resolution electrohydrodynamic jet printing. Small (Weinheim der Bergstrasse, Germany) 11 (34), 4237–4266.

Ozbolat, I., 2015a. Scaffold-based or scaffold-free bioprinting: competing or complementing approaches? Journal of Nanotechnology in Engineering and Medicine 6 (2), 1–6.

Ozbolat, I.T., 2015b. Bioprinting scale-up tissue and organ constructs for transplantation. Trends in Biotechnology 33 (7), 395–400.

Ozbolat, I.T., Chen, H., Yu, Y., 2014. Development of "Multi-arm Bioprinter" for hybrid biofabrication of tissue engineering constructs. Robotics and Computer-Integrated Manufacturing 30 (3), 295–304.

Ozbolat, I.T., Hospodiuk, M., 2016. Current advances and future perspectives in extrusion-based bioprinting. Biomaterials 76, 321–343.

Ozbolat, I.T., Khoda, A.K.M., 2014. Design of a new parametric path plan for additive manufacturing of hollow porous structures with functionally graded materials. Journal of Computing and Information Science in Engineering 14 (4), 41005.

Ozbolat, I.T., Koc, B., 2010. Modeling of spatially controlled biomolecules in three dimensional porous alginate structures. ASME Transactions, Journal of Medical Devices 4 (4), 041003(1)–041003(11).

Ozbolat, I.T., Koc, B., 2011. Multi-function based modeling of 3D heterogeneous wound scaffolds for improved wound healing. Computer-Aided Design and Applications 8 (1), 43–57.

Ozbolat, I.T., Yu, Y., 2013. Bioprinting toward organ fabrication: challenges and future trends. IEEE Transactions on Bio-Medical Engineering 60 (3), 691–699.

Pati, F., et al., 2015. Biomimetic 3D tissue printing for soft tissue regeneration. Biomaterials 62, 164–175.

Pati, F., et al., 2014. Printing three-dimensional tissue analogues with decellularized extracellular matrix bioink. Nature Communications 5 (3935).

Pavillon, N., Hobro, A.J., Smith, N.I., 2013. Cell optical density and molecular composition revealed by simultaneous multimodal label-free imaging. Biophysical Journal 105 (5), 1123–1132.

Pfister, A., et al., 2004. Biofunctional rapid prototyping for tissue-engineering applications: 3D bioplotting versus 3D printing. J.ournal of Polymer Science Part A: Polymer Chemistry 42 (3), 624–638.

Phillippi, J.A., et al., 2008. Microenvironments engineered by inkjet bioprinting spatially direct adult stem cells toward muscle- and bone-like subpopulations. Stem Cells 26 (1), 127–134.

Poellmann, M.J., et al., 2011. Patterned hydrogel substrates for cell culture with electrohydrodynamic jet printing. Macromolecular Bioscience 11 (9), 1164–1168.

Poldervaart, M.T., et al., 2013. Sustained release of BMP-2 in bioprinted alginate for osteogenicity in mice and rats. PloS One 8 (8), e72610.

Regemat3D. Available at: <http://regemat3d.com/versions> (12.03.16.).

Regenhu Biosystems Architects. Available at: <http://www.regenhu.com> (27.02.16.).

Regenovo Biotechnology Co, Ltd. <http://regenovo.com/english/index.aspx> (27.02.16.).

Renn, M., Pastel, R., Lewandowski, H., 1999. Laser guidance and trapping of mesoscale particles in hollow-core optical fibers. Physical Review Letters 82 (7), 1574–1577.

Ringeisen, B.R., et al., 2006. Jet-based methods to print living cells. Biotechnology Journal 1 (9), 930–948.

Ringeisen, B.R., et al., 2004. Laser printing of pluripotent embryonal carcinoma cells. Tissue Engineering 10 (3–4), 483–491.

Ringeisen, B.R., et al., 2002. Picoliter-scale protein microarrays by laser direct write. Biotechnology Progress 18 (5), 1126–1129.

Robbins, J.B., et al., 2013. Bioprinted three-dimensional (3D) human liver constructs provide a model for interrogating liver biology. FASEB Journal 27, 6275.

Rodríguez-Dévora, J.I., et al., 2012. High throughput miniature drug-screening platform using bioprinting technology. Biofabrication 4 (3), 035001.

Root Analysis, 2014. 3D Bioprinting Market, pp. 2014–2030.

Roskos, K., et al., 2015. Essentials of 3D Biofabrication and Translation. Elsevier.

Roth, E., et al., 2004. Inkjet printing for high-throughput cell patterning. Biomaterials 25 (17), 3707–3715.

Seraph Robotics. Scientis 3D Printer. Available at: <http://www.scientist3d.com> (12.03.16.).

Seyednejad, H., et al., 2011. Preparation and characterization of a three-dimensional printed scaffold based on a functionalized polyester for bone tissue engineering applications. Acta Biomaterialia 7 (5), 1999–2006.

Sheshadri, P., Shirwaiker, R.A., 2015. Characterization of material–process–structure interactions in the 3D bioplotting of polycaprolactone. 3D Printing and Additive Manufacturing 2 (1), 20–31.

Shim, J.-H., et al., 2012. Bioprinting of a mechanically enhanced three-dimensional dual cell-laden construct for osteochondral tissue engineering using a multi-head tissue/organ building system. Journal of Micromechanics and Microengineering 22, 085014.

Singh, M., et al., 2010. Inkjet printing-process and its applications. Advanced Materials 22 (6), 673–685.

Skardal, A., Atala, A., 2015. Biomaterials for integration with 3-D bioprinting. Annals of Biomedical Engineering 43 (3), 730–746.

Smith, C.M., et al., 2004. Three-dimensional Bioassembly tool for generating viable tissue-engineered constructs. Tissue Engneering 10 (9), 1566–1576.

Song, S.J., et al., 2010. A three-dimensional bioprinting system for use with a hydrogel-based biomaterial and printing parameter characterization. Artificial Organs 34, 1044–1048.

Suntivich, R., et al., 2014. Inkjet printing of silk nest arrays for cell hosting. Biomacromolecules 15 (4), 1428–1435.

Sutanto, E., et al., 2012. A multimaterial electrohydrodynamic jet (E-jet) printing system. Journal of Micromechanics and Microengineering 22 (4), 045008.

SYS+ENG. Available at: <http://www.syseng.de/produkte/index.html> (12.03.16.).

Tan, E.Y.S., Yeong, W.Y., 2015. Concentric bioprinting of alginate-based tubular constructs using multi-nozzle extrusion-based technique. International Journal of Bioprinting 1, 49–56.

Tasoglu, S., Demirci, U., 2013. Bioprinting for stem cell research. Trends Biotechnology 31 (1), 10–19.

Visser, J., et al., 2013. Biofabrication of multi-material anatomically shaped tissue constructs. Biofabrication 5, 035007.

Wang, L., et al., 2016. Automated quantitative assessment of three-dimensional bioprinted hydrogel scaffolds using optical coherence tomography. Biomedical Optics Express 7 (3), 894.

Wijshoff, H., 2010. The dynamics of the piezo inkjet printhead operation. Physics Reports 491 (4–5), 77–177.

Wilson, W.C., Boland, T., 2003. Cell and organ printing 1: protein and cell printers. The Anatomical Record Part A: Discoveries in Molecular, Cellular, and Evolutionary Biology 272 (2), 491–496.

Workman, V.L., et al., 2014. Controlled generation of microspheres incorporating extracellular matrix fibrils for three-dimensional cell culture. Advanced Functional Materials 24 (18), 2648–2657.

Wu, C., et al., 2011. Three-dimensional printing of hierarchical and tough mesoporous bioactive glass scaffolds with a controllable pore architecture, excellent mechanical strength and mineralization ability. Acta Biomaterialia 7 (6), 2644–2650.

Xie, J., Wang, C.-H., 2007. Electrospray in the dripping mode for cell microencapsulation. Journal of Colloid and Interface Science 312 (2), 247–255.

Xiong, R., et al., 2015a. Freeform drop-on-demand laser printing of 3D alginate and cellular constructs. Biofabrication 7 (4), 045011.

Xiong, R., Zhang, Z., Huang, Y., 2015b. Identification of optimal printing conditions for laser printing of alginate tubular constructs. Journal of Manufacturing Processes 20, 450–455.

Xu, C., et al., 2012. Scaffold-free inkjet printing of three-dimensional zigzag cellular tubes. Biotechnology and Bioengineering 109 (12), 3152–3160.

Xu, F., et al., 2010. A droplet-based building block approach for bladder smooth muscle cell (SMC) proliferation. Biofabrication 2 (1), 014105.

Xu, F., et al., 2011. A three-dimensional in vitro ovarian cancer coculture model using a high-throughput cell patterning platform. Biotechnology Journal 6 (2), 204–212.

Xu, J., Grant, S.A., Pastel, R.L., 2003. Laser-guided direct writing: a novel method to deposit biomolecules for biosensors arrays. IEEE Transactions on Biomedical Engineering 50 (1), 126–128.

Xu, T., et al., 2013a. Complex heterogeneous tissue constructs containing multiple cell types prepared by inkjet printing technology. Biomaterials 34 (1), 130–139.

Xu, T., et al., 2009. Fabrication and characterization of bio-engineered cardiac pseudo tissues. Biofabrication 1 (3), 035001.

Xu, T., et al., 2008. High-throughput production of single-cell microparticles using an inkjet printing technology. Journal of Manufacturing Science and Engineering 130 (2), 021017.

Xu, T., et al., 2013b. Hybrid printing of mechanically and biologically improved constructs for cartilage tissue engineering applications. Biofabrication 5 (1), 015001.

Xu, T., et al., 2005. Inkjet printing of viable mammalian cells. Biomaterials 26 (1), 93–99.

Xu, T., et al., 2006. Viability and electrophysiology of neural cell structures generated by the inkjet printing method. Biomaterials 27 (19), 3580–3588.

Yamaguchi, S., et al., 2012. Cell patterning through inkjet printing of one cell per droplet. Biofabrication 4, 045005.

Yan, J., Huang, Y., Chrisey, D.B., 2013. Laser-assisted printing of alginate long tubes and annular constructs. Biofabrication 5, 015002.

Yanez, M., et al., 2014. In vivo assessment of printed microvasculature in a bilayer skin graft to treat full-thickness wounds. Tissue Engineering Part A 21 (1–2), 224–233.

Yu, Y., Zhang, Y., Ozbolat, I.T., 2014. A hybrid bioprinting approach for scale-up tissue fabrication. Journal of Manufacturing Science and Engineering 136 (6), 61013.

Yusof, A., et al., 2011. Inkjet-like printing of single-cells. Lab on a chip 11 (14), 2447–2454.

Zhang, A.P., et al., 2012. Rapid fabrication of complex 3D extracellular microenvironments by dynamic optical projection stereolithography. Advanced Materials 24 (31), 4266–4270.

Zhang, Y., et al., 2015. In vitro study of directly bioprinted perfusable vasculature conduits. Biomaterials Science 3 (1), 134–143.

Zou, F., et al., 2016. Enhanced osteogenic differentiation and biomineralization in mouse mesenchymal stromal cells on a β-TCP robocast scaffold modified with collagen nanofibers. RSC Advances 6 (28), 23588–23598.

Further Reading

Akkouch, A., Yu, Y., Ozbolat, I.T., 2015. Microfabrication of scaffold-free tissue strands for three-dimensional tissue engineering. Biofabrication 7 (3), 31002.

Dolati, F., et al., 2014. In vitro evaluation of carbon-nanotube-reinforced bioprintable vascular conduits. Nanotechnology 25 (14), 145101.

Jayasinghe, S.M., Edirisinghe, M.J., De Wilde, T., 2002. A novel ceramic printing technique based on electrostatic atomization of a suspension. Materials Research Innovations 6 (3), 92–95.

MicroFab Technologies Inc. Available at: <http://microfab.com> (03.03.16.).

8 Roadmap to Organ Printing

CHAPTER OUTLINE

8.1 Introduction

Despite the increase in donors, organ shortage continues to be problematic. For example, in 2008, more than 28,000 patients received transplants in the United States and 50,463 new patients were added to transplantation wait list 1 year later; nearly half of them received a transplant but quarter of them died while waiting for a suitable organ (Saidi and Hejazii Kenari, 2014). The long-term solution to this problem, as with the solutions to other grand engineering challenges, requires building or manufacturing living organs from an individual's own cells. For the past three decades, tissue engineering has emerged as a multidisciplinary field involving scientists, engineers, and physicians, for the purpose of creating biological substitutes mimicking native tissue to replace damaged tissues or restore malfunctioning organs (Langer and Vacanti, 1993). The traditional tissue engineering strategy is to seed cells onto scaffolds, which can then proliferate and differentiate, and remodel three-dimensional (3D) functional tissues. Tissues and organs that are anatomically thin or avascular, such as skin, cartilage, bone, bladder, etc., have been successfully engineered (Fisher and Mauck, 2012). Although significant progress has been made in the past decade both in research and clinical applications, it is obvious that complex 3D organs require more precise multicellular structures with vascular network integration, which cannot be accomplished by traditional methods (Ozbolat, 2015).

3D bioprinting processes have emerged to deposit living cells for 3D tissue and organ fabrication using extrusion-based bioprinting (EBB) (Ozbolat and Hospodiuk, 2016), droplet-based bioprinting (DBB) (Gudapati et al., 2016), and laser-based bioprinting (LBB) (Piqué, 2011), as detailed in Chapters 4–6, respectively. Bioprinting offers great precision for the spatial placement of cells, rather than merely providing scaffold support. Although still in its infancy, this technology appears to be a promising avenue for advancing tissue engineering toward organ fabrication, ultimately mitigating organ shortage and saving lives. Fig. 8.1 demonstrates the concept of futuristic 3D direct organ printing technology, where multiple living cells with supportive media stored in cartridges are printed layer by layer using DBB technology. It offers a controllable fabrication process, which allows precise placement of various biomaterial and/or cell types simultaneously according to the natural arrangement within the target tissue or organs. Multiple cell types, including organ-specific cells from both stroma (i.e., fibroblasts,

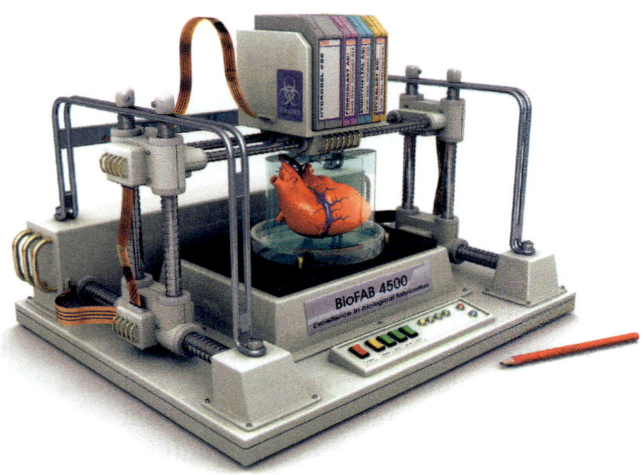

FIGURE 8.1 Organ Printing Concept. 3D functional organs are printed bottom-up using living cells in a supportive medium *(Image courtesy of Christopher Barnatt, www.explainingthefuture.com).*

smooth muscle, and endothelial cells) and parenchyma (i.e., hepatocytes, stellate, Kupffer, and liver sinusoidal endothelial cells for liver) constitute the entire organ. Although the concept seems to be trivial considering the complexity and functionality of the parts that can be manufactured using contemporary 3D printing technology, several challenges impede the evolution of organ printing (Ozbolat and Yu, 2013).

Despite the progress in tissue engineering, several issues must be addressed for organ printing to become a reality. The most critical challenge in organ printing is the integration of a vascular network, a problem that faces the majority of tissue engineering technologies. Without vascularization, engineered 3D thick tissue or organs cannot get enough nutrients or efficiently exchange gasses, and remove waste, all of which are needed for tissue maturation during perfusion. This results in low cell viability and malfunction of artificial organs. Systems must be developed to transport nutrients, growth factors, and oxygen to cells while extracting metabolic waste products such as lactic acid, carbon dioxide, and hydrogen ions so the cells can grow and organize to form the organ. Cells in a large 3D organ structure cannot maintain function without a transport system traditionally provided by blood vessels. Blood vessels are an intraorgan branched vascular tree that is a part of the circulatory system in the human body. Fluid and media transport as well as oxygenation takes place at the capillary level. Bioprinting technology, on the other hand, currently does not allow organ fabrication where bifurcated vessels are manufactured with capillaries to mimic natural vascular anatomy. Although several researchers have investigated the development of vascular trees using computer models (Mondy et al., 2009), only a few attempts have been made toward fabricating bifurcated or branched channels so far (Norotte et al., 2009). Successful tissue maturation with a functional mechanically integrated bifurcated blood vessel network is still not a reality.

8.2 State-of-the-Art in Organ Printing

Bioprinting of organs of the clinically relevant dimensions has yet to be performed (Ozbolat, 2015). Up to now, there are two major strategies followed for organ printing including scaffold-free and scaffold-based approaches.

Using scaffold-free approach, Forgacs and his coworkers at the University of Missouri, Columbia, bioprinted heterocellular tissue spheroids, producing scaffold-free vascular constructs (Norotte et al., 2009). Upon fusion of tissue spheroids followed by a tissue maturation process of 3 days postbioprinting, the support material was removed manually to generate the lumen. Multiple cell types, including human umbilical vein smooth muscle cells and human skin fibroblast cells, were printed together to fabricate multicellular constructs. The same group also demonstrated bioprinting of cell pellets, instead of tissue spheroids, for fabrication of blood vessels (see Fig. 8.2A1-A3) and nerve conduits using a similar approach, where the pellet was deposited between strands of agarose, which were inert to cell adhesion facilitating aggregation of cells in 3D (Norotte et al., 2009; Owens et al., 2013). The bioprinting platform used in this study, called

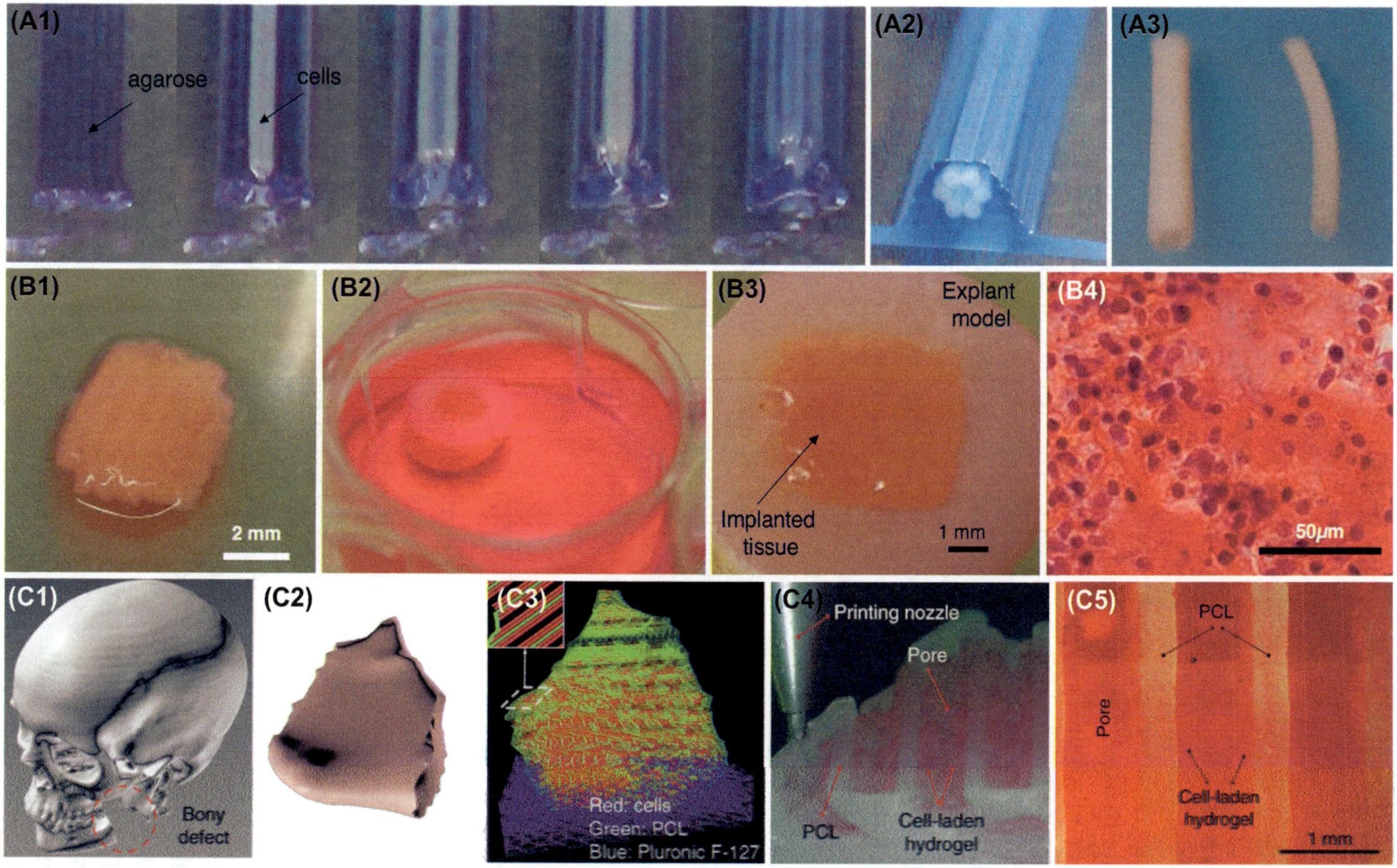

FIGURE 8.2 Examples of Organ Printing. (A1) Step-by-step demonstration of scaffold-free bioprinting of cell pellet along with agarose support, (A2) where the bioprinted construct facilitated aggregation of pig smooth muscle cells in 3 days (A3) followed by removal of the agarose support *(Reproduced/adapted with permission from Norotte et al. (2009))*. (B1) Multilayer bioprinting of free-standing cartilage tissue strands facilitated complete fusion of strands in a week followed by (B2–B3) implantation on a bovine osteochondral explant with a 4 mm × 4 mm defect. (B4) Further cultivation of the bioprinted patch resulted in cartilage that was histologically close to the native bovine cartilage *(Reproduced/adapted from Yu et al. (2016))*. (C1–C2) A computer-aided design (CAD) model of a human mandible bone generated for a defect captured using CT images. (C3) Toolpath plan was generated for the cell-laden bioink, polycaprolactone (PCL), and fugitive Pluronic F-127, and (C4) 3D printing was performed accordingly. (C5) Alizarin Red staining demonstrated osteogenic differentiation of human amniotic fluid derived stem cells (hAFSCs) in a long-term cultured mandible bone construct *(Reproduced/adapted with permission from Kang et al. (2016))*.

Novogen MMX Bioprinter™, has been specialized for bioprinting a broad array of cell types to create functional 3D tissues that can recapitulate in vivo biology for human disease research, drug discovery and development, and toxicology testing. One of the major challenges of this technology is the use of a mold, which restricts the geometry of the tissues into thin tubular shapes. In this regard, the author's group recently used tissue strands as building blocks for larger-scale cartilage patches (Yu et al., 2016). Using 8-cm-long cartilage tissue strands, cartilage patches that were histologically close to native bovine cartilage, were 3D bioprinted without the need for a mold thus allowing scale-up bioprinting (see Fig. 8.2B1–B4). As cartilage is avascular, the use of tissue strands produced large cartilage patches that can be used for human joint repair in the future. Despite these efforts, further research and development is needed to scale-up the constructs to clinically relevant volumes. When building large-scale organ constructs, mechanical integrity as well as the integration of the vascular network with the rest of the organ seems to be the major obstacle to expanding the technology for further clinical applications.

Recently, scaffold-based bioprinting approach has been utilized to generate larger-scale tissue constructs (Kang et al., 2016). Using polycaprolactone (PCL) as a 3D-printed thermoplastic frame along with Pluronic as a fugitive ink, mechanically strong and stable cell-laden tissue constructs were printed with a porous architecture prior to implantation. The concept was successfully tested for various tissue types such as cartilage, bone, and muscle on murine models. A similar concept was previously attempted (Pati et al., 2014), where decellularized matrix components of various tissue types, such as adipose and cartilage, were bioprinted along with PCL fibers to fabricate larger-scale tissue constructs. Although larger-scale constructs were 3D printed with better structural and mechanical integrity, use of PCL in tissue construct remains a major drawback due to its slow degradation rate that may interfere with soft tissue regeneration.

8.3 Roadmap to Organ Printing

Organ printing is a computer-aided process in which cells and/or cell-laden biomaterials are placed according to a blueprint model that serves as building blocks that are further assembled into 3D constructs and matured toward functional organ formation. It is an automated approach that offers a pathway for scalable, reproducible mass production of engineered living organs, where multiple cell types can be positioned precisely to mimic their natural counterparts. Developing a functional organ requires advances in integration of three types of technology (Ozbolat and Yu, 2013; Lanza et al., 2007): (1) *cell technology*, which addresses the procurement of functional cells at the level needed for clinical applications, (2) *biofabrication technology*, which involves combining the cells with biomaterials in a functional 3D configuration, and (3) *technologies for in vivo integration*, which addresses the issue of bioprinted organ immune acceptance, in vivo safety and efficacy, and monitoring of organ integrity and function postimplantation. To successfully realize organ printing in practice at the clinical level, robust automated protocols and procedures should be established. Fig. 8.3 illustrates the roadmap to organ printing, which is composed of three major steps including (1) preorgan printing stage, (2) organ printing stage, and (3) postorgan printing stage.

In preorgan printing stage, the required raw materials consisting of patient-specific cells, nonimmunological biomaterials, growth factors, and cytokines for the organ printing process are prepared. Patient-specific cells can be obtained from stem cells such

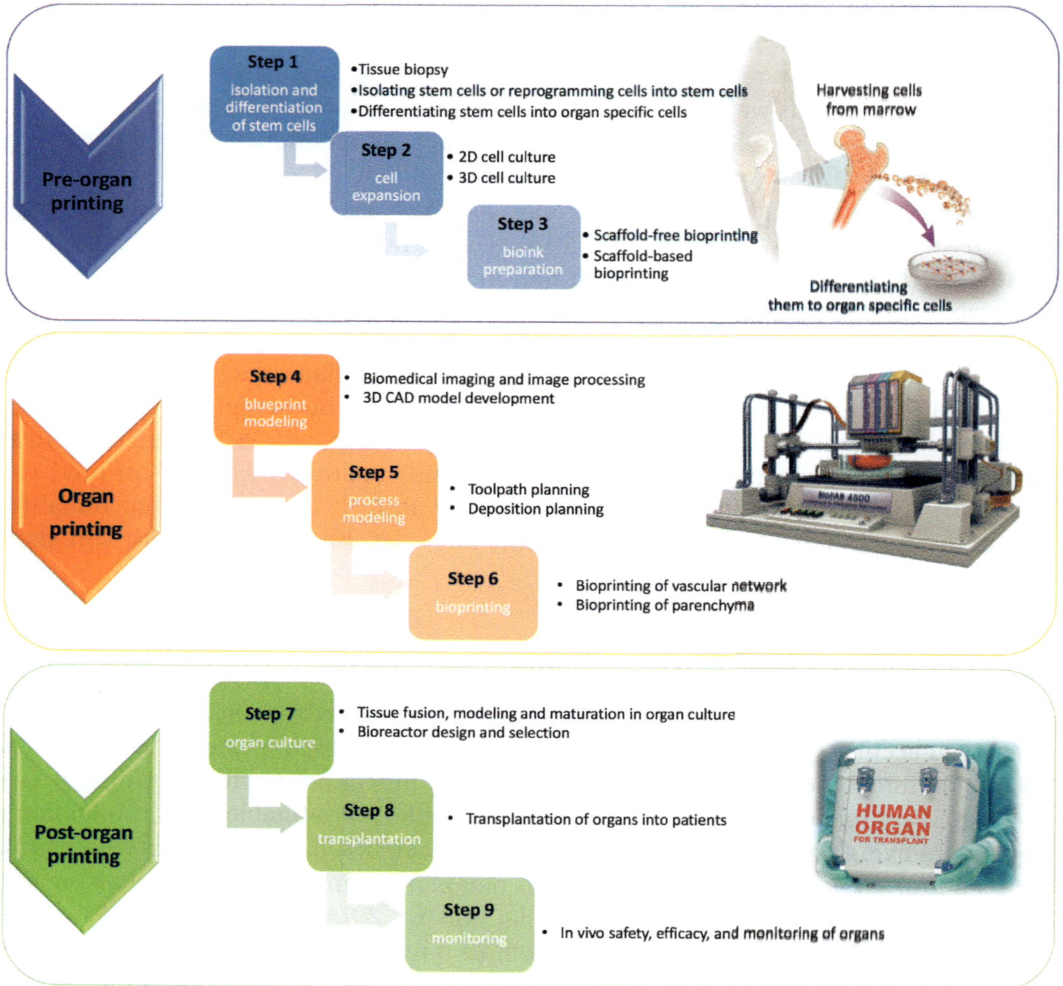

FIGURE 8.3 Roadmap to organ printing process *(Image courtesy of Elsevier for stem cell isolation image Lanza et al. (2007); Christopher Barnatt from www.explainingthefuture.com for bioprinter image; Elsevier for organ transplant image).*

as bone marrow stem cells. Ideally, stem cells should be harvested with minimum invasion; for example, skin fibroblasts can be reprogrammed into induced pluripotent stem cells (iPSCs). Once stem cells are isolated, the next step is to differentiate stem cells into organ-specific cells that are essential to reconstruct the highly heterocellular nature of complex organs. After expansion of cells in sufficient numbers for the scale-up organ printing mission, cells can be cultured in two-dimensional (2D) or 3D depending on the organ to be printed. For example, in the case of the pancreas, islets of Langerhans need to be fabricated in the form of spheroids (Fennema et al., 2013; Bernard et al., 2012). Next, the bioink material, with the cell density comparable to the cell density in natural organs, is prepared using one of the approaches presented in Chapter 3.

In organ printing stage, anatomically correct models of organs should be acquired for the target organ. Currently, there exist several noninvasive medical imaging techniques, as discussed in Section 2.3, to capture the 3D geometry of human organs. Then, the CAD blueprint model can be prepared using one of the appropriate blueprint modeling techniques, discussed in Section 2.4, and imported to machine control software (see Section 7.2.1) to run the bioprinter. At this step, the bioprinter needs two major pieces of information including (1) what to deposit, and (2) where and when to print. During the organ printing process, both the parenchymal and stromal part of the organ should be printed in tandem along with any support or temporary structural elements needed.

After the organ printing process, the bioprinted construct is highly fragile and not structurally coherent or integrated at a sufficient level to facilitate transplantation. Therefore the postorgan printing stage is critical to obtain functional, mechanically stable, and innervated organs for transplantation. The cultivation period necessitates proper bioreactor technologies to enable mechanical and chemical stimulation and signaling to regulate organ remodeling and growth. Upon sufficient maturation and testing of organs, the organs can be transplanted to the patient, and the functionality and in vivo safety parameters monitored for a significant period of time. The following section discusses in detail each of the three major stages for the roadmap to organ printing.

8.3.1 Isolation and Differentiation of Stem Cells

Successful organ printing relies heavily upon advancements in stem cell technology as native tissues and organs are heterocellular. Acquisition of functional primary cells from patients with visceral dysfunction such as liver or heart failure or other devastating diseases such as type I diabetes as autologous beta (β) cells is not possible. Stem cells, which are found in several tissues in human body, can self-renew to produce more stem cells and have the remarkable potential to differentiate into diverse specialized cell types to form various organs. A variety of cell types can be used for this application, such as embryonic stem (ES) cells (Thomson et al., 1998), adult stem cells (ASCs) (Baglioni et al., 2009), iPSCs (Takahashi et al., 2007), human adipocyte stem cells (ADSCs) (Gimble et al., 2007), and tissue-specific cell lines (Pan et al., 2009). Although ES cells are pluripotent, their availability has been hampered by controversial ethical concerns due to their derivation from early embryos (Wert, 2003). Induced pluripotent stem cells have eliminated those issues, as somatic cells from patients can be easily isolated with minimally invasive procedures such as skin biopsy. The obtained skin fibroblasts can be reprogrammed into adult cells from all three germ layers in vitro, which have a great potential in regenerative medicine for cell therapy applications or tissue or organ fabrication. Reprogramming of somatic cells to obtain iPSCs, depending on the method used, may pose substantial risk and thus limit their clinical translation. Human adipocyte stem cells also eliminate the ethical concerns as abundant amount of adipose tissue can be easily isolated from subcutaneous adipose deposits with safe, minimal invasive procedures in an outpatient setting. Additionally, adipocyte stem cells retain pluripotency in vitro (Bunnell et al., 2008). Thus these stem cell types provide a wide range of cell sources for organ printing; however, there are still some impediments with their use. Although autologous stem cells can be differentiated into organ-specific cells for organ printing, there is still a risk of tissue rejection by the recipient (Lanza et al., 2007). Phenotypic behavior of stem cells can even change during the bioprinting process. In addition, organ fabrication requires various types of organ-specific cells, which is not currently feasible with current stem cell isolation and differentiation technologies. Although stem cells offer great promise as an unlimited source of cells for organ printing, a greater understanding of and control over the differentiation process is required to generate expandable organ-specific cells of consistent quality with the desired phenotype and genotype thereby minimizing organ rejection by the recipient posttransplantation. In addition, immunobarrier devices or molecular level interventions in the form of DNA modifications are essential to overcome immunologic rejection of organs. Moreover, imaging modalities such as positron emission tomography and nuclear magnetic resonance (NMR) imaging should be used to monitor the functionality of seeded stem cells noninvasively; NMR offers a unique advantage in monitoring organ integrity and cell function without the need to modify the cells genetically (Stabler et al., 2005).

8.3.2 Cell Expansion

Although current stem cell technologies can expand stem cells into adequate numbers for laboratory experiments, future organ printing technologies will require scale-up manufacturing of stem cells for larger-scale human tissues for transplantation and generation of tissue samples for pharmaceutical use. To attain sufficient numbers of cells for human organ printing, advanced bioprocessing technologies should be implemented to enable practical expansion of stem cells in compliance with good manufacturing practices with appropriate quality assurance measures, bioprocess monitoring control, and automation (Placzek et al., 2009). Each stem cell type has a different expansion potential. Embryonic stem cells have unlimited expansion capacity; however, other stem cells do not. For example, mesenchymal stem cells (MSCs) from young donors have 40 population doubling; whereas MSCs from older donors are limited to 25 population doubling (Stenderup et al., 2003). As previously discussed, the use of ES cells have other issues such as ethical considerations while MSCs have other limitations such as the need for an invasive procedure to obtain a limited sample volume as they are primarily isolated from bone marrow. Therefore other stem cells such as iPSCs and ADSCs stand as promising cell sources that can be obtained in large quantities from abundant tissue volumes isolated using minimally invasive procedures. After isolation, stem cells should be plated and expanded in appropriate culture conditions. In general, expansion culture environments are maintained at 5% carbon dioxide (CO_2), 20% oxygen, 37°C, and pH 7.4; however, growth and differentiation of different stem cells may vary under different conditions. For example, it has been demonstrated that a lower pH level of 7.1 increased the expansion of megakaryocyte progenitor cells (Yang et al., 2002). Large volumes of cells need to be expanded in a bioreactor culture with appropriate nutrient and waste exchange, accommodations for high cell density, and a continuous monitoring and feedback mechanism. For organ printing, two different strategies can be used in loading stem cells including (1) bioprinting differentiated stem cells during the organ printing process or (2) bioprinting predifferentiated stem cells followed by differentiation into organ-specific cell lineages within appropriate sectors of the printed organ constructs. The former approach is preferred over the latter one, in general, as differentiation of multiple cell types into different lineages is extremely challenging requiring spatiotemporal delivery of growth factors or plasmid DNA (Ozbolat and Hospodiuk, 2016).

8.3.3 Bioink Preparation

Upon expansion to sufficient numbers, cells are processed for bioink preparation. Depending on the bioink type utilized, such as hydrogels, cell aggregates, microcarriers, or decellularized matrix components as discussed in Chapter 3, different cell quantities are required. Quality assessment of the cells is essential to ensure that their purity, phenotype, genotype, and functionality are acceptable.

As hydrogels are primarily used in tissue construct biofabrication, appropriate hydrogel bioink materials should be selected based on the target organ type as well as the utilized bioprinting modality. Hydrogel-based bioink materials can be processed while the cells are in culture for expansion as some hydrogels require prolonged preparation times. For example, if collagen type I is used as a bioink component, it should be screened for the presence of any contaminants and immunoreactive components; its protein profile and molecular structure should match that of standard collagen type I. Such screening should be performed for each component of the bioink solution. As composite bioink materials may have several components, the sequence of adding each one should be based on well-established protocols as slight variations at the preparation stages may result in substantial differences in the performance of the bioink solution. Then, cells need to be added and homogenously mixed into the bioink solution at a sufficient density to facilitate tissue formation. Although different tissue types require different cell densities, higher cell densities enable better cell–cell interactions and induce successful tissue formation. As the hydrogel-based bioink solutions, in their precursor form, possess a nonporous liquid microenvironment for cells, cells should be added at the latest stage of the bioink preparation. If possible, some media should be added to the bioink solution to minimize any cellular necrosis. In addition, precursor forms of the bioink solution components can also be toxic to cells; therefore it is ideal to bioprint and crosslink the precursor solution in shortest possible period of time.

For other bioink types, such as cell aggregate–based bioink materials, different preparation procedures are required. The cell pellet is relatively easy to process; however, sufficient cohesiveness should be achieved by retaining the pellet for a period of time (15 min–1 h) in glass capillaries (Owens et al., 2013). Extending this time can adversely affect the cell viability due to oxygen insufficiency. In addition, high-precision instruments should be used to economize on bioink material during the process. For tissue spheroid preparation, various methods [i.e., mold culture, microfluidics-based or magnetic assembly techniques (see Chapter 3)] can be used for high-throughput fabrication. Tissue spheroids should be harvested after sufficient cohesiveness and mechanical properties are attained. If neovascularization within spheroids is crucial, such as in the case of pancreatic islets or tumor models, then cocultured spheroids should be harvested after a single day in culture as further culture reduces angiogenic potential. For tissue strands, a minimum culture period should be provided to facilitate sufficient cell aggregation (Yu et al., 2016). As there is no hydrogel or other exogenous materials, cells need to be cultured in specialized reagents, such as serum and growth factors, that are conducive to maintaining cell viability. As these reagents are expensive, future organ bioprinting technologies will need to devise cost-effective scale-up production strategies to increase the availability of humanized reagents with a wide range of commercial availability.

After preparation of the bioink materials, they are loaded into the bioprinter. As native tissues and organs are heterocellular in their organization, careful loading of multiple bioink solutions is essential and adequate calibration should be performed before running the bioprinter. For extended bioprinting processes, additional bioink materials may be needed therefore manual/automatic unloading and loading needs to be performed to complete the entire construct.

8.3.4 Blueprint Modeling

To bioprint an organ construct, a blueprint model is essential to guide the bioprinting process. Organ bioprinting processes are complex compared to the bioprinting of cells within bulk- or lattice-shaped hydrogel scaffolds. These endeavors include scaffold-free bioprinting (Yu et al., 2016; Norotte et al., 2009), integration of scaffold-free approach with vascular network (Yu et al., 2014), a scaffold-based approach with integrated vascular network (Zhang et al., 2013a), and the use of a hard polymeric frame to support cell-laden hydrogel sections (Kang et al., 2016). All these approaches are highly complicated in their construction, where multiple materials need to be bioprinted, hence requiring a complex blueprint model. Such complex blueprint models can be developed using one or more of available techniques such as CAD-based systems, image-based design, freeform design, implicit surfaces, and space filling curves as discussed in Section 2.3. For scaffold-free approaches, particularly, where the bioprinting process guide the tissue self-assembly, tissue remodeling, fusion, and contraction are commonly observed, resulting in significant deviations from the originally bioprinted construct. Therefore the blueprint model and the associated toolpath plan should compensate for the postbioprinting changes.

8.3.5 Process Planning

Upon generation of the blueprint model for the target organ, a process plan should be performed to determine how to bioprint the organ construct including its compartments and components, such as stromal, parenchyma, blood vessels, and support material. An appropriate toolpath plan is thus essential to provide the bioprinter with information about the robot motion and the deposition patterns so that exact deposition of different bioink constituents can be determined. This information is then transferred from toolpath planning software to the machine control software via digital signals that control the motion and dispensing mechanisms, such as actuation of motors and air pressure, respectively (Ozbolat et al., 2014). For toolpath planning, both Cartesian- and parametric-based approaches, as discussed in Section 2.5, can be considered. As organ printing may necessitate bioprinting multiple bioink materials or even the support material, Cartesian-based toolpath planning is preferred due to its simplicity.

8.3.6 Bioprinting of Vascularized Organs

At this step of organ fabrication, organ constructs can be 3D bioprinted using any single or combinations of existing bioprinting modalities including EBB, DBB, and LBB as presented in Chapters 4–6, respectively. As EBB modality facilitates fabrication of 3D constructs at the clinically relevant volumes, it is currently preferred over other methods, but can also be integrated with others if required. To print organs at clinically relevant volumes, robust technologies and protocols should be developed to enable bioprinting of vascular constructs in multiple-scale ranges from arteries and veins down to capillaries. Since it is difficult to print capillaries at submicron scale using the current bioprinting technology, one alternative strategy can be bioprinting the macrovasculature with the expectation that the interconnecting capillaries will be formed on their own (Yu et al., 2014). In this regard, two alternative approaches have been considered in the literature including indirect bioprinting utilizing a fugitive ink that is removed by thermally induced decrosslinking leaving a vascular network behind (Kolesky et al., 2014; Lee et al., 2014a,b) and direct bioprinting of vasculature network in tandem with the rest of the tissue constructs (Yu et al., 2014).

8.3.6.1 Indirect Bioprinting of Vascular Network

In the last few years, several researchers have attempted bioprinting with a fugitive bioink to create vascular channels including Bertassoni and his coworkers (see Fig. 8.4A1–A2) (Bertassoni et al., 2014), Chen's group (see Fig. 8.4B1-B2) (Miller et al., 2012), and Lewis and her coworkers (see Fig. 8.4C) (Kolesky et al., 2014). In these studies, cell-laden hydrogels were used as the base material to fabricate the tissue construct where a vascular network was created by 3D printing a sacrificial material, such as Pluronic F-127, agarose, and gelatin, followed by its removal after complete gelation of the hydrogel. Such a construct displayed sufficient structural integrity. The integrated vascular network resulted in increased cell viability inside the construct; regions near the channels exhibited significant differences in cell viability compared to regions away from the channels.

The majority of researchers have attempted to create vascular networks in macroscale by generating an endothelial lining inside the lumen via colonization of endothelial cells through perfusion. Dai et al. took one step forward and have successfully achieved angiogenesis by sprouting endothelial cells within a fibrin network loaded with other support cells (see Fig. 8.4D1–D2) (Lee et al., 2014a,b). Their study demonstrated that creating a vascular channel with the luminal surface covered with endothelial cells improved the diffusion of plasma protein and dextran molecules. Similar angiogenesis models have already been developed in lab-on-a-chip models, where several types of support cells have been used in cancer metastasis studies lead by Kamm's and George's groups (Chung et al., 2009; Sheng et al., 2014). Despite the great flexibility in bioprinting channels and the ability to initiate angiogenesis, this technology still faces with several challenges. First of all, loading cells in hydrogels does not support cell–cell interactions, and limited phenotypic stability and activity of cells are observed during in vitro incubation. Fibrin demonstrated a superior environment for angiogenesis while fibrin plays a crucial role in blood clotting (Janmey et al., 2009); however, fibrin is not a hospitable environment for all support cell types (cells that are considered tissue-specific cell types) and does not preserve the construct integrity for long periods of time. With further advancements in these technologies, vascularization that provides an efficient media exchange system for thick tissue fabrication will be a reality in the near future.

8.3.6.2 Direct Bioprinting of Vascular Network

In addition to efforts using temporary sacrificial materials to generate channels, vascular network bioprinting has been demonstrated using various direct bioprinting approaches. For example, scaffold-free bioprinting of vascular networks has been performed using tissue spheroids as building blocks as shown in Fig. 8.5A1–A3 (Norotte et al., 2009). Six days after deposition, tissue spheroids made of human skin fibroblasts (HSFs) completely fused and maturated into a vascular tissue with branches demonstrating the ability of spheroids to self-assemble. In addition to the scaffold-free approach, scaffold-based approaches have been extensively studied by the author's research group through the use of a coaxial nozzle apparatus (see Fig. 8.5B1–B2), which allows direct bioprinting

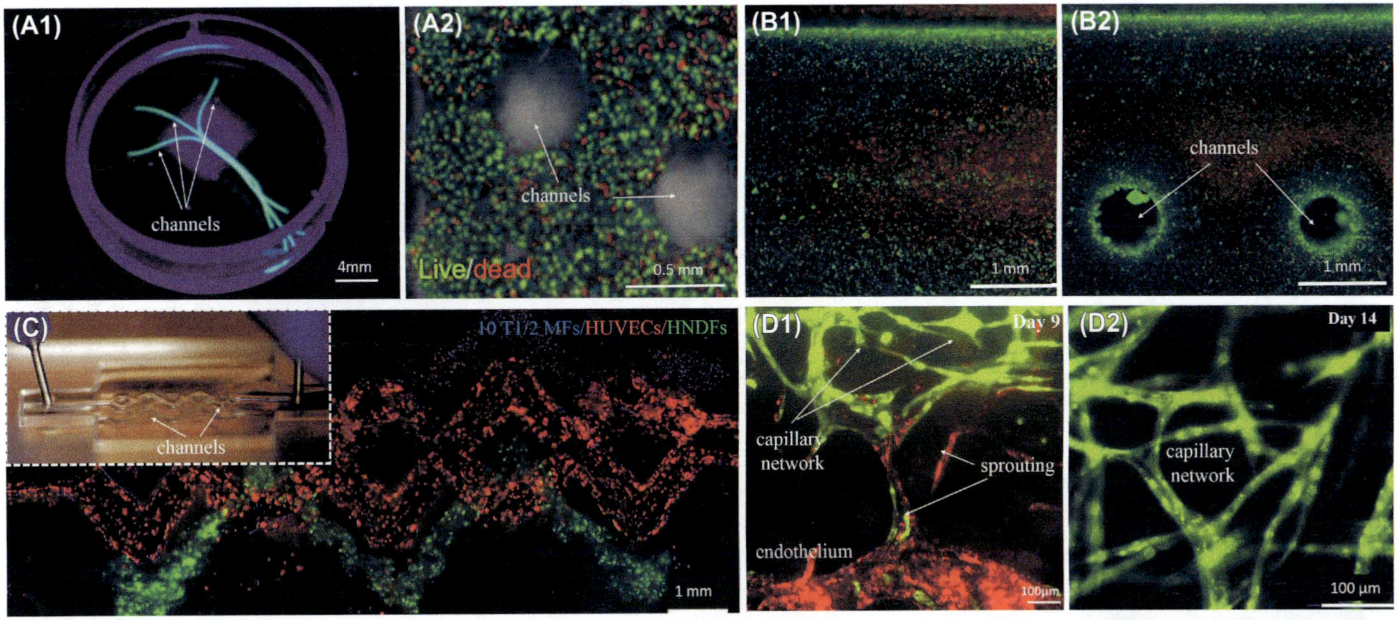

FIGURE 8.4 Indirect Bioprinting of Vascular Channels Using Fugitive Ink. (A1) A photograph of bioprinted agarose hydrogel filaments as fugitive ink representing branched vascular network in a gelatin methacryloyl (GelMA) hydrogel block and (A2) a high resolution cross-sectional view of GelMA block stained for live and dead cells *(Reproduced/adapted with permission from Bertassoni et al. (2014))*; 3D printing carbohydrate glass as a fugitive ink leaving vascular channels in agarose gel loaded with primary rat hepatocytes and stromal fibroblast were stained with a fluorescent live/dead assay (green, Calcein AM; red, Ethidium Homodimer) (B1) showing a considerable percentage of death cells in slab gels without channels compared to (B2) high viability of cells in channeled gels, particularly around the perfused channels *(Reproduced/adapted with permission from Miller et al. (2012))*; (C) an image acquired during evacuation of the fugitive ink showing channels in GelMA scaffold (upper-left), which were later glued with $10T^1/_2$ fibroblasts, human umbilical vein endothelial cells (HUVECs), and human dermal fibroblasts *(Reproduced/adapted with permission from Kolesky et al. (2014))*; and (D1) sprouting of endothelium (stained with *red fluorescent protein*) into capillary network (stained with *green fluorescent protein*) within fibrin gel on day 9 and (D2) a high resolution image of the capillary network on day 14. *(Reproduced/adapted with permission from Lee et al. (2014a,b)).*

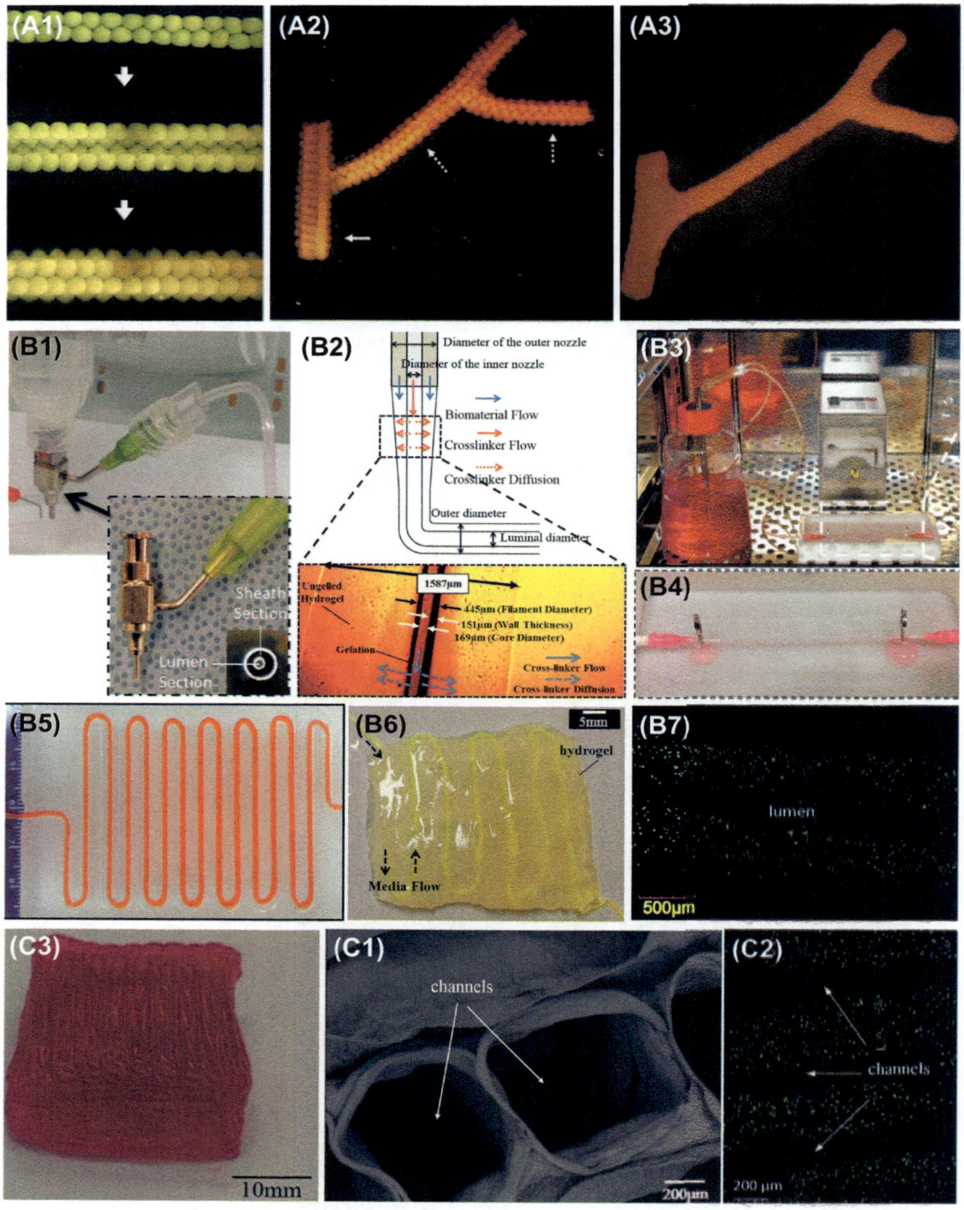

FIGURE 8.5 Direct Bioprinting of Vascular Network. (A1) Scaffold-free bioprinting of a branched vascular network using 300 μm human skin fibroblast spheroids (solid and broken arrows show 1.2 and 0.9 mm in vascular diameter, respectively), where spheroids (A2) fuse and maturate into tissue after 6 days of deposition (A3) *(Reproduced/adapted with permission from Norotte et al. (2009))*; (B1–B2) Coaxial extrusion setup for bioprinting vascular network, where the crosslinker solution flowing through the core facilitates rapid gelation of alginate vascular tubes, (B3–B4) which are perfusable over prolonged pulsatile flow. (B5) Complex patterns could be easily generated *(Reproduced from Zhang et al. (2015))* and (B6) vascular network embedded within bulk hydrogel solutions *(Reproduced with permission from Zhang et al. (2013a))*. (B7) Cells kept their high viability over time. The similar concept was further enhanced to (C1–C2) bioprinted vascular channels embedded in a large alginate construct (C3) showing L929 mouse fibroblasts in green. *(Reproduced/adapted with permission from Gao et al. (2015))*.

of the vasculature with immediate crosslinking of sodium alginate bioink generating a smooth and continuous lumen of any desired length (Zhang et al., 2015). The anatomy can be determined by controlling the bioprinting parameters and the shape of the vascular network can be mediated by bioprinting where the vasculature can be loaded with cells such as fibroblast and smooth muscle cells and cultured in perfusion chamber prolonged times (see Fig. 8.5B3–B4). Complex patterns were bioprinted and the vascular network was easily integrated with larger-scale bulk hydrogels with cell viability over 95% retained over a week culture (see Fig. 8.5B5-B7) (Zhang et al., 2013a). The coaxial nozzle bioprinting was further used to demonstrate the embedding of vascular channels in hydrogel constructs increasing the viability of cells compared to cells in bulk hydrogels (Gao et al., 2015).

8.3.6.3 Integration of Vascular Network With Parenchymal Tissue

The ultimate goal of tissue engineering techniques is the generation of a functional tissue or organ with an integrated vascular network. To successfully create multiscale vascularization within organ constructs, the constructs need be placed in a custom-made perfusion bioreactor, where vascular pedicles are connected to facilitate continuous medium flow in vitro. The perfusion bioreactor not only ensures sufficient structural support for the printed organ construct, but also provides an environment similar to in vivo conditions. Essential growth factors such as vascular endothelial growth factor, fibroblast growth factor, and epidermal growth factor (EGF) are supplemented within the circulating culture media. The printed constructs mature over time, creating an organ at the clinically relevant size enclosing the vasculature during in vitro incubation. More importantly, upon the formation of the 3D organ constructs, the previously mentioned angiogenesis growth factors continue to be supplied during in vitro culture to drive the natural process of vascularization between the main vasculature and prevascularized constructs. Ultimately, thick 3D constructs can be fabricated with a biomimetic vasculature system and be readily available for transplantation, disease modeling, or drug screening. This will be a major breakthrough toward fabrication of larger-scale organs.

Studies have demonstrated perfusable blood vessel network embedded in thick tissues using bioprinting and traditional fabrication approaches. For example, a recent study (Yu et al., 2014) demonstrated hybrid bioprinting of vasculature in tandem with tissue strands using a Multi-Arm BioPrinter (Ozbolat et al., 2014), where fibroblast tissue strands quickly fuse to each other, mature and form the tissue around the vasculature. Tissue strands were comprised only of cells and their extracellular matrix (ECM). They were used as building blocks to construct the scale-up organ due to their quick fusion, folding, and maturation capabilities. Using traditional fabrication approaches, scientists integrated vascularization with 3D cell sheet fabrication technology, where endothelial cells within a cardiac cell sheet sprouted and connected to the main blood vessel upon perfusion of growth factor–rich culture media (Sekine et al., 2013). Another study demonstrated that a prevascularized hepatic bud, when transplanted in vivo, can successfully **anastomose** to the main blood vessel and survive for a long period of time, performing its original function (Takebe et al., 2014). All of these findings offer the potential for organ printing to have a similar nature-driven effect upon perfusion. When the media is perfused through a continuous vascular network within the vascularized tissue constructs, the biological signals as well as the media gradient along the perfusion direction would guide endothelial cell reorganization, migration, and facilitate angiogenesis within the organ and orchestrate capillary network formation toward the media supply.

Newly generated capillaries within the organ constructs are expected to anastomose to the main vasculature, so that media supplied through these newly formed capillaries would guarantee the survival of the organ constructs for longer periods of time. Continuous media circulation within the newly generated constructs would also accelerate the tissue maturation process by supplying sufficient growth factors, which drive tissue-specific cells to secrete ECM and further facilitate tissue or organ maturation, producing a functional vascularized perfusable organ. Later, the matured organ could be used for drug testing by directly delivering different drugs via the perfusion system to evaluate the organ response. Moreover, 3D-printed organ constructs could be implanted in vivo by suturing the main vasculature to the host to replace damaged or diseased tissues or organs.

8.3.7 Advanced Bioreactor Technologies for Organ Culture

After the organ bioprinting process, as discussed previously, the fabricated construct needs to be transferred to a bioreactor for long-term culture to facilitate cell growth and proliferation, vascularization, and organ maturation. A bioreactor can be defined as a system in which the conditions are closely controlled with respect to physiological conditions to induce certain behavior in living cells, tissues, and organs (Korossis et al., 2005). Three major bioreactor types have been used in culturing engineered tissue constructs including static and mixed flasks, rotating wall, and perfusion bioreactors (Gaspar et al., 2012). Mixed flask culture or rotating wall utilizes a convection mass transfer mechanism; however, perfusion bioreactors enable both convection and diffusion-mediated mass transfer. Complex-organ systems such as decellularization-based approaches or bioprinted vascularized organ constructs require perfusion culture that forces culture medium through the vascular inlets and collects it from outlets using a suction mechanism. The ideal bioreactor should provide the appropriate physical stimulation to cells, a continuous supply of nutrients (e.g., glucose, amino acids) and removal of by-products of cellular metabolism. The bioreactor should also facilitate sufficient convection and diffusion of biochemical factors and oxygen, as well as provide mechanical stimuli to induce mechanotransduction and the appropriate deposition of ECM proteins with controlled orientation and structure. In addition, such a bioreactor should maintain aseptic conditions, allow for a high media volume to tissue construct volume ratio, fail to generate any toxic products, and be easy to clean after the culture period. In general, different organ and tissue types, possessing different anatomical, biological, mechanical, and structural characteristics, may need specialized bioreactor designs; however, the three major requirements for bioreactor design include (1) mass transport, (2) mechanical, and (3) electrical stimulation

Mass transport through a bioreactor system is by far the most essential requirement for successful cultivation of printed organs. As organ constructs possess micro- or macrosize pore, mass transport of oxygen, nutrients, and regulatory molecules is highly limited under static conditions. In addition, metabolites, CO_2, and lactic acid need to be removed from the organ constructs. As solubility of oxygen within media is low, exposure of cells to oxygen in organ constructs is reduced. Therefore the bioreactor system should support circulation of the fresh media throughout the entire organ construct and facilitate efficient convection.

Mechanical stimulation of organ constructs, via mechanical compression or stretch, hydrodynamic pressure, and fluid flow (Salehi-Nik et al., 2013), is a crucial factor for successful maturation of bioprinted organ constructs (see Fig. 8.6). Mechanical stimulation can improve adhesion and stretching of cells, mediates the deposition direction of ECM proteins, triggers the secretion of biological factors, and determines whether cells aggregate or detach from the organ constructs. For example, adhesion strength and orientation of endothelial cells are highly dependent on shear stress, where cells orient and elongate in the direction of the flow and facilitates the formation of tight intercellular junctions, and the release of more nitric oxide (Li et al., 2015). On the other hand, chondrocytes grown in an organ construct under cyclic compression test demonstrated better mechanical properties and deposition of ECM proteins such as proteoglycans (Kisiday et al., 2004). Cell aggregates are more sensitive to mechanical stimuli compared to cells alone due to their large volume (Henzler, 2000); therefore the likelihood of detachment of cell aggregates from tissue constructs is higher than that of individual cells.

Electrical stimulation is another important factor to enhance the functionality of particular tissue constructs such as cardiac or muscle tissue or the innervation of

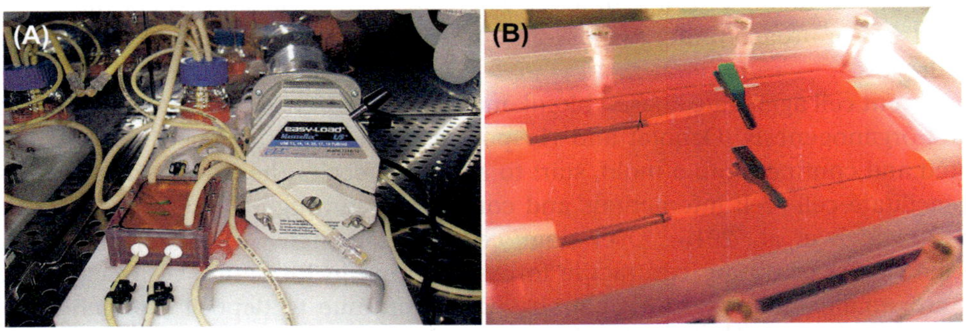

FIGURE 8.6 (A) A perfusion bioreactor (B) for cultivation of bioprinted blood vessels for further tissue maturation, and deposition of collagen and elastin proteins *(Reproduced/adapted with permission from Norotte et al. (2009)).*

composite tissues with nerves. For example, bioprinted cardiomyocytes in alginate constructs demonstrated better contractile properties under electrical stimulation (Xu et al., 2009). In addition, electrical stimuli can be integrated with mechanical stimuli to initiate appropriate functionalities. For example, engineered muscle tissues demonstrated higher contractile properties along with better elongation of muscle cells along the tissue construct when the tissue is exposed to optimal electromechanical stimuli (Liao et al., 2008).

In addition to its stimulatory function, the ideal bioreactor should also possess the capability of controlling the tissue quality of each and every printed organ over time. In this regard, noninvasive and nondestructive approaches should be developed to monitor the quality of organs or the metabolic states of cells, such as measurement of glucose uptake or oxygen consumption using embedded sensors. In addition, mechanical quality of load-bearing organs such as bone and cartilage is also important; bioreactors should advance the mechanical stimulation over time to increase the mechanical properties of the developing tissue. Advanced monitoring capabilities should be integrated to read the mechanical parameters from the construct and direct adjustment of the stimulation automatically. All these monitoring capabilities will increase the efficiency of post-bioprinting organ culture processes and increase the quality and replicability of organs within predetermined biofabrication specifications (Korossis et al., 2005). This will be crucial for printed organs used in pharmaceutical and drug testing.

In addition to bioreactor considerations, postbioprinting of organs is another important step toward successful transplantation. The transfer of a printed organ to the bioreactor should be performed with extreme care to prevent degradation in quality and function of the organ. Thus future bioprinters can be enclosed in a bioreactor system that will allow direct and rapid connection of printed structures to perfusion channels.

8.3.8 Organ Remodeling and Maturation

During the bioreactor culture, bioprinted organ constructs exhibit different biological and morphological changes over time depending on the bioink and bioprinting strategy utilized in the organ printing process. For example, organ constructs made using a scaffold-free approach undergo a different process than cells suspended and bioprinted in hydrogels.

Different cell aggregate—based bioink materials experience a different series of events during organogenesis (Ozbolat and Hospodiuk, 2016). Cells in pellet form, when bioprinted and confined into a mold, start to adhere to each other to minimize free energy and facilitate cell—cell interactions and connections through cadherin-mediated adhesion (Akkouch et al., 2015). Over time, cells deposit their own ECM, promoting cell adhesion and generating contractile forces resulting in formation of intact neotissues that are smaller than their original size. Cells continue to deposit parenchymal ECM components such as elastin and collagen, where the cohesion and mechanical properties of the tissue increases and the tissue matures and eventually attains a morphology and physiology close to the native tissues. When sufficient structural cohesion is achieved, the mold structure can be removed from the construct to allow better perfusion and diffusion. If other cell aggregate–based bioink materials are used such as tissue spheroids (Mironov et al., 2016) and strands (Yu et al., 2016), tissue fusion starts immediately through cross-migration of cells and deposition of ECM components into the space in aggregates. To minimize the configurational energy during fusion, fused aggregates assume a more rounded geometry followed by deposition of ECM components and maturation of the tissue toward a nativelike morphology.

Cells bioprinted in hydrogel matrix, on the other hand, are exposed to a different environment and exhibit different chain of events during organogenesis. As cells loaded in hydrogels, they first attach to the scaffold matrix, and proliferate and deposit their own ECM. Meanwhile, they express proteinases including matrix metalloproteinases (MMPs), which causes the degradation of the bioink material. For example, MMP-1 and MMP-13 cleave collagen type I in skin and bone tissue, respectively (Nagase et al., 2006). As cells grow and increase in number, and the matrix around them starts to degrade, slow changes are observed in the morphology and physiology of the organ construct.

In addition to these events, neovascularization is another important factor, where endothelial cells form into tubular organization followed by incorporation of pericyte-like supporting cells, such as human normal lung fibroblasts and smooth muscle cells, surrounding the endothelial structures, stabilizing their growth, and improving the mechanical integrity of developing capillaries. Later, these tubes anastomose to each other forming a larger vascular network that can be connected to larger-scale vascular network (Ozbolat, 2015). Depending on the target organ type, its morphology, structural and mechanical properties, function and physiology, different types of strategies, and bioink materials can be utilized.

8.3.9 Transplantation, Immunosurveillance, and In Vivo Safety, Efficacy, and Monitoring of Organs

Bioprinted organs, depending on their type, may pose difficulties associated with transplantation such as cellular ischemia requiring the printed organ to be transported on ice, the need for various flush solutions to prevent cellular edema, delay cell destruction, and maximize functions of organs after perfusion is reestablished. Once a bioprinted organ arrives in the operating room, it needs to be implanted in the appropriate site and attached to an uninjured intact vascular pedicle so that the organ can be perfused. Larger organs require larger vascular pedicles for immediate parenchymal perfusion; however, as the bioprinted organs need to be fully engrafted with the host, angiogenic integration with the recipient microcirculation is also essential. Since it is challenging to bioprint capillaries within bioprinted organ using current bioprinting technologies, one alternative approach is to bioprint endothelial cells within the construct and have the microcirculatory system developed naturally within the host postimplantation (Ozbolat, 2015). Ischemic resilient organs, such as kidney, may be more amenable to this strategy than other visceral organs such as liver and pancreas. In addition, the vascular network within bioprinted organs should be lined with an endothelium layer to prevent blood coagulation. Tight junctions of endothelial cells can be achieved in vitro or such organization can be performed in vivo post-implantation if the size of the printed organs is small (Itoh et al., 2015). The other important requirement for bioprinted organs is their innervation capability depending on their type and function. During transplantation, it has been shown that transplants denervate for a period and recover nerve function over time posttransplantation. For example, histological staining of transplanted kidneys demonstrated evidence of nerve function restoration after weeks posttransplant; recovery continues for years (Mulder et al., 2013). Similar recovery of nerve function can be seen in other organs such as heart (Murphy et al., 2000). Thus nerve tissue should be incorporated into bioprinted organs as one of the future goals to augment currently existing allogeneic transplants.

After the operation, transplant patients are placed in the intensive care unit to manage fluid shifts and electrolyte balance. As 3D-printed organs are envisioned to be fabricated using autologous cells, the need for immunosuppressive agents may be minimal; however, if needed, transplant patients should be treated with immunosuppressive agents as early as possible and their dose should be adjusted based on the blood levels and functional status of the transplanted organ. One of the major post-operative issues is the nosocomial infections that are the fourth leading cause of morbidity and mortality (Kaye, 2011). Such infections arise due to biofilm formation on implants by *Staphylococcus epidermidis*. During in vitro bioprinting processes and long-term organ culture, bioprinted organs can be contaminated leading to a unique type of nosocomial infection. Therefore postoperative monitoring for clinical signs of infection (i.e., increased/decreased white blood cell count, fever, edema) and bio-printed organ failure is absolutely vital. Infection may require aggressive antimicrobial therapy. Postoperative status of organs can be monitored using noninvasive imaging techniques (i.e., computed tomography or magnetic resonance imaging) for connective tissues. For visceral organs, such as liver and kidney, different analyses can be informative such as serum bilirubin and INR to assess liver function, and creatinine and blood urea nitrogen to assess kidney function. As bioprinted organs are still in their infancy in terms of clinical translation, there might be many other unforeseeable issues and uncertainties. Patients receiving bioprinted implants may require more aggressive monitoring than traditional transplant patients.

Although autologous cells are envisioned to be used in organ printing, the bioink materials used from other species may elicit a host immune response after reimplantation as they acquire a layer of host protein, inducing immune response by interactions with inflammatory cells. Macrophages play an important role in adhesion of foreign body giant cells and release degradation factors, which could decompose the bioprinted organ. This can be mitigated by the use of antioxidants (Christenson et al., 2006).

Thus monitoring of cytokine proinflammatory cytokine levels, such as interleukin-1 beta (IL-1β) and IL-6, might be essential in measuring cellular response and bioimplantation success.

8.4 Limitations

Despite the great progress in the last decade, whole-organ bioprinting is still a major roadblock. Current organ models are comprised of very small volumes that are appropriate for drug testing and disease modeling applications providing the appropriate physiological response has been realized; however, bioprinting of human scale organs has yet to be achieved (Ozbolat et al., 2016). There are a few major limitations requiring further investigation. One is to bioprint a multiscale vascular network from arteries and veins down to capillaries. Recent efforts demonstrated bioprinting larger-scale vessels using scaffold-based (Zhang et al., 2015) or scaffold-free (Norotte et al., 2009) approaches successfully. In addition, bioprinting-induced capillary network growth has been demonstrated in scaffold-based systems such as fibrin and collagen hydrogels (Lee et al., 2014a,b). Despite these advances, a vascular network in multiple scales has yet to be produced. Recent attempts in bioplotting in thermally reversible hydrogel bath demonstrated the fabrication of complex vascular network (Hinton et al., 2015); however, the use of limited cell densities hampers further efforts to connect them to capillaries.

Recently demonstrated efforts using fugitive ink for creation of perfusable channels present a suitable approach for fabrication of tissue models for drug testing and pharmaceutical purposes, or cancer or disease models (Peng et al., 2016). Such a system, on the other hand, is not convenient for transplant applications as cells are primarily embedded in hydrogels. Such an approach can support a small gel-based scaffold that can be implanted in connective tissues such as bone or subcutaneous tissue. For internal organs, this strategy can perhaps be used as a patch for solid organ repair, but may not be suitable for whole-organ bioprinting. As vascular networks are used as perfusable channels only and do not actually possess a native blood vessel anatomy, little experimentation has been done. It is expected that these channels will deteriorate in vivo due to biodegradation and may not maintain their morphology.

Recent work demonstrated the use of a thermoplastic-based frame utilizing PCL, which retains its shape upon printing due to its thermoplastic nature (Kang et al., 2016). Hydrogel-based composite bioink was reinforced within porous network along with fugitive Pluronic to generate porosity. Although larger-scale tissue construction was demonstrated, use of PCL, which has a prolonged degradation time, represents a major drawback in the proposed effort. Although PCL supports the structural integrity of hydrogel-based bioink materials, which might be crucial for load-bearing organs, its use for soft tissues may be inappropriate as it can interfere with the soft tissue regeneration.

The volume of PCL material can possibly be minimized to reduce the effect of long-term existence of thermoplastic materials.

Use of hydrogel-based bioink currently entails a significant number of challenges as already described in the limitations section of Chapter 3 but the author prefers to detail some crucial points related to organ printing. One of the major drawbacks is the lack of cell—cell contact as cells cannot proliferate to a tissue-level density and this can interfere with the degradation process. Degradation brings significant challenges such as toxicity of by-products, elevated production of lactic acid, and lack of synchronicity between tissue regeneration and degradation of the hydrogel matrix. Therefore scaffold-free bioprinting is a promising approach in advancing tissue regeneration toward morphologically and physiologically relevant tissues; however, it may be dependent on the target organ type as well as the ultimate application such as pharmaceutical or transplantation use. For transplantation applications, there are further issues to be considered if the construct is for direct transplantation or transplantation following a prolonged in vitro culture.

One of the other current limitations is the lack of available organ-specific cells along with their differentiation protocols. For example, pancreas is a highly complex organ with endocrine and exocrine portions, where the endocrine portion is in charge of insulin production. In this regard, a replacement endocrine organ is vitally important for type I diabetes patients. The endocrine portion of an average human pancreas is made of approximately a million cell clusters called islets of Langerhans consisting of four main cell types including alpha (α), β, delta, and gamma cells secreting glucagon, insulin, somatostatin (regulates/stops α and β cells), and pancreatic polypeptide, respectively (Ozbolat and Yu, 2013). As human islets do not survive in vitro for longer periods and β cells die when they are disassociated from islets, successful differentiation of these cells is essential. Although there are a few seminal studies demonstrating the differentiation of functional beta cells (Pagliuca et al., 2015), there is a consensus that alpha cells also regulate the function of beta cells, therefore differentiation of other cell types is also important for proper function of engineered islets. Currently, the differentiation of these cells has not yet been achieved.

The lack of appropriate perfusion bioreactor systems for different organ type is also another obstacle. Although bioreactor technologies are available for geometrically simple organs such as irrigation dripping perfusion bioreactor for tubular tissues [i.e., blood vessels (Mironov et al., 2009)], other complex organs may possess different anatomies and printed organs may have additional special requirements such as a stepwise increase in the mechanical stress applied to the construct as the coherency of the tissue increases. In addition to limitations in bioreactor technologies, there are major limitations with the existing imaging techniques to quantify or establish the quality of bioprinted tissues. As organ printing necessitates the fabrication of larger-scale organ constructs, existing optical imaging technologies, such as confocal images or two-photon microscopy, are not capable of efficiently imaging the cells in solid organs when the cell density is high (Nam et al., 2014). Therefore multimodel imaging, such as using optical imaging along with nuclear medicine and radiographic imaging, can be used to demonstrate functionality, cell incorporation, and anatomy of the regenerating organs at high resolution.

8.5 Future Directions

In vitro fabrication of physiologically relevant tissues is a highly sophisticated phenomenon comprised of a hierarchical arrangement of multiple cell types, including a multiscale network of vasculature in stroma and parenchyma, along with lymphatic vessels and, occasionally, neural and muscle tissue, depending on the tissue type. In vitro–engineered organs that incorporate all of these components are still far out on the horizon. The major roadblock toward this ambitious goal is multiscale vascularization and the plethora of research that is required to further improve the alternative approaches previously presented. As larger vasculatures can be bioprinted using EBB systems, a controllable capillary network can be created naturally as demonstrated in hydrogels (Chung et al., 2009; Sheng et al., 2014). Since the timescale of neovascularization and the postbioprinting maturation of tissue construct is not the same, where neovascularization takes place in 10 days to 2 weeks; printed parenchymal cells require media and oxygen support immediately and therefore macrovascular network should be created with a diffusion distance of 200–300 μm (Zhang et al., 2013b) depending on the biomaterial and its interstitial flow capabilities. In addition, biomaterials with high microporosity can overcome the previously mentioned issues in some extent. Bioprinting technology offers a great benefit in the hierarchical arrangement of cells or construction of tissue blocks in a 3D microenvironment, but the bioink and the postbioprinting maturation phase are as important as the bioprinting process itself. Although hydrogels such as fibrin, collagen, and GelMA support neovascularization, they may not provide the ideal microenvironment and signaling for survival, motility, and differentiation of a wide array of tissue-specific cells; additionally, hydrogel stability over a prolonged in vitro culture period is weak (Aper et al., 2004; Nichol et al., 2010). Thus tissue-specific cell types can be bioprinted in scaffold-free manner. For example, pancreatic islets or lymphatic follicles in prevascularized form can be printed within a very small hydrogel coated on them, which can support growth of contiguous vascular network within spheroids along with capillaries sprouting into the hydrogel coating. These sprouts can further elongate and anastomose with sprouts from other spheroids (Peng et al., 2016). In addition, successful sprouting of these capillaries from spheroids to the macrovascular network is also crucial to make a fully contiguous vascular network. The postbioprinting process is also crucial and necessitates mechanical and chemical stimulation and signaling to regulate tissue remodeling and growth, development of new bioreactor technologies enabling rapid maturation of tissues, multiscale vascularization for survivability of printed organs, and mechanical integrity and innervation for transplantation.

In addition to efforts in printing organs at the clinically relevant dimensions, monitoring of these organs, postprinting as well as establishment of quality and regulatory standards for the entire process from stem cell isolation to posttransplantation monitoring during follow-up care is also essential. Thus involvement from other disciplines, such as quality assurance, economics, and law, will be highly beneficial to enable rapid and cost-effective fabrication of organs that meet stringent quality and safety standards.

8.6 Summary

This chapter presents the roadmap to organ printing technology that requires a sequence of interrelated processes spanning from isolation of stem cells to transplantation into a human; seamlessly automated protocols and systems are essential for customized functional organ fabrication. This pathway includes (1) isolation and differentiation of stem cells, (2) cell expansion, (3) bioink preparation, (4) blueprint modeling, (5) process planning, (6) bioprinting process, (7) organ remodeling and maturation in a bioreactor, (8) transplantation, and (9) posttransplantation monitoring. Although the technology shows a great deal of promise, there is still a long way to go to practically realize this ambitious vision. Overcoming current impediments in cell and biomanufacturing technologies, and innovative technologies for in vivo integration are essential for developing seamlessly automated platforms from stem cell isolation to transplantation.

References

Akkouch, A., Yu, Y., Ozbolat, I.T., 2015. Microfabrication of scaffold-free tissue strands for three-dimensional tissue engineering. Biofabrication 7 (3), 31002.

Aper, T., et al., 2004. Use of a fibrin preparation in the engineering of a vascular graft model. European Journal of Vascular and Endovascular Surgery: the Official Journal of the European Society for Vascular Surgery 28 (3), 296–302.

Baglioni, S., et al., 2009. Characterization of human adult stem-cell populations isolated from visceral and subcutaneous adipose tissue. FASEB 23 (10), 3494–3505.

Bernard, A.B., Lin, C.-C., Anseth, K.S., 2012. A microwell cell culture platform for the aggregation of pancreatic β-cells. Tissue Engineering Part C: Methods 18 (8), 583–592.

Bertassoni, L.E., et al., 2014. Direct-write bioprinting of cell-laden methacrylated gelatin hydrogels. Biofabrication 6 (2), 024105.

Bunnell, B.A., et al., 2008. Adipose-derived stem cells: isolation, expansion and differentiation. Methods 45 (2), 115–120.

Christenson, E.M., Anderson, J.M., Hiltner, A., 2006. Antioxidant inhibition of poly(carbonate urethane) in vivo biodegradation. Journal of Biomedical Materials Research—Part A 76 (3), 480–490.

Chung, S., et al., 2009. Cell migration into scaffolds under co-culture conditions in a microfluidic platform. Lab on a chip 9, 269–275.

Fennema, E., et al., 2013. Spheroid culture as a tool for creating 3D complex tissues. Trends in Biotechnology 31 (2), 108–115.

Fisher, M.B., Mauck, R.L., 2012. Tissue engineering and regenerative medicine: recent innovations and the transition to translation. Tissue Engineering Part B: Reviews 19 (1), 1–13.

Gao, Q., et al., 2015. Coaxial nozzle-assisted 3D bioprinting with built-in microchannels for nutrients delivery. Biomaterials 61, 203–215.

Gaspar, D.A., Gomide, V., Monteiro, F.J., 2012. The role of perfusion bioreactors in bone tissue engineering. Biomatter 2 (4), 167–175.

Gimble, J.M., Katz, A.J., Bunnell, B.A., 2007. Adipose-derived stem cells for regenerative medicine. Circulation Research 100 (9), 1249–1260.

Gudapati, H., Dey, M., Ozbolat, I., 2016. A comprehensive review on droplet-based bioprinting: past, present and future. Biomaterials 102, 20–42.

Henzler, H.J., 2000. Particle stress in bioreactors. Advances in Biochemical Engineering/Biotechnology 67, 35–82.

Hinton, T.J., et al., 2015. Three-dimensional printing of complex biological structures by freeform reversible embedding of suspended hydrogels. Science Advances 1 (9).

Itoh, M., et al., 2015. Scaffold-free tubular tissues created by a Bio-3D printer undergo remodeling and endothelialization when implanted in rat aortae. PLoS One 10 (9), e0136681.

Janmey, P.A., Winer, J.P., Weisel, J.W., 2009. Fibrin gels and their clinical and bioengineering applications. Journal of the Royal Society Interface 6 (30), 1–10.

Kang, H., et al., 2016. A 3D bioprinting system to produce human-scale tissue constructs with structural integrity. Nature Biotechnology 34 (3), 312–319.

Kaye, D., 2011. Copper kills 97 percent of hospital bacteria. Clinical Infectious Diseases 53 (7), i–ii.

Kisiday, J.D., et al., 2004. Effects of dynamic compressive loading on chondrocyte biosynthesis in self-assembling peptide scaffolds. Journal of Biomechanics 37 (5), 595–604.

Kolesky, D., et al., 2014. Bioprinting: 3D bioprinting of vascularized, heterogeneous cell-laden tissue constructs. Advanced Materials 26 (19), 3124–3130.

Korossis, S., et al., 2005. Bioreactors in tissue engineering. In: Ashammakhi, N., Reis, R.L. (Eds.), Topics in Tissue Engineering, pp. 1–23.

Langer, R., Vacanti, J.P., 1993. Tissue engineering. Science 260 (5110), 920–926.

Lanza, R., Langer, R., Vacanti, J. (Eds.), 2007. Principles of Tissue Engineering. Elsevier.

Lee, V., et al., 2014a. Generation of multi-scale vascular network system within 3D hydrogel using 3D bio-printing technology. Cellular and Molecular Bioengineering 7 (3), 460–472.

Lee, V.K., et al., 2014b. Creating perfused functional vascular channels using 3D bio-printing technology. Biomaterials 35 (28), 8092–8102.

Li, X., et al., 2015. Vitro recapitulation of functional microvessels for the study of endothelial shear response, nitric oxide and $[Ca^{2+}]_i$. PLoS One 10 (5), e0126797.

Liao, I.-C., et al., 2008. Effect of electromechanical stimulation on the maturation of myotubes on aligned electrospun fibers. Cellular and Molecular Bioengineering 1 (2), 133–145.

Miller, J.S., et al., 2012. Rapid casting of patterned vascular networks for perfusable engineered three-dimensional tissues. Nature Materials 11 (9), 768–774.

Mironov, V., et al., 2009. Organ printing: tissue spheroids as building blocks. Biomaterials 30 (12), 2164–2174.

Mironov, V., et al., 2016. Patterning of Tissue Spheroids Biofabricated From Human Fibroblasts on the Surface of Electrospun Polyurethane Matrix Using 3D Bioprinter.

Mondy, W.L., et al., 2009. Computer-aided design of microvasculature systems for use in vascular scaffold production. Biofabrication 1 (3), 035002.

Mulder, J., et al., 2013. Renal sensory and sympathetic nerves reinnervate the kidney in a similar time-dependent fashion after renal denervation in rats. American Journal of Physiology. Regulatory, Integrative and Comparative Physiology 304 (8), R675–R682.

Murphy, D.A., et al., 2000. The heart reinnervates after transplantation. Annals of Thoracic Surgery 69 (6), 1769–1781.

Nagase, H., Visse, R., Murphy, G., 2006. Structure and function of matrix metalloproteinases and TIMPs. Cardiovascular Research 69 (3), 562–573.

Nam, S.Y., et al., 2014. Imaging strategies for tissue engineering applications. Tissue Engineering. Part B, Reviews 21 (1), 1–44.

Nichol, J.W., et al., 2010. Cell-laden microengineered gelatin methacrylate hydrogels. Biomaterials 31 (21), 5536–5544.

Norotte, C., et al., 2009. Scaffold-free vascular tissue engineering using bioprinting. Biomaterials 30 (30), 5910–5917.

Owens, C.M., et al., 2013. Biofabrication and testing of a fully cellular nerve graft. Biofabrication 5 (4), 045007.

Ozbolat, I.T., 2015. Bioprinting scale-up tissue and organ constructs for transplantation. Trends in Biotechnology 33 (7), 395–400.

Ozbolat, I.T., Chen, H., Yu, Y., 2014. Development of "Multi-arm Bioprinter" for hybrid biofabrication of tissue engineering constructs. Robotics and Computer-Integrated Manufacturing 30 (3), 295–304.

Ozbolat, I.T., Hospodiuk, M., 2016. Current advances and future perspectives in extrusion-based bioprinting. Biomaterials 76, 321–343.

Ozbolat, I.T., Peng, W., Ozbolat, V., August 2016. Application areas of 3D bioprinting. Drug Discovery Today 21 (8), 1257–1271.

Ozbolat, I.T., Yu, Y., 2013. Bioprinting toward organ fabrication: challenges and future trends. IEEE Transactions on Bio-medical Engineering 60 (3), 691–699.

Pagliuca, F.W., et al., 2015. Generation of functional human pancreatic β cells in vitro. Cell 159 (2), 428–439.

Pan, C., et al., 2009. Comparative proteomic phenotyping of cell lines and primary cells to assess preservation of cell type-specific functions. Molecular and Cellular Proteomics : MCP 8 (3), 443–450.

Pati, F., et al., 2014. Printing three-dimensional tissue analogues with decellularized extracellular matrix bioink. Nature Communications 5, 3935.

Peng, W., Unutmaz, D., Ozbolat, I.T., 2016. Bioprinting towards physiologically relevant stissue models for pharmaceutics. Trends in Biotechnology (in press).

Piqué, A., 2011. The matrix-assisted pulsed laser evaporation (MAPLE) process: origins and future directions. Applied Physics A 105 (3), 517–528.

Placzek, M.R., et al., 2009. Stem cell bioprocessing: fundamentals and principles. Journal of the Royal Society Interface 6 (32), 209–232.

Saidi, R.F., Hejazii Kenari, S.K., 2014. Challenges of organ shortage for transplantation: solutions and opportunities. International Journal of Organ Transplantation Medicine 5 (3), 87–96.

Salehi-Nik, N., et al., 2013. Engineering parameters in bioreactor's design: a critical aspect in tissue engineering. BioMed Research International, 762132, 2013.

Sekine, H., et al., 2013. In vitro fabrication of functional three-dimensional tissues with perfusable blood vessels. Nature Communications 4, 1399.

Sheng, W., et al., 2014. Capture, release and culture of circulating tumor cells from pancreatic cancer patients using an enhanced mixing chip. Lab on a Chip 14, 89–98.

Stabler, C.L., et al., 2005. In vivo noninvasive monitoring of a tissue engineered construct using 1H NMR spectroscopy. Cell Transplantation 14 (2–3), 139–149.

Stenderup, K., et al., 2003. Aging is associated with decreased maximal life span and accelerated senescence of bone marrow stromal cells. Bone 33 (6), 919–926.

Takahashi, K., et al., 2007. Induction of pluripotent stem cells from adult human fibroblasts by defined factors. Cell 131 (5), 861–872.

Takebe, T., et al., 2014. Generation of a vascularized and functional human liver from an iPSC-derived organ bud transplant. Nature Protocols 9 (2), 396–409.

Thomson, J.A., et al., 1998. Embryonic stem cell lines derived from human blastocysts. Science 282 (5391), 1145–1147.

Wert, G.D., 2003. Human embryonic stem cells: research, ethics and policy. Human Reproduction 18 (4), 672–682.

Xu, T., et al., 2009. Fabrication and characterization of bio-engineered cardiac pseudo tissues. Biofabrication 1 (3), 035001.

Yang, H., Miller, W., Papoutsakis, E., 2002. Higher pH promotes megakaryocytic maturation and apoptosis. Stem Cell 20, 320–328.

Yu, Y., et al., 2016. Three-dimensional bioprinting using self-assembling scalable scaffold-free “tissue strands” as a new bioink. Scientific Reports 6, 28714.

Yu, Y., Zhang, Y., Ozbolat, I.T., 2014. A hybrid bioprinting approach for scale-up tissue fabrication. Journal of Manufacturing Science and Engineering 136 (6), 61013.

Zhang, Y., Yu, Y., Chen, H., et al., 2013a. Characterization of printable cellular micro-fluidic channels for tissue engineering. Biofabrication 5 (2), 025004.

Zhang, Y., et al., 2015. In vitro study of directly bioprinted perfusable vasculature conduits. Biomaterials Science 3 (1), 134–143.

Zhang, Y., Yu, Y., Ozbolat, I.T., 2013b. Direct bioprinting of vessel-like tubular microfluidic channels. Journal of Nanotechnology in Engineering and Medicine 4 (2), 020902.

9

Applications of 3D Bioprinting*

CHAPTER OUTLINE

There are no such things as applied sciences, only applications of science
Louis Pasteur

*With minor contributions by Dr. Weijie Peng, The Pennsylvania State University.

9.1 Introduction

Bioprinting is a growing field that makes a revolutionary impact on medical and pharmaceutical sciences, and it has gained significant attention worldwide. It is a computer-aided transfer process for simultaneous writing of living cells and biomaterials with a prescribed layer-by-layer stacking organization to fabricate bioengineered constructs (Ozbolat, 2015b). It offers great precision on spatial placement of cells, proteins, DNA, drug particles, grow factors, and biologically active particles to better guide tissue generation and formation. This powerful technology appears to be more promising for advancing tissue fabrication toward physiologically relevant tissue constructs, tissue models, tissues and organs, and organs-on-a-chip models for a broad spectrum of application areas (Ozbolat and Hospodiuk, 2016).

Bioprinting technology has a broad utility in various application areas such as tissue engineering and regenerative medicine (Jakab et al., 2010; Moroni et al., 2006), transplantation and clinics (Ozbolat, 2015a), drug screening and high-throughput assays (Snyder et al., 2011), and cancer research (Perkins, 2007) as depicted in Fig. 9.1.

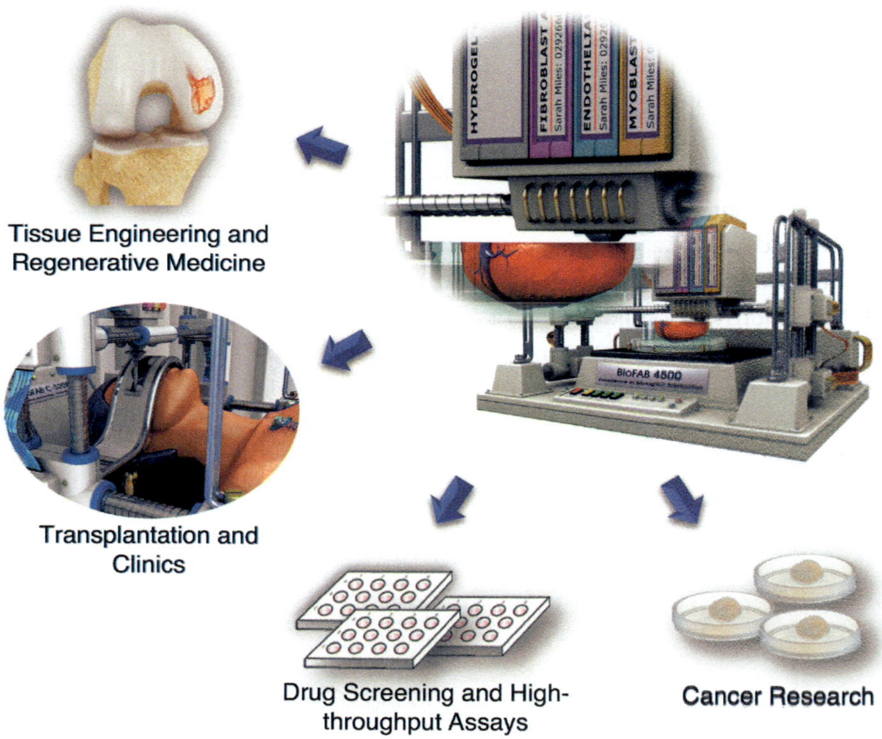

FIGURE 9.1 Application areas of bioprinting technology including tissue engineering and regenerative medicine, transplantation and clinics, drug screening and high-throughput assays, and cancer research *(Image courtesy of Christopher Barnatt, www.explaningthefuture.com).*

Bioprinting for tissue engineering and regenerative medicine fields has been around for more than a decade, and anatomically correct cell-laden constructs and scaffolds have been fabricated for various tissue types from connective and epithelial tissues to muscle and nervous tissues. With its great advantage in patterning and precisely positioning multiple cell types, bioprinting has circumvented one of the major shortcomings of traditional scaffold fabrication techniques and has enabled fabrication of nativelike tissues with heterocellular microenvironment. Although the vast majority of the efforts have been geared toward the fundamental science behind major bioprinting techniques such as extrusion-based bioprinting (EBB) (see Chapter 4), droplet-based bioprinting (DBB) (see Chapter 5), and laser-based bioprinting (LBB) (see Chapter 6), a substantial focus has recently been given to bioprinting for functional tissue fabrication (Ozbolat, 2015a). Particularly, considerable work has been dedicated to bioprinting for animal transplantation, where bioprinted tissues have been implanted to various associated sites in vivo. With the latest advances in in situ bioprinting, bioprinting technology has become a highly attractive approach to build body parts in operating rooms. As further progress taking place in biomaterials, cells, and transplantation technologies, bioprinting will translate from bench to bedside when approved for human use and has a myriad of advantageous in operating rooms in the near future. Before transitioning into clinical practice, bioprinting has already made a great leap in pharmaceutical use as it does not entail any regulatory approvals and there is currently an emerging bioprinting market for tissue fabrication for drug testing and high-throughput assays. With the inclusion of multiple cell types and facilitated complex heterocellular physiologically relevant environment, bioprinted tissue models (i.e., liver) have been used in drug screening. In addition, bioprinting has recently been used in cancer research to investigate cancer pathology, growth, and metastasis in a physiologically relevant microenvironment (Knowlton et al., 2016).

In this chapter, application areas of bioprinting technology are presented with an in-depth discussion on successfully bioprinted tissue types in tissue engineering and regenerative medicine, transplantation and clinics, drug screening and high-throughput assays, and cancer research. For each application, limitations of existing technologies are discussed, and future prospects are provided to the reader.

9.2 Tissue Engineering and Regenerative Medicine

Bioprinting of functional organs at clinically relevant dimensions still remains elusive as there are several challenges such as but not limited to the integration of vascular network from arteries and veins down to capillaries, incorporation of various cell types to recapitulate complex organ biology, and limited structural and mechanical integrity and long-term functionality (Ozbolat and Yu, 2013). Despite these difficulties, a wide variety of tissues have been successfully bioprinted such as thin or hollow tissues [i.e., blood vessel (Itoh et al., 2015)] or tissues that do not need vascularization, i.e., cartilage (Yu et al., 2016).

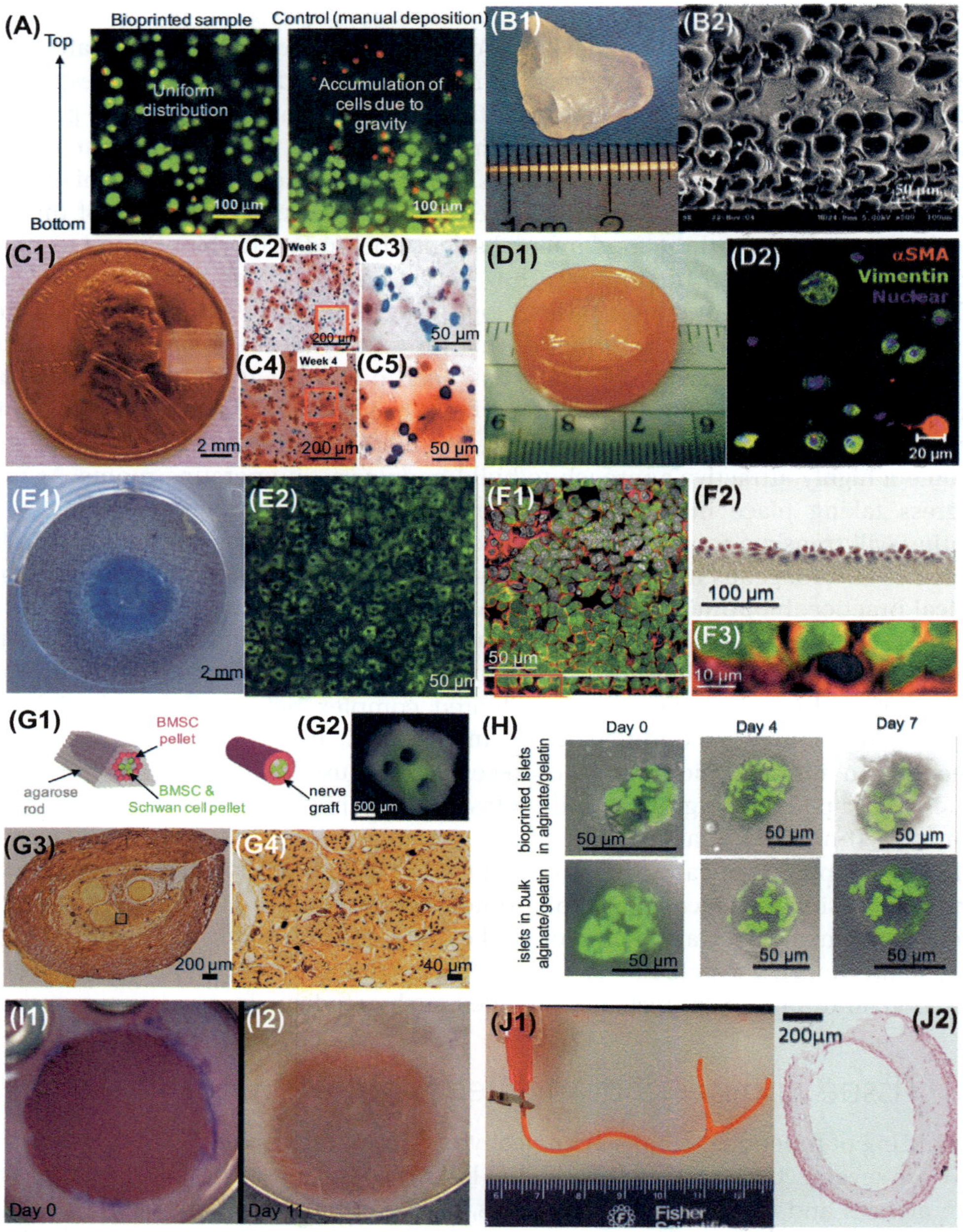

FIGURE 9.2 Bioprinted tissue constructs for tissue engineering and regenerative medicine. (A) Inkjet bioprinting of human mesenchymal stem cells (hMSCs) in hydrogels for bone tissue engineering, where bioprinting resulted in uniform distribution of hMSCs in oppose to accumulated hMSCs at the bottom of the scaffold due to gravity when hMSCs were manually pipetted *(Reproduced/adapted with permission from Gao et al. (2014)).* (B1) Bioprinting of cardiac tissue constructs with connected ventricles using a modified-HP printer. (B2) SEM image

9.2.1 Bone Tissue

Bone tissue engineering has been widely studied using bioprinting as bioprinting has the ability to fabricate anatomically correct patient-specific tissue constructs. In a recent study (Gao et al., 2014), a thermal inkjet bioprinter was used to fabricate poly(ethylene glycol) dimethacrylate (PEGDMA) scaffolds. Bone marrow–derived human mesenchymal stem cells (hMSCs) were coprinted with nanoparticles of bioactive glass and hydroxyapatite (HA) under simultaneous polymerization. Bioprinting in that study enabled uniform distribution of hMSCs compared to manually pipetted hMSCs, which accumulated at the bottom of the scaffold due to gravity (see Fig. 9.2A). The results revealed that the bioprinted constructs encapsulating hMSCs and HA demonstrated the highest cell viability, collagen production, and alkaline phosphate activity with increased compressive modulus after 21-day culture in vitro. Bioprinting HA particles were also performed for in situ bioprinting purposes, where an LBB system was used to deposit HA nanoparticles (n-HAs) into mouse calvarial defects in a framework study (Keriquel et al., 2010), as detailed in Section 9.3.

In another study, Fedorovich et al. (2008) bioprinted heterocellular tissue constructs made of Matrigel™ and alginate hydrogels. Endothelial progenitor and multipotent stromal cells were bioprinted in a spatially controlled manner, and the bioprinted constructs were subcutaneously implanted into immune-deficient mice. By

of the cross section of the scaffold showing loaded cells *(Reproduced/adapted with permission from (Xu et al. (2009a,b))*. (C1) Bioprinting of a 4 mm-PEG cartilage tissue construct with (C2–C5) Safranin-O staining with limited glycosaminoglycan deposition without transforming growth factor beta-1 and fibroblast growth factor-2 treatment even if high density (20 million cells per mL) was used *(Reproduced/adapted with permission from Cui et al. (2012b))*. (D1) A bioprinted heart valve with encapsulated human aortic valvular interstitial cell and (D2) a representative immunohistochemistry image showing αSMA (*green*) and vimentin (*red*) expression *(Reproduced/adapted with permission from (Duan et al. (2014))*. (E1) A bioprinted 40-layer alginate ring-shape construct, where (E2) human embryonic stem cells differentiated toward hepatocyte-like cells showing positive for albumin expression *(Reproduced/adapted with permission from Faulkner-Jones et al. (2015))*. (F1) Bioprinted four-layer lung tissue model with highly organized distribution of a 549 cells (*green*) and endothelial cells (labeled with VE-cadherin in pink), where F-actin and nuclei were labeled in *red* and *white*, respectively. (F2) Histological cross section stained with Masson–Goldner trichrome coloration showing highly uniform thickness of a tissue sample. Cytoplasm, collagen fibers, and cell nuclei were stained in *red*, *green*, and *dark brown*, respectively. (F3) Sagittal cross section demonstrates uniform epithelial layer on the top and endothelial cell layer at the bottom *(Reproduced/adapted with permission from Horváth et al. (2015))*. (G1) Scaffold-free bioprinting of nerve tissue using bone marrow stem cell (BMSC) pellet and coculture of BMSC and Schwan cell pellet, where cell pellet was bioprinted within printed agarose mold for aggregation of cells (G2) for fabrication of multiluminal nerve grafts. (G3–G4) Bielschowsky's staining of histological sections showing axons in *black dots (Reproduced/adapted with permission from Owens et al. (2013))*. (H) Green fluorescent protein–transduced islets plotted in alginate/gelatin scaffolds kept their morphology over a week culture compared to the encapsulated counterparts in bulk hydrogels (control) *(Reproduced/adapted with permission from Marchioli et al. (2015))*. (I1) A bioprinted skin substitute consisting of 20-layer of fibroblasts and 20-layer of keratinocytes on the top of Matriderm® was implanted on dorsa of a mice (I2) resulted in complete wound closure on Day 11 *(Reproduced/adapted from open-access source Michael et al. (2013))*. (J1) Bioprinted vascular tissue constructs using a coaxial nozzle apparatus, where (J2) loaded human umbilical vein smooth muscle cells (HUVSMCs) generated smooth muscle matrix under 6-week differentiation period, particularly in the luminal and outer surface of the tissue constructs *(Reproduced/adapted from Zhang et al. (2015))*.

incorporating osteoinductive biphasic calcium phosphate microparticles, multipotent stromal cells were differentiated into osteogenic lineage and facilitated bone formation in 6 weeks. In addition to osteoinductive materials, incorporation of growth factors is also crucial in stem cell differentiation in bone tissue engineering. Phillippi et al. (2008) demonstrated the effect of bone morphogenetic protein (BMP-2) on stem cell fate. Using inkjet bioprinting of patterned BMP-2 on fibrin-coated coverslips, primary muscle-derived stem cells were differentiated toward osteogenic lineage on the pattern even if they were treated with myogenic differentiation conditions.

9.2.2 Cardiac Tissue

Cardiac tissue engineering has been a growing interest as heart failure is a devastating disease (Hirt et al., 2014). While myocardium tissue has a limited regeneration capability as myocytes proliferation rapidly ceases after birth (Eulalio et al., 2012), tissue engineering of such a structurally and functionally complicated organ is essential. In the literature, limited attempt has been made in bioprinting of cardiac tissue models. Jakab et al. (2008) demonstrated EBB of tissue spheroids comprising human vascular endothelial cells (HUVECs) and cardiac cells isolated from myocardial tubes of chicken embryos. Tissue spheroids, which were adhesive and scaffold-free and which possessed rapid self-assembly capabilities, were bioprinted next-to-each other on collagen type-I biopaper in a single-layer grid pattern. Upon bioprinting, tissue spheroids were fused together in approximately 70 h and formed a single cardiac tissue patch that can synchronously beat. In addition to the scaffold-free approach undertaken in the above-mentioned work, scaffold-based bioprinting has been investigated in a few studies. Xu et al. (2009a,b) bioprinted cardiac tissue constructs in a half-heart shape with connected ventricles using inkjet-based bioprinting as shown in Fig. 9.2B1–B2. In their study, primary feline adult and H1 cardiomyocytes were encapsulated in alginate/gelation composite hydrogels, and the cross-linker (calcium chloride solution) was selectively sprayed layer by layer. The resulting tissue construct with connected ventricles was electrically stimulated, and functional excitation–contraction coupling was successfully demonstrated. In addition to these studies, patterning of cells was also applied in cardiac tissue engineering. Gaebel et al. (2011) utilized a laser-induced forward transfer (LIFT) technique to pattern HUVECs and hMSCs in a geometrically defined pattern on polyester urethane urea (PEUU), and the fabricated samples were transplanted to the infarcted zone of rat hearts after LAD ligation. In 8 weeks posttransplantation, samples with LIFT-derived patterns facilitated increased vessel formation compared to randomly bioprinted cells as control groups, and the resulted myocardium patch provided significant functional improvement. Besides primary cells, human cardiac–derived cardiomyocyte progenitor cells (hCMPCs) were also bioprinted in mesh pattern made of alginate hydrogel (Gaetani et al., 2012). Bioprinted hCMPCs demonstrated phenotypic properties of cardiac lineage with enhanced expression of early cardiac transcription factors Nkx2.5, Gata-4, and Mef-2c.

9.2.3 Cartilage Tissue

Current tissue engineering techniques for cartilage regeneration cannot produce cartilage tissue that is indistinguishable from native tissue in terms of zonal properties and architectures (Makris et al., 2015). Thanks to its great potential for precise spatial and temporal deposition of cells and biomaterials with sophisticated patterns, bioprinting has recently gained increasing attention for engineering cartilage tissues that can closely mimic native tissues with zonally differentiated cells and extracellular matrix (ECM) composition (Kesti et al., 2015). Due to absence of blood vessels, cartilage tissue bioprinting has been extensively studied using various bioprinting modalities. LBB of stem cell–differentiated chondrocytes was attempted by Gruene et al. (2010) in which a computer-aided biofabrication technique was used with the assistance of LIFT. They successfully bioprinted porcine bone marrow–derived mesenchymal stem cells (MSCs) with high viability, where cells maintained their functionality and differentiation ability into osteogenic and chondrogenic lineage.

Inkjet-based bioprinting has also been used in cartilage tissue engineering as well as for cartilage defect repair. Cui et al. (2012a) modified an HP desktop printer into a bioprinter, where they were able to bioprint human chondrocytes loaded in PEGDMA hydrogel in a layer-by-layer manner. The bioprinted cartilage construct had mechanical properties and biochemical composition close to native cartilage. Also by implanting bioprinted cartilage constructs into articular cartilage defects, integration with the native tissue was observed with enhanced interface strength, which significantly improved the quality of the repaired cartilage tissue. In another study using the above experimental setup, the same group fabricated PEG scaffolds (see Fig. 9.2C1) and investigated the effect of combined transforming growth factor beta-1 (TGF-β1) and fibroblast growth factor-2 (FGF-2) on cell proliferation and differentiation capability, and demonstrated that samples treated with TGF-β1 and FGF-2 facilitated the highest glycosaminoglycan (GAG) content (Cui et al., 2012b) and samples without growth factor treatment did not secrete GAG even in 4-week culture (see Fig. 9.2C2–C5). Most recently, Xu et al. (2013) created a hybrid bioprinting method to fabricate mechanically improved cartilage tissue constructs by combining three-dimensional (3D) bioprinting and electrospinning techniques. In that study, electrospinning of polycaprolactone (PCL) fibers together with inkjet bioprinting of rabbit elastic chondrocytes in fibrin–collagen hydrogel was demonstrated. After printing, cell viability was well maintained and fabricated constructs formed cartilage tissues both in vitro and in vivo. Furthermore, the printed structures showed improved mechanical properties compared to printed hydrogels alone.

In addition to above hydrogels, sodium alginate has been widely used for cartilage tissue bioprinting. The author's group demonstrated hybrid bioprinting of chondrocytes loaded in bioprinted filaments in tandem with bioprinting of chondrocyte spheroids to increase the cell density of the tissue constructs (Ozbolat et al., 2014). A Multi-Arm BioPrinter was used to facilitate such a complex hybrid architecture. Using sodium alginate and silver nanoparticles, McAlpine's group (Mannoor et al., 2013) successfully printed bionic ear models, which were composed of chondrocyte-loaded alginate in ear shape and a conductive coil with the ability to translate sound waves into digital data. In addition to bioprinting cartilage tissue constructs, there have been studies to improve the bioink capabilities as well. In this regard, Bonassar's group presented a mixing chamber to increase the homogeneity of crosslinked sodium alginate loaded with chondrocytes (Cohen et al., 2010). The presented study revealed that as mixing of cell-loaded precrosslinked alginate increased, the fidelity and mechanical properties of the bioprinted constructs improved in addition to the enhancement in their cell viability. Recently, Markstedt et al. (2015) demonstrated mixing alginate with nanocellulose, which has outstanding shear thinning properties enabling fabrication of anatomically correct ear and meniscus constructs. Apart from hydrogels mainly used as bioink, Cho and his coworkers (Pati et al., 2014) recently used Taylor's organ decellularization approach (Ott et al., 2008) to remove cells from native cartilage and chopped it into smaller fragments leaving gel-like material behind. The material was then loaded with chondrocytes and bioprinted in tandem with PCL supporting frame to generate cartilage tissue constructs. The new bioink demonstrated highly suitable environment for growth and proliferation of loaded chondrocytes.

Despite the great progress in bioprinting for cartilage tissue regeneration, bioprinting of zonally stratified articular cartilage tissues with different structural, biomechanical, and biological properties is still a challenge and further progress is needed to achieve articular cartilage tissue constructs with zonal differentiation including more horizontal and thinner collagen fibers with high cell density in superficial zone, and relatively vertical and thicker collagen fibers with less cell density in deeper zones.

9.2.4 Heart Valve

In addition to cardiac tissue engineering, engineering heart valves is also important as heart valves do not possess regeneration capability and dysfunctional heart valves, if the damage or disease is detrimental, need to be replaced by mechanical or biological prosthetic counterparts (Hockaday et al., 2014). Such replacement valves, however, are limited by thrombogenicity and calcification (Jana and Lerman, 2015). Despite its critical role in cardiovascular system, only a very limited number of work has been demonstrated in bioprinting of heart valves. Butcher's group at Cornell University demonstrated the bioprinting of a heart valve for the first time (Hockaday et al., 2012) using a dual-head bioprinter modified from a Fab@Home printer (Malone and Lipson, 2007). In that work, a dual crosslinking mechanism, consisting of ionic and physical crosslinking, was used to print polyethylene glycol diacrylate (PEGDA) mixed with sodium alginate. After printing, porcine aortic valve interstitial cells were seeded and cultured for up to 21 days. In their study, anatomically accurate axisymmetric aortic valve geometries, composed of a root wall and trileaflets, were demonstrated. Although the first-time presented work does not fall under bioprinting as cells were not involved during the printing process, the group later demonstrated bioprinting of aortic valves using different hydrogels and cell phenotypes. In another study by that group (Duan et al., 2013), dual-nozzle bioprinting of composite alginate/gelatin hydrogel was performed to fabricate thin hydrogel discs. Aortic root sinus smooth muscle cells (SMCs) and aortic valve interstitial cells (VICs) were spatially bioprinted, and samples were incubated for a week. The results revealed a cell viability of $81.4 \pm 3.4\%$ and $83.2 \pm 4.0\%$ SMCs and VICs, respectively. Acellular aortic valve constructs, on the other hand, exhibited reduced modulus, ultimate strength, and peak strain. In a recent study (Duan et al., 2014), the same group presented bioprinting of composite hydrogels using methacrylated hyaluronic acid (Me-HA) and methacrylated gelatin (Me-Gel) loaded with human aortic valvular interstitial cells (HAVICs). Fabricated samples (see Fig. 9.2D1) represented the designed trileaflet valve shape accurately, and the cells bioprinted with increased Me-Gel concentration exhibited better spreading. HAVICs encapsulated within the composite hydrogel expressed alpha smooth muscle actin (α-SMC) and vimentin (see Fig. 9.2D2) and remodeled ECM with deposition of collagen and GAGs.

9.2.5 Liver Tissue

Although liver has excellent regenerative and recuperative properties, liver tissue engineering has been a growing interest while liver failure, in association with failure of multiple organs, is a significant cause of morbidity and mortality (Yoon No et al., 2015). Engineering liver tissues stands as a promising direction for future organ transplantation needs in addition to the great potential of bioprinted liver tissue models in drug testing and high-throughput screening as liver tissue is highly sensitive to drug toxicity. Faulkner-Jones et al. (2015) demonstrated the bioprinting of human-induced pluripotent stem cells (hiPSCs), where bioprinted hiPSCs were stimulated and differentiated into hepatocytes for liver microorgan engineering. The presented work systematically analyzed the effect of the bioprinting process and parameters on stem cell fate and the influence of pressure and nozzle length on the viability of hiPSC and human embryonic stem cells, concluded that the utilized inkjet bioprinting process was gentle enough to maintain viability and pluripotency of cells, and directed their differentiation into hepatic lineage. A dual-head valve-based inkjet bioprinter was used to deposit sodium alginate and calcium chloride to fabricate multilayer tissue constructs (see Fig. 9.2E1), and the results demonstrated that bioprinted stem cells differentiated into hepatic lineages successfully after a 17-day differentiation period and expressed hepatocyte markers including HNF4α, albumin, and ZO-1, where albumin secretion peaked on day 21 (see Fig. 9.2E2).

In addition to bioprinting liver tissue constructs, liver carcinoma HepG2 immortal cells were bioprinted in larger tissue models. Bertassoni et al. utilized a modified NovoGen MMX Bioprinter™ and bioprinted HepG2 cells, and fibroblast within gelatin-methacrylamide (GelMA) hydrogel strands along with agarose strands. Upon printing, agarose solidified immediately due to rapid drop in the temperature, and UV light was applied to photo-crosslink GelMA precursor under 6.9 mW/cm^2 of UV light (360–480 nm) up to a minute (Bertassoni et al., 2014a). After complete gelation of GelMA, agarose was completely removed to create perfusable channels. The study revealed that cells preserved their viability up to 8 days. The similar work was then extended using other hydrogels such as star poly(ethylene glycol-co-lactide) acrylate (SPELA), PEGDMA, and PEGDA hydrogels at different concentrations (Bertassoni et al., 2014b).

This section presented liver tissue bioprinting attempts for tissue engineering only, and further discussion on bioprinting of liver tissue models for drug testing and high-throughput screening will be provided to the reader in Section 9.4.

9.2.6 Lung Tissue

Bioprinting for lung tissue engineering is highly new as there is only a recent work attempted to fabricate a lung tissue model using bioprinting. Horváth et al. (2015) demonstrated bioprinting of an in vitro air–blood barrier model using BioFactory® by regenHU Ltd. In this regard, they bioprinted a zonally stratified tissue construct layer by layer. First, a thin layer of Matrigel™ was bioprinted as a basement membrane followed by bioprinting of a single layer of EA.hy926 endothelial cells to facilitate attachment of cells on the Matrigel™ layer. Later, on day 2, a new layer of Matrigel™ was bioprinted on the top of the previously built construct followed by bioprinting of a single layer of A549 epithelial cells. Manually deposited layers were also constructed as control samples. On day 5, the samples were fixed for characterization, and cell viability of >95% and ≥86% were achieved for epithelial and endothelial cells, respectively. As can be seen in Fig. 9.2F1 and F3, epithelial and endothelial cells were uniformly distributed with epithelial cells on the top and endothelial cells at the bottom. Sagittal histological sections also confirmed formation of a highly thin, packed, and uniform tissue layer (see Fig. 9.2F2) compared to manually pipetted control samples. The barrier quality, such as tightness of the constructs, was investigated through measuring the translocation of blue Dextran molecules from the apical to the basolateral compartment of the samples after 3 days of culture, and results revealed that the tightness of the bioprinted samples was better than that of the manually pipetted samples.

9.2.7 Neural Tissue

Engineering tissues for nervous system offers tremendous promise to replace diseased, aged, or injured components of nervous system; however, there is limited work done in the context of bioprinting nerve grafts. Lee et al. (2010) studied the effect of vascular endothelial growth factor (VEGF) release on proliferation and migration of murine neural stem cells (C17.2). In their study, C17.2 cells were bioprinted on a collagen layer next to a fibrin disk loaded with VEGF. The study showed that cells migrated toward VEGF-releasing fibrin gel and proliferated successfully in contrast to the cells that could not proliferate in collagen matrix. Recently, Hsieh et al. (2015) demonstrated bioprinting of a thermo-responsive polyurethane (PU) hydrogel with tunable stiffness and gelation ability at 37°C without need for a crosslinker. They showed the effectiveness of the bioink by loading it with neural stem cells and injecting it into a zebrafish embryo neural injury model. The results revealed that the injected gel rescued the function of impaired nervous system in 6 days.

Owens et al. (2013) used a scaffold-free approach, where pellet of Schwann cells and bone marrow stem cells were extruded within a 3D-printed agarose mold (see Fig. 9.2G1 for the schematic of the process). Cells in agarose mold aggregated and formed nerve tissue graft with three lumina in each as shown in Fig. 9.2G2. The fabricated grafts were then implanted into mice, and their histology (see Fig. 9.2G3–G4) and functionality were evaluated 10 months after implantation and compared with the functionality of autologous grafts and hollow collagen grafts. Although the number of samples was not enough to draw a definitive conclusion about the performance of the 3D-bioprinted grafts with respect to commercially available collagen grafts, the presented case demonstrated a proof-of-concept for bioprinting nerve grafts.

9.2.8 Pancreas Tissue

As primary pancreatic β-cells do not easily survive in vitro and only a very few attempts were taken place in differentiation of β-cells from human stem cells, regeneration of pancreas tissues is primarily embodied to the extent that only β-cells from mouse lines or insulinoma cells have been used to fabricate pancreatic islets (Pagliuca and Melton, 2013; Pagliuca et al., 2015; Raikwar et al., 2015). A very few work has been done in the context of bioprinting for pancreatic tissues. Recently, Marchioli et al. (2015) encapsulated human and mouse islets as well as rat insulinoma INS1E β-cells within alginate or alginate/gelatin hydrogels and bioprinted them in dual-layer scaffolds. The scaffolds were later implanted in diabetic mice and explanted 7 days thereafter. Although the viability and morphology of islets were not impaired by encapsulation and bioprinting processes in both alginate and alginate/gelatin hydrogels (see Fig. 9.2H), bioprinted islets and INS1E β-cells lost their functionality in 7 day as they were not responsive to the change in glucose level. This can be attributed to the high level of presence of calcium (Ca^{2+}) ions within crosslinked alginate because transmembrane calcium ion gradient, mediated by voltage-gated calcium channels, stimulated higher insulin secretion at low glucose level (Proks and Ashcroft, 1995). In addition, a recent work demonstrated the microfabrication of scaffold-free tissue strands (with strong expression of insulin) for EBB (Akkouch et al., 2015), where tissue strands were made of rat fibroblasts and mouse insulinoma TC-3 β-cells in the core and shell, respectively. The authors envisioned to use the demonstrated tissue strands for scale-up tissue bioprinting purposes.

9.2.9 Skin Tissue

Several tissue engineering approaches have been applied in skin tissue fabrication and tissue substitutes including autologous split-thickness skin graft (gold standard) (Coruh and Yontar, 2012), allografts (Leon-Villapalos et al., 2010), acellular dermal substitutes, and cellularized graft-like commercial products (Leon-Villapalos et al., 2010), i.e., Dermagraft and Apligraf (Organogenesis Inc.) (Metcalfe and Ferguson, 2007). Recently, bioprinting technology has been adopted for skin tissue fabrication as well. Lee et al. (2013) presented bioprinting of skin tissue using an 8-channel valve-based bioprinter, where a 13-layer tissue construct was bioprinted layer by layer using collagen hydrogel. Keratinocytes were bioprinted on the top of alternating layers of human foreskin fibroblasts and acellular collagen layers, and the resulting constructs demonstrated densely packed cells in epidermis layers in oppose to the dermis with low density of cells and less ECM deposition. In addition to DBB, LBB has also been used for biofabrication of skin tissue substitutes (Koch et al., 2012). Cells from human immortalized keratinocyte cell line and NIH 3T3 fibroblasts were bioprinted in collagen matrix in alternating layers on a sheet of Matriderm™. Histological results demonstrated high density of keratinocytes and fibroblasts with expression of laminin protein, which is a major component of basement membrane in skin. The same group extended their work (Michael et al., 2013) and demonstrated implantation of the tissue constructs on dorsa of mice as shown in Fig. 9.2I1. Results revealed that the bioprinted tissues were engrafted with the hosts in 11 days (see Fig. 9.2I2) with stratified epidermis with early sign of differentiation and formation of *stratum corneum* as well as some blood vessels. Control samples at the air–liquid interface in vitro culture, on the other hand, demonstrated proliferation of cells with limited differentiation. In a recent study (Yanez et al., 2014), Boland's group demonstrated the effect of bioprinting endothelial cells within skin substitutes on formation of macrovasculature during new tissue remodeling. In this regard, they encapsulated neonatal human dermal fibroblast and neonatal human epidermal keratinocytes (NHEKs) in collagen and laid down the dermis layer followed by patterning human dermal microvascular endothelial cells (HMVECs) on dermis layer of the construct by selectively bioprinting thrombin-laden HMVECS on manually deposited fibrinogen layer. The process was completed by covering the fibrin layer with collagen-laden NHEK cells. Then, the fabricated skin substitutes were implanted on dorsa of mice and compared with implanted commercially available skin substitutes (control). The results revealed that bioprinted HMVECs formed microvessels and the bioprinted constructs barely generated contraction compared to the control groups. In abovementioned studies, tissue constructs were bioprinted in vitro and implanted to a host; however, Skardal et al. (2012) demonstrated in situ bioprinting of stratified skin substitutes by alternating layer of fibrinogen/collagen and thrombin loaded with amniotic fluid–derived stem cells due to their lack of immunogenicity. With in situ bioprinting, skin substitutes were 3D bioprinted directly onto full thickness wounds on pigs and recapitulated the native skin more closely than control groups including the bioink loaded with MSCs and acellular hydrogels. Despite the efforts in skin tissue bioprinting, biofabrication of skin substitutes that virtually mimic native skin is still a challenge as integrating sweat glands is remained elusive.

9.2.10 Vascular Tissue

Bioprinting of scale-up tissues and organs vitally depends on vascularization as integration of vascular network will essentially provide oxygen and media supply to cells for their survival and function (Ozbolat, 2015b). Vascular tissue fabrication has been performed by various bioprinting modalities including EBB (Zhang et al., 2013a,b; Yu et al., 2013; Norotte et al., 2009), DBB (Xu et al., 2012; Christensen et al., 2015; Blaeser et al., 2013), and LBB (Xiong et al., 2015b). In EBB, a wide variety of extrusion techniques have been utilized. The author's group used coaxial-nozzle extrusion, where hydrogels including sodium alginate and chitosan were bioprinted directly in tubular form with encapsulated cells (Zhang et al., 2013a,b). During coaxial (core–shell) flow, ejected crosslinker (flowing through the core) contacted the precursor hydrogel solution (flowing through the shell) and facilitated rapid gelation and formation of tubular constructs (Fig. 9.2J1). Six-week-cultured HUVSMC-laden samples demonstrated deposition of smooth muscle matrix (Fig. 9.2J2). That approach enabled direct bioprinting of vascular constructs in a practical manner. In addition, there are other direct vascular tissue bioprinting approaches, such as bioprinting droplets of cell-laden hydrogels layer by layer using inkjet-based bioprinting performed by Nakamura et al. (Nishiyama et al., 2008), Huang's group (Xu et al., 2012; Christensen et al., 2015), and Blaeser et al. (2013). With the ability of bottom-up construction, inkjet-based bioprinting enabled branched tubes built in both horizontal and vertical directions. A similar approach was also performed using LBB demonstrated by Huang's group (Xiong et al., 2015a,b). In abovementioned studies, scaffold-based approaches were utilized; however, Forgacs and his coworkers followed a scaffold-free approach in bioprinting vascular tissues, where tissue spheroids were bioprinted one by one and self-assembled into larger tissue units (Norotte et al., 2009). As agarose is inert to cell adhesion, the printed agarose mold facilitated rapid fusion of tissue spheroids and maturation of the tissue.

In addition to direct bioprinting of tubular vascular tissues, indirect bioprinting of perfusable tissue constructs has been performed using various hydrogels including fibrin (Lee et al., 2014), collagen (Zhao et al., 2012), and GelMA (Bertassoni et al., 2014a). In indirect approach, a fugitive ink [that is dissolvable or reversibly crosslinkable such as agarose (Bertassoni et al., 2014b), sugar (Miller et al., 2012), Pluronic (Wu et al., 2011), and gelatin (Zhao et al., 2012)] was used to create open channels. Upon removing the fugitive ink, endothelial cells were perfused and glued to create endothelium within open channels (Miller et al., 2012). This approach enables bioprinting of highly complex vascular constructs that can be perfused over long time depending on the degradation profile of the matrix. Although both approaches can be utilized, the former one is more appropriate in generating vascular grafts for transplantation and the second one is more appropriate for fabrication of perfusable channels for in vitro tissue engineering applications (Ozbolat, 2015a). Bioprinted vascular tissues should be designed and fabricated in a way that they can be easily sutured to a blood vessel in a host, and possess certain properties such as enough mechanical strength to satisfy suture retention and burst pressure, sufficient intactness of endothelium to prevent thrombosis, and a high patency rate to support occlusion-free circulation (Quint et al., 2011).

9.2.11 Composite Tissues

In addition to single tissue types, efforts have been geared toward bioprinting composite tissues to recapitulate the complex biology, anatomy, and functionality of organ-level structures. Merceron et al. (2015) recently demonstrated fabrication of muscle–tendon units by bioprinting hybrid constructs using a multihead nozzle assembly. In this regard, PCL and PU was 3D printed to construct a frame to support cellular constructs, where half of the unit was printed using PCL and the other half was printed using PU (Fig. 9.3A1–A4). A composite hydrogel-based bioink, comprising 3 mg/ml hyaluronic acid, 35 mg/ml gelatin, and 25 mg/ml fibrinogen in calcium-free high-glucose Dulbecco's Modified Eagle Medium (DMEM), was used to 3D bioprint 3T3 fibroblasts and myoblasts into the PCL and PU frames to construct tendon and muscle units, respectively. The results revealed cell viability of >80% with differentiated cells at the end of a 7-day culture. The final muscle–tendon units were elastic on the PU-C1C12 muscle section with an elastic modulus of 0.39 ± 0.05 MPa and stiff on the PCL-3T3 tendon side with an elastic modulus of 46.47 ± 2.67 MPa.

In addition to muscle–tendon units, bioprinting of osteochondral models has been an interest in tissue engineering. Fedovorich et al. (2011) demonstrated bioprinting of MSCs and chondrocytes using alginate in mesh pattern with two different cell types

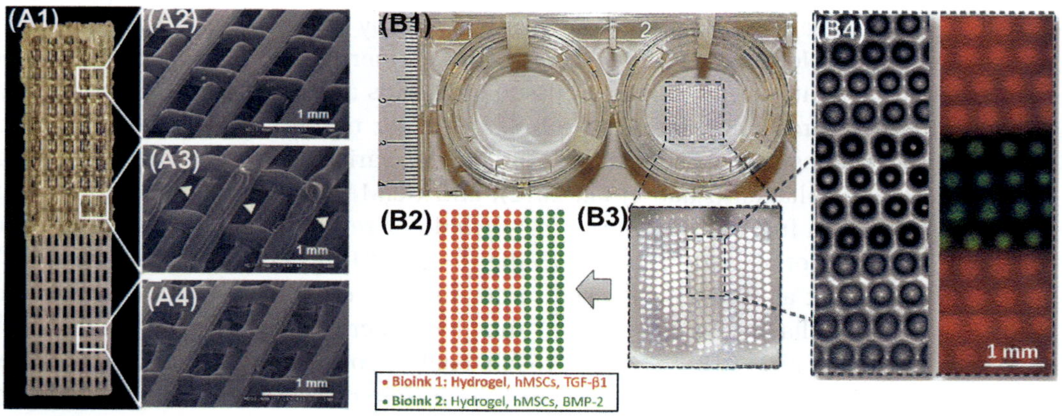

FIGURE 9.3 Bioprinted composite tissue constructs. (A1) A muscle–tendon unit frame made of polyurethane (PU) (upper-half) and polycaprolactone (PCL) (lower-half) at a higher magnification view of (A2) printed PU filaments, (A2) filaments at the interface, and (A3) printed PCL filaments *(Reproduced/adapted with permission from Merceron et al. (2015))*. (B1) Bioprinted fibrocartilage samples (B2–B3) patterned by selectively depositing human mesenchymal stem cell (hMSC)–laden methacrylated gelatin droplets loaded with either transforming growth factor beta-1 or bone morphogenetic protein (BMP-2). (B4) Bioprinted precursor gel droplets were photo-crosslinked, and droplets were demonstrated using Rhodamine B (*red*) and Dextran-Alexa Fluor 488 (*green*) *(Reproduced/adapted from open source Gurkan et al. (2014))*.

bioprinted within two opposite ends of the scaffold. MSCs were coextruded with osteoinductive biphasic calcium phosphate particles, HA, and β-tricalcium phosphate. The bioprinted samples were cultured with a mixture of chondrogenic and osteogenic medium up to 21 days. The results revealed that bioprinted osteochondral tissue constructs demonstrated differentiated characteristics of cells into both osteogenic and chondrogenic lineages along with related ECM deposition in vitro and in vivo. A similar approach was performed by Park et al. (2014), where a systematic analysis was performed to understand the effect of native ECM components on the fate of osteoblasts and chondrocytes. In this regard, they bioprinted osteoblasts in collagen type-I and chondrocytes in hyaluronic acid and compare the performance of bioprinted osteoblasts and chondrocytes when they were bioprinted in hyaluronic acid and collagen type-I, respectively. Fourteen-day culture in vitro suggested that osteochondral tissue regeneration could be successfully attained when proper hydrogel type was selected. The same group demonstrated another osteochondral model by depositing alginate hydrogel loaded with human chondrocytes and human MG63 osteoblasts within a PCL frame (Shim et al., 2012). Osteoblasts and chondrocytes were supplemented with osteogenic and chondrogenic growth factors loaded in hydrogels for differentiation purposes. Another approach was conducted using acoustic-based bioprinting for the same purpose, where bioprinted nanodroplets of MSCs in TGF-β1 and BMP-2 patterns (see Fig. 9.3B1–B4) resulted in localized differentiation of MSCs toward osteogenic and chondrogenic lineages shown by the gene expression study (Gurkan et al., 2014).

In addition to osteochondral models, Yu and Ozbolat (2014) demonstrated hybrid bioprinting of macrovascularized stromal tissue, where scaffold-free tissue strands made of fibroblasts were assembled around a perfusable macrovasculature loaded with SMCs extruded through a coaxial nozzle unit (Yu et al., 2014). Tissue strands quickly fused and assembled around the macrovasculature in a week, which can be further scaled-up by extending the macrovascular network.

9.2.12 Other Tissue Types

In addition to the presented tissue types, there is a few other work at the early fundamental study level for bioprinting of retinal and brain tissues. Lorber et al. (2014) presented piezoelectric inkjet bioprinting of retinal ganglion cells (RGCs) and glia and investigated the effect of bioprinting parameters on the viability of cells and their growth-promoting properties. They concluded that inkjet bioprinting did not adversely affect the cell viability and RGC neurite outgrowth, rather RGCs demonstrated further neurite growth when bioprinted on a glial substrate. Recently, Lozano et al. (2015) presented manual deposition of primary cortical neuron-laden gellan gum-RGD for brainlike tissue fabrication. Three-layer constructed tissue models, with cortical neurons encapsulated in the top and bottom layers, demonstrated axon growth and penetration toward the cell-free middle layer in 5 days. Although no computer-control motion system was applied, the presented work unveiled the first-time demonstration of layer-by-layer fabrication for brain tissue engineering.

9.3 Transplantation and Clinics

Bioprinting of living tissue and organ constructs has been widely studied, and performance of these constructs was assessed via animal transplantation. Several bioprinted tissue types, including but not limited nerve (Owens et al., 2013), cardiac (Gaebel et al., 2011), blood vessel (Itoh et al., 2015), bone (Keriquel et al., 2010), and skin (Yanez et al., 2014), have been implanted into associated locations on animals to evaluate their functionality, neovascularization, and anastomosis and engraftment with the host (Ozbolat, 2015a). In addition, various tissue constructs have been bioprinted and implanted subcutaneously to assess in vivo differentiation of cells and functionality of implanted tissue constructs (Fedorovich et al., 2011). Despite these attempts, none of bioprinted tissues has been clinically used for humans as no approval has been granted from Food and Drug Administration (FDA) yet. There are no regulations laid down for bioprinters or bioprinted products; however, with the increasing global interest and emerging businesses in the growing bioprinting market, the success with the first technology going through FDA regulations will be exemplary for preceding technologies and products. For details of the regulatory concerns of bioprinting, the reader is referred to Chapter 10.

While bioprinting technology is still in its infancy in clinics, 3D-printed plastic, ceramic, or metallic implants for bone tissue replacement (Bose et al., 2013) have been successfully transplanted into humans. In addition to permanent implants, a recent work published in *the New England Journal of Medicine* (Zopf et al., 2013) demonstrated a unique case of transplantation of a 3D-printed bioresorbable airway splint into an infant. The institutional review board of the University of Michigan consulted with FDA and approved the use of 3D-printed device under the emergency-use exemption and the written consent of the patient's parents. No unforeseen problems have been observed with the splint, and full degradation of the device is expected to take around 3 years. This was an exemplary case for clinical use of 3D-printed scaffolds and hopefully will open up similar success with the bioprinted tissues and organs. Despite the accomplishments in bioprinting research, bioprinting for transplantation in a clinical setting for humans requires further advances and translational efforts (Ozbolat, 2015a). Organs and tissues that do not need significant vascularization (i.e., skin and cartilage) are expected to be translated into clinical use sooner. Tissues and organs that are metabolically highly active (i.e., heart, pancreas, and liver) are immensely challenging. No bioprinting technology so far facilitated fabrication of a vascular hierarchical network spanning arteries and veins down to capillaries. Since it is difficult to bioprint capillaries at the submicron scale using the current technology, an alternative could be to bioprint macrovasculature and then leave the nature to

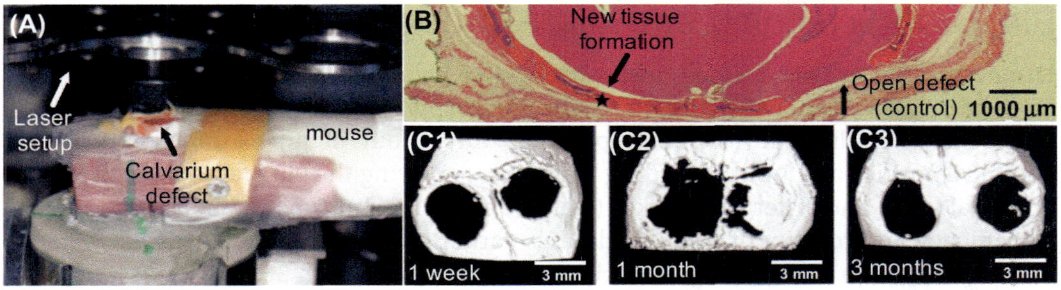

FIGURE 9.4 (A) Laser-assisted bioprinting setup for in situ bone printing of hydroxyapatite nanoparticles into critical-size calvarium defects in mice model. (B) Histology results of three-month in vivo culture revealing new tissue formation (*marked with star*) in oppose to an empty defect. (C1) X-ray microtomography images of bone tissue formation (C1) in 1 week, (C2) 1 month, and (C3) 3 months *(Reproduced/adapted with permission from Michael et al. (2013)).*

create capillaries by itself. The other approach in facilitating vascularization is in situ bioprinting of tissue and organ constructs directly into the defect sites in surgery settings rather than bioprinting tissue constructs and maturating and assessing them in vitro before transplantation. With in situ bioprinting, bioprinted tissue constructs can recruit endothelial cells from the host and facilitate neovascularization followed by anastomosis of newly formed vessels with the vascular network of the host. Therefore, in situ bioprinting has a great advantage over traditional two-step bioprinting approach and can be applied for regeneration of a wide array of tissues and organs (i.e., maxillo- and craniofacial reconstruction, plastic surgery, skin tissue, and flap tissue). In situ bioprinting has been recently used in skin regeneration for large wounds on pig models (Skardal et al., 2012) and calvarium defects in rodents (Ozbolat, 2015a; Keriquel et al., 2010). Fig. 9.4A demonstrates laser-assisted printing of n-HA particles into critical size defects on a mouse model, where one of the defects left empty for the control group. The histology and microtomography results for bone regeneration were not consistent (see Fig. 9.4B–C), which was due to immobilization of printed n-HA particles within the defects. Although the ink in the demonstrated work did not comprise any biologics, it unveiled the application of LBB systems in operating rooms, which will enable translation of bioprinting technologies from bench to bedside.

One of the controversies of the clinical translation potential of bioprinted tissues and organs originates from the bioprinting technology itself as bioprinting involves living cells in bioink and the use of patient-specific cells is fairly new in bioprinting. Stem cells, such as embryonic stem cells and induced-pluripotent stem cells (Yoshida and Yamanaka, 2010), have been potential unlimited sources of patient-specific cells for fabrication of tissues and organs. Patient-specific cells can be differentiated, then bioprinted or bioprinted, and then differentiated toward multiple lineages to fabricate tissues and organs that will have minimum immunogenicity risk as discussed in Chapter 8.

9.4 Drug Screening and High-Throughput Assays

Drug discovery entails a time-consuming and costly endeavor that requires substantial investment in financial and human resources. Despite continuing efforts to improve the productivity of drug development process, only 1 out of an estimated 10,000 new chemical entities and 1 out of 10 drug candidates entering the clinical trial reach the final approval stage and enter the market (Nam et al., 2015). Improving the ability to predict the efficacy and toxicity of drug candidates earlier in drug discovery process will speed up the translation of new drugs into clinics. Recent attempts in 3D in vitro assay systems is an ideal way to resolve this bottleneck since 3D-printed tissue models can closely mimic the native tissue and have the capability to be used in high-throughput assays as they can be bioprinted in microarrays. Bioprinted tissue and organ models have been increasingly considered for the potential of pharmaceutics use such as drug toxicology and high-throughput screening (Peng et al., 2016). Among the three different modalities discussed in previous chapters, DBB has been most common for pharmaceutical use due to its simplicity, versatility, and high-throughput capability (Gudapati et al., 2016). Table 9.1 shows the major strengths and limitations of each modality, within the application domain of pharmaceutics.

In the literature, liver and tumor tissues have been a primary focus in fabrication of tissue models for pharmaceutics. Sun's group investigated the fabrication of a bioprinted liver microorgan model for drug metabolism (Chang et al., 2008) (see Fig. 9.5A1). In that study, an automated syringe-based direct cell writing process was applied for extrusion of hepatocyte (HepG2) cell–encapsulated alginate strands as demonstrated in Fig. 9.5A2. Polydimethylsiloxane (PDMS) elastomer soft lithography was combined with a micromolding technique to fabricate 3D microfluidic chambers housing aforementioned constructs. The presented 3D liver microorgan with a sinusoidal flow pattern was an in vitro 3D microfluidic, microanalytical, microorgan (3DM) device for simulation of the physiological liver response to drug administrations and toxic chemical exposure. Effective drug metabolism in microliver chamber was demonstrated by metabolizing a nonfluorescent prodrug, 7-ethoxy-4-trifluoromethyl coumarin, to an effluent fluorescent metabolite 7-hydroxy-4-trifluoromethyl coumarin. Additionally, they schemed and created dual-microtissue microfluidic chips, which were connected to facilitate multicellular interaction and downstream effects of metabolism on the target tissue (Chang et al., 2010; Snyder et al., 2011). Epithelial cells and hepatocytes encapsulated in Matrigel™ were used to show the path of drug diffusing from blood stream to the tissue as epithelial cells are the cells lining along the lumen through which the drugs pass from blood stream to the target, where hepatocytes were used as the target cell type. The antiradiation drug amifostine was used as a prodrug, which can be converted to an active form by epithelial cells. The results showed that the percentage of radiation-damaged cells for the single tissue was more than twice the dual tissue. Based on the presented tissue model, researchers developed a computational macroscale model for such in vitro tissue models using a convection–diffusion–cell kinetics numerical framework, which is

Table 9.1 Bioprinting Modalities and Their Performance Comparison in Pharmaceutical Applications

	Background	Strengths	Limitations	Applications in Pharmaceutics	References
Extrusion-based Bioprinting (EBB)	• Introduced in early 2000s • The most common and affordable bioprinting modality • Driven by pneumatic or mechanical forces • Print materials in the form of filaments • Compatible with a wide range of bioink properties	• Compatibility with viscosities in a wide range (30 mPa/s to >6 × 10^7 mPa/s) • Enables bioprinting of scaffold-free bioink such as tissue spheroids, which is not currently feasible using other modalities • Facilitates vascularization using direct or indirect (with fugitive ink) bioprinting • Suitable to extrude three-dimensional tissue constructs or organ-on-a-chip for drug testing and toxicity analysis • Commercially available with moderate cost	• Substantial cell damage due to shear stress of highly viscous fluids, small nozzle diameter and high dispensing pressure • Not practical for high-throughput bioprinting of tissue models • Limited bioprinting resolution preventing direct fabrication of micro-capillary network • Limited control on cell—cell and cell—matrix interactions	• Liver-on-a-chip on a polydimethylsiloxane (PDMS) bioreactor for testing hepatic toxicity of acetaminophen • Valve- and pneumatic-based extrusion of liver microorgan on a PDMS chamber for assaying drug metabolic properties • Extrusion of breast cancer neotissues in a multiwell plate to test antitumor drugs	Chang et al. (2010); King et al. (2014); Bhise et al. (2016); Snyder et al. (2011)
Droplet-based Bioprinting (DBB)	• First introduced in early 2000s • Inkjet printers are the most commonly used type of DBB • Driven by thermal, piezoelectric, or acoustic forces • Print materials in the form of liquid droplets	• Compatibility with small viscosities in the range of 3.5–12 mPa/s • High speed (1–10,000 droplets/s), high resolution (1–300 picoliter in volume) • Compatibility with many biological materials including living cells, DNA, RNA, biochemicals • Suitable to drop cell populations on microarrays or organ-on-a-chip for HTS • Affordable, versatile, and commercially available	• No uniformity in droplet size • Inconstancy in encapsulating a single cell in each droplet on microarrays for high throughput screening (HTS) • Nozzle clogging in high cell densities and fibrous bioink solutions • Cross-contamination when bioprinting of multiple bioink solutions takes place simultaneously	• Thermal inkjet bioprinting *Escherichia coli*—laden alginate for high-throughput antibiotics screening • Piezoelectric jetting of Sac6-EGFP yeast cells as microarrays for analysis of drug dose—response of latrunculin A	Rodríguez-Dévora et al. (2012); Saunders and Derby, (2014)

Continued

Table 9.1 Bioprinting Modalities and Their Performance Comparison in Pharmaceutical Applications—cont'd

	Background	Strengths	Limitations	Applications in Pharmaceutics	References
Laser-based Bioprinting (LBB)	• First introduced in 1999 • Less popular than DBB or EBB • Consists of a pulsed laser beam with a focusing system, a donor slide including two layers (energy-absorbing layer and biological material layer), and a collector substrate • Stereolithography and its modifications also enable bioprinting of cells • Driven by laser generated shock waves	• Compatibility with viscosities in range of 1–300 mPa/s • Nozzle-free • Generating negligibly cell damage • Facilitates deposition of cells in the densities of 10^8 cells/ml with a resolution of one cell per droplet • High-resolution feature of stereolithography and its modifications enables integration of vascular channels within tissue constructs	• Labor intensive and time-consuming preparation • Difficulty of accurately targeting and depositing cells • High cost and no commercial availability • Not practical to bioprint heterocellular models	• LBB has not been applied to pharmaceutical use yet	Peng et al., (2016)

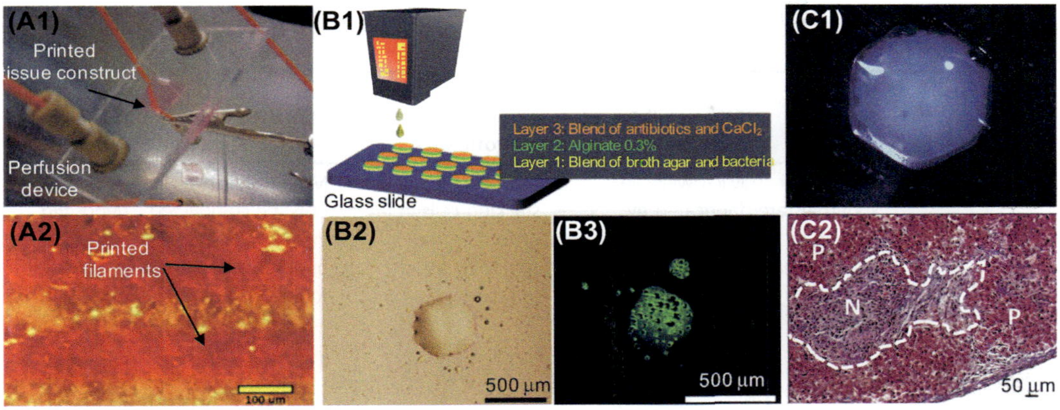

FIGURE 9.5 Bioprinted tissue models for drug testing and high-throughput screening: (A1) bioprinted liver tissue model loaded into a perfusion chamber *(Reproduced/adapted with permission from Chang et al. (2010))*, (A2) where HepG2-laden alginate filaments were patterned allowing media flow for drug testing *(Reproduced/adapted with permission from Tourlomousis and Chang (2015))*. (B1) A schematic showing inkjet-bioprinting of three-layer constructs, where agar and bacteria were bioprinted on a glass slide followed by printing of alginate and blend of antibiotics and $CaCl_2$, (B2) light microscopy, and (B3) fluorescence imaging of the bioprinted samples *(Reproduced/adapted with permission from Ref Rodríguez-Dévora et al. (2012))*. (C1) A 3 × 3 mm bioprinted liver tissue model for drug testing with (C2) hematoxylin and eosin stain showing parenchymal (P) and non-parenchymal (N) regions *(Image courtesy of Organovo Holdings, Inc.)*.

helpful for future research in 3D microorgan pharmacokinetics and toxicity (Tourlomousis and Chang, 2015).

Emerging microengineering technologies enable versatile fabrication of 3D cell-based microarrays including soft lithography, surface patterning, microfluidic-based manipulation, and bioprinting (Feng et al., 2011). Among them, bioprinting technology has numerous advantages, including high precision control over size, microarchitecture and cellular composition, high-throughput capability, coculture and vascularization ability, and low risk of cross-contamination, where multiple tissue types need to be located separately with minimum cross-migration of cells (see Table 9.2 for the comparison) (Peng et al., 2016). A recent study developed a novel inkjet-based bioprinting method for assembling a high-throughput miniature drug-screening platform as presented in Fig. 9.5B1 (Rodríguez-Dévora et al., 2012). The authors applied a modified Hewlett Packard model 5360 compact disk printer with picoliter per droplet resolution and bioprinted *Escherichia coli*–laden alginate to array a chip on coverslips (see Fig. 9.5B2–B3). Droplets of three antibiotics were printed on the spots of cells in a layer-by-layer fashion. Results demonstrated similar cell viability, functionality, and antibacterial effects of antibiotics in both inkjet-bioprinted and micropipetted samples, which confirmed that inkjet-bioprinted high-throughput array is an effective method to minimize the typical drug screening test. Demirci's group presented cell-based biosensors (CBBs), where acoustic-based bioprinting, studied by the same group earlier for high-throughput screening purposes with various cells (including mouse embryonic

Table 9.2 Comparison of Bioprinting With Other Three-Dimensional In Vitro Technologies

Methods	Hanging Drop Method	Microwell-Based Method	Microfluidics	Magnetic Force–Based Patterning	Bioprinting
Mechanisms	Cellular spheroids are formed by gravitational force	Microwells are fabricated by nonadhesive materials to forming cellular spheroids	Microflow mediates stacking cells in layers or forming cell spheroids using trapping	Magnetically labeled cells are compacted in spheroids form under magnetic forces	Cells are deposited in scaffold-based or scaffold-free manner
Size uniformity	++	+++	+++	+++	+++
Microarchitectural controllability	+	++	+++	+++	+++
Scalability	++	+	+	++	+++
Coculture ability	++	++	++	+	+++
High-throughput capability	+	+++	+++	+++	+++
Low risk of cross-contamination	+	+	++	++	+++

+++, high;++, medium;+, low.

stem cells, fibroblasts, AML-12 hepatocytes, human Raji cells, and HL-1 cardiomyocytes) (Demirci and Montesano, 2007), was used to create microarray of SMC droplets in collagen. The bioprinted microarray was then stimulated with different environmental conditions (e.g., temperature), and the effect of the applied stimuli as well as the bioprinting process parameters on cell viability was evaluated. With the bioprinted CBBs, the effects of analytes, such as pathogens, contaminants, toxins, and drug candidates, on living systems can be obtained (Xu et al., 2009a,b). Besides 3D bioprinting of high-throughput cell microarrays, controlled delivery of drug candidates into cell microarrays is also a key factor for successful drug screening. Various methods have been developed for controlled drug delivery onto cell microarrays, including drug patterning, drug stamping, aerosol sprays, and microfluidic drug loading (Feng et al., 2011).

Recently, bioprinting companies have developed bioprinted tissue models for high-throughput drug screening (Vaidya, 2015; Nelson, 2015). In November 2014, Organovo began offering its 3D-printed "exVive3D" liver tissue models to screen drugs for liver toxicity. A scaffold-free tissue bioprinting approach was performed using NovoGen MMX Bioprinter™, where pellet of cocultured human hepatocytes, hepatic stellate, and endothelial cells were bioprinted into a temporary mold structure with building units in hexagonal shape (see Fig. 9.5C1) (Roskos et al., 2015). After bioprinting, cells further aggregated and the tissue construct matured toward a nativelike tissue model (see Fig. 9.5C2), which maintains normal function for at least 42 days. Formation of micro-capillaries took place at certain locations. The bioprinted tissues were characterized by

ATP production and secretion of liver-specific albumin protein. The results revealed that ATP production increased over time during 4-week culture period, and the enzyme-linked immunosorbent assay (ELISA) results showed that albumin secretion increased after fabrication and stabilized in 21 days. Organovo's system demonstrated very clear signals confirming the commercial drug's safety and the failed drug's toxicity. Other companies, including Aspect Biosystems from Vancouver, Canada, and Texas-based Nano3D Biosciences, are also developing technology for the similar purpose.

9.5 Cancer Research

Two-dimensional (2D) tumor models have been widely used in cancer research; however, they do not represent the physiologically relevant environment of cancer tissues as they lack cell–cell and cell–matrix interactions in 3D. Thus, bioprinting has offered great advantages to recapitulate cancer microenvironment to precisely locate various cell types and microcapillaries to study cancer pathogenesis and metastasis; however, bioprinting for cancer research is new, and only a few research work has been performed in this emerging application area (Knowlton et al., 2015).

Demirci's group was the first to demonstrate bioprinting of tumor tissue models for in vitro assays (Xu et al., 2011). In their study, human ovarian cancer (OVCAR-5) cells and MRC-5 fibroblasts were bioprinted using an inkjet-based bioprinting platform with dual ejectors. Multiple cell types were spontaneously bioprinted on Matrigel™ to form multicellular acini in a high-throughput and reproducible manner with a spatially mediated microenvironment with controlled cell density and cell–cell distance. The presented approach did not only demonstrate a tool for cancer research but also provided a great platform for high-throughput screening. Sun's group recently demonstrated bioprinting of HeLa cells to form cervical tumor models (Zhao et al., 2014). In this regard, HeLa cells were extruded and bioprinted in a gelatin/alginate/fibrinogen composite hydrogel in patterned form with >90% cell viability. In 5–8 days, HeLa cells migrated toward each other and formed cell aggregates within hydrogel filaments (see Fig. 9.6) in oppose to the control groups, where cells in 2D culture formed cell sheets with lower chemoresistance and lower level expression of metalloproteinase. Although these two studies presented biofabrication of tumor spheroids using bioprinting technology, biofabrication of a larger tissue model to study cancer cell migration and metastasis is also important. Huang et al. (2014) demonstrated a laser-based 3D projection printing system to bioprint HeLa cells and noncancerous 10 T1/2 fibroblasts in PEGDA along with microvascular network with channel widths of 25, 45, and 120 μm to reflect blood vessel diameters. The results revealed that bioprinted fibroblasts were not affected by the morphology of the channel width; however, HeLa cells migrated significantly when the channel diameter decreased. In addition to scaffold-based approaches, Organovo company demonstrated scaffold-free bioprinting of breast cancer model using NovoGen Bioprinting™ platform, where cancer cells were surrounded by a

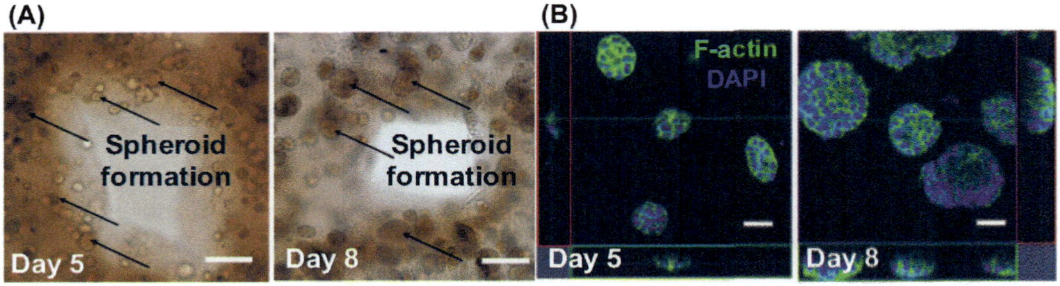

FIGURE 9.6 Bioprinted cervical tumor model. (A) Phase-contrast images showing bioprinted HeLa cells forming spheroids within gelatin/alginate/fibrinogen on day 5, where spheroids got larger with further aggregation and proliferation of cells on day 8. (B) Immunofluorescence images showing f-actin and DAPI (nuclei) of the forming aggregates on days 5 and 8 *(Reproduced/adapted with permission from Zhao et al. (2014)).*

physiologically relevant stromal milieu comprising of MSC-differentiated adipose cells, mammary fibroblasts, and endothelial cells (see Fig. 9.6B1) (King et al., 2014). Histomorphological analysis revealed that bioprinted neotissues were viable for 2 weeks in vitro with a clear compartmentalization of adipose, stromal, and epithelial components with localized signs of microcapillary formation. The effects of chemotherapeutic drug tamoxifen were assessed for viability by ATP luciferase assay and concluded that isolated 2D cancer cells were more susceptible to tamoxifen-induced toxicity than cells incorporated into 3D tissue models when treated with same dose of the drug for the same period in vitro. Despite the recent attempts in engineering cancer microenvironment using bioprinting technology, further advancements are needed for fabrication of philologically relevant complete microenvironment, comprising tumor site, healthy site, and microvascular network in between, to study cancer metastasis research.

Table 9.3 summarizes the application areas of bioprinting technology and lists the tissue types that have been successfully bioprinted along with the information of cell and bioink types, bioprinting modalities, and bioprinters used in fabrication of each tissue type.

9.6 Limitations

Despite the great progress in the field of bioprinting and its benefits in the presented application areas, there are several challenges to be circumvented for fabrication of functional tissues. Bioprinted tissues and bioprinting technologies entail different shortcomings for each distinct application as discussed in detail below.

9.6.1 Limitations in Bioprinting for Tissue Engineering and Regenerative Medicine

Bioprinting for bone tissue fabrication has been extensively studied as bone is one of the most widely engineered tissue types in regenerative medicine. The majority of bone

Table 9.3 Applications of Bioprinting Technologies

Application	Tissue Type	Cell Types Bioprinted	Bioink or Substrate Used	Bioprinting Modalities Used	Bioprinters Used	Remarks
Tissue engineering and regenerative medicine	Bone	Bone marrow–derived human mesenchymal stem cells (Gao et al., 2014); endothelial progenitor and multipotent stromal cells (Fedorovich et al., 2008); primary muscle-derived stem cells (Phillippi et al., 2008)	PEGDMA (Gao et al., 2014); n-HA slurry (Keriquel et al., 2010); Matrigel™ and alginate (Fedorovich et al., 2008); bone morphogenetic protein (BMP-2) and fibrin (substrate) (Phillippi et al., 2008)	Thermal inkjet (Gao et al., 2014); laser-induced droplet ejection (Keriquel et al., 2010); EBB (pneumatic) (Fedorovich et al., 2008); piezoelectric drop-on-demand (Phillippi et al., 2008)	Hewlett–Packard deskjet (Gao et al., 2014); HT-BioLP workstation (Keriquel et al., 2010); Bioplotter (Fedorovich et al., 2008); MicroJet™ (Phillippi et al., 2008)	Bioprinting bone tissue for critical-size defects is currently feasible, but bioprinting of scale-up vascularized bone tissues still remains elusive.
	Cardiac	Cardiac cells and HUVECs (Jakab et al., 2008); primary feline adult cardiomyocytes and HL1 cardiac muscle cells (Xu et al., 2009a,b); HUVEC and human mesenchymal stem cell (Gaebel et al., 2011); human cardiac–derived cardiomyocytes progenitor cells (Gaetani et al., 2012)	Tissue spheroids and collagen type-I (biopaper) (Jakab et al., 2008); alginate (Xu et al., 2009a,b; Gaetani et al., 2012); PU (Gaebel et al., 2011)	EBB (mechanical) (Jakab et al., 2008; Gaetani et al., 2012); thermal inkjet (Xu et al., 2009a,b); LIFT (Gaebel et al., 2011)	nScrypt (Jakab et al., 2008); HP DeskJet 550 printers (Xu et al., 2009a,b); custom laser bioprinter (Gaebel et al., 2011); BioScaffolder (Gaetani et al., 2012)	As cardiac cells do not have proliferation capability, scaffold-free bioprinting with high cell density is advantageous.
	Cartilage	Human chondrocytes (Cui et al., 2012a); rabbit elastic chondrocytes (Xu et al., 2013); bovine articular chondrocytes (Ozbolat et al., 2014); calve articular chondrocytes (Mannoor et al., 2013); human nasoseptal chondrocytes (Markstedt et al., 2015)	PEGDMA (Cui et al., 2012a); fibrin–collagen type I (Xu et al., 2013); alginate[25,26]; alginate/nanocellulose (Markstedt et al., 2015)	Thermal inkjet (Cui et al., 2012a); solenoid inkjet (Xu et al., 2013); EBB (pneumatic) (Ozbolat et al., 2014); EBB (microvalve) (Markstedt et al., 2015); EBB (mechanical) (Mannoor et al., 2013)	HP Deskjet 500 printer (Cui et al., 2012a); XYZ plotter (Xu et al., 2013); MABP (Ozbolat et al., 2014); Fab @ home[26]; regenHU (Markstedt et al., 2015)	Considerable work has been performed; however, zonally stratified articular cartilage is still a challenge and a great need in clinical use.

Continued

Table 9.3 Applications of Bioprinting Technologies—cont'd

Application	Tissue Type	Cell Types Bioprinted	Bioink or Substrate Used	Bioprinting Modalities Used	Bioprinters Used	Remarks
	Heart valve	Aortic root sinus smooth muscle cells and aortic valve interstitial cells (Duan et al., 2013); aortic valvular interstitial cells (Duan et al., 2014)	PEGDA and alginate (Hockaday et al., 2012); alginate and gelatin (Duan et al., 2013); methacrylated gelatin (Duan et al., 2014)	EBB (mechanical) (Hockaday et al., 2012; Duan et al., 2013; Duan et al. 2014)	Fab@home (Hockaday et al., 2012; Duan et al., 2013; Duan et al. 2014)	Although anatomically accurate tissue models have been bioprinted, no performance evaluation has been done in vivo.
	Liver	Human-induced pluripotent stem cells and human embryonic stem cells (Faulkner-Jones et al., 2015); HepG2 (Bertassoni et al., 2014a)	Alginate (Faulkner-Jones et al., 2015); GelMA (Bertassoni et al., 2014a)	Valve-based inkjet (Faulkner-Jones et al., 2015); EBB (mechanical) (Bertassoni et al., 2014a)	Custom cell printer (Faulkner-Jones et al., 2015); NovoGen MMX Bioprinter™ (Bertassoni et al., 2014a)	Limited progress has been made in bioprinting of liver tissues for regenerative medicine and patient-specific cells with long-term viability are still a concern.
	Lung	Endothelial and epithelial cells (Horváth et al., 2015)	Matrigel™ (substrate) (Horváth et al., 2015)	Valve-based inkjet (Horváth et al., 2015)	BioFactory® (Horváth et al., 2015)	Although lung is hollow and reasonable easy to survive compared to some other organ types, human airway models for cytotoxicity testing seem to be in the near horizon.
	Neural	Murine neural stem cells (Lee et al., 2010; Hsieh et al., 2015); Schwann cells and bone marrow stem cells (Owens et al., 2013)	Collagen type I (substrate) (Lee et al., 2010); polyurethane (Hsieh et al., 2015); cell pellet and agarose (support) (Owens et al., 2013)	Microvalve-based inkjet (Lee et al., 2010); EBB (mechanical) (Owens et al., 2013; Hsieh et al., 2015)	Custom 4-head dispenser (Lee et al., 2010); NovoGen MMX Bioprinter™ (Owens et al., 2013)	Nerve grafts are commercially available for short damages, but bioprinting has the capability to generate longer counterparts.
	Pancreas	INS1E β-cells, mouse islets and human islets (Marchioli et al., 2015)	Alginate and alginate/gelatin (Marchioli et al., 2015)	EBB (pneumatic) (Marchioli et al., 2015)	BioScaffolder (Marchioli et al., 2015)	Beta cell source, its long-term functionality and viability, and availability of associated cells are still a challenge.

Skin	Human foreskin fibroblast and HaCaT keratinocytes (Lee et al., 2013); HaCaT keratinocyte cells and NIH 3T3 fibroblasts (Koch et al., 2012; Michael et al., 2013); human dermal microvascular endothelial cells (Yanez et al., 2014); amniotic fluid–derived stems (Skardal et al., 2012)	Collagen type-I (Lee et al., 2013); collagen type-I on Matriderm ™ (substrate) (Koch et al., 2012; Michael et al., 2013); thrombin (Yanez et al., 2014); collagen/fibrinogen and thrombin (Skardal et al., 2012)	Microvalve-based inkjet (Lee et al., 2013; Skardal et al., 2012); LIFT (Koch et al., 2012; Michael et al., 2013); thermal inkjet (Yanez et al., 2014)	Custom 8-head dispenser (Lee et al., 2013); LaBP (Koch et al., 2012; Michael et al., 2013); Modified HP Deskjet 340 (Yanez et al., 2014); skin printer (Skardal et al., 2012)	Great progress has been made in skin bioprinting, but advancements are needed for further improvement in scarless tissue formation and integration of sweat glands.
Vascular	HUVSMCs (Zhang et al., 2015; Dolati et al., 2014; Norotte et al., 2009); chondrocytes (Zhang et al., 2013b; Yu et al., 2013); 3T3 mouse fibroblasts (Christensen et al., 2015); HUVEC (Lee et al., 2014; Zhao et al., 2012) and normal human lung fibroblast (Lee et al., 2014); human skin fibroblasts (Norotte et al., 2009)	Alginate (Zhang et al., 2015; Christensen et al., 2015); alginate and chitosan (Zhang et al., 2013b; Yu et al., 2013), alginate with carbon nanotubes (Dolati et al., 2014); fibrin (Lee et al., 2014); collagen (Zhao et al., 2012); GelMA (Bertassoni et al., 2014a); tissue spheroids (Norotte et al., 2009)	Coaxial nozzle extrusion (Zhang et al., 2013b; 2015; Yu et al., 2013; Dolati et al., 2014) piezo-inkjet (Christensen et al., 2015); valve-based inkjet (Lee et al., 2014; Zhao et al., 2012)	Nordson (Zhang et al., 2013b; 2015; Yu et al., 2013; Dolati et al., 2014); Microfab (Christensen et al., 2015); custom multihead dispenser (Lee et al., 2014; Zhao et al., 2012); NovoGen MMX Bioprinter™(Bertassoni et al., 2014a; Norotte et al., 2009)	Long-term in vivo efficacy of bioprinted blood vessel has not been tested yet. For organ fabrication, enabling technologies are needed to bioprint vascular network in multiscale.
Composite	3T3 fibroblasts and myoblasts (Merceron et al., 2015); MSCs (Feng et al., 2011; Fedorovich et al., 2011) and chondrocytes (Fedorovich et al., 2011); osteoblast and chondrocytes (Park et al., 2014; Shim et al., 2012); HUVSMCs and fibroblasts (Yu et al., 2014)	Hyaluronic acid/gelatin/ fibrinogen and PU (Merceron et al., 2015); alginate (Fedorovich et al., 2011; Shim et al., 2012; Yu et al., 2014); collagen type I and hyaluronic acid (Park et al., 2014); tissue strands (Yu et al., 2014)	EBB (pneumatic) (Merceron et al., 2015; Fedorovich et al., 2011; Park et al., 2014; Shim et al., 2012; Yu et al., 2014); acoustic-based droplet (Feng et al., 2011)	Custom multinozzle head (Merceron et al., 2015; Fedorovich et al., 2011; Feng et al., 2011); MtoBS (Park et al., 2014; Shim et al., 2012); MABP (Yu et al., 2014)	Bioprinting of composite tissues is highly vital, and a substantial progress is needed to generate organ-level constructs by integrating tissues such as bone, muscle, tendon, nerve, blood vessels, and skin together.

Continued

Table 9.3 Applications of Bioprinting Technologies—cont'd

Application	Tissue Type	Cell Types Bioprinted	Bioink or Substrate Used	Bioprinting Modalities Used	Bioprinters Used	Remarks
Pharmaceutics and drug testing	Liver	HepG2 (Chang et al., 2010; 2008); epithelial cells and hepatocytes (Snyder et al., 2011); human hepatocytes, hepatic satellite cells, and endothelial cells (Roskos et al., 2015)	Alginate (Chang et al., 2010; 2008); Matrigel™ (Snyder et al., 2011); cell pellet (Roskos et al., 2015);	EBB (valve) (Snyder et al., 2011)·(Chang et al., 2010; 2008); EBB (mechanical) (Roskos et al., 2015)	Multinozzle system (Snyder et al., 2011)· (Chang et al., 2010; 2008); NovoGen MMX Bioprinter™ (Roskos et al., 2015)	Bioprinted liver tissue models have a great potential in early drug discovery, but a standard model is yet to be developed.
	Cell droplets for high-throughput arrays	*Escherichia coli* (Rodríguez-Dévora et al., 2012); primary smooth muscle cells from rat bladder (Xu et al., 2009a); mouse embryonic stem cells, fibroblasts, AML-12 hepatocytes, human Raji cells, and HL-1 cardiomyocytes (Demirci and Montesano, 2007)	Alginate and soy agar (substrate) (Rodríguez-Dévora et al., 2012); collagen (Xu et al., 2009a); sucrose and dextrose (Demirci and Montesano, 2007)	Thermal inkjet (Rodríguez-Dévora et al., 2012); acoustic-based (Xu et al., 2009a; Demirci and Montesano, 2007)	Modified-HP (Rodríguez-Dévora et al., 2012); A custom acoustic bioprinter (Xu et al., 2009a; Demirci and Montesano, 2007)	Picoliter size of droplets can be generated with high accuracy in droplet size and location, which is highly efficient for high-throughput arrays for drug testing.
Transplantation and clinics	Bone, cartilage and skin	Amniotic fluid–derived stem cells and Bone marrow–derived MSCs (Skardal et al., 2012); bone marrow stem cells (Ozbolat, 2015a)	Polycaprolactone (Zopf et al., 2013); nHA (Keriquel et al., 2010); collagen–fibrin (Skardal et al., 2012); alginate and Pluronic collagen (Ozbolat, 2015a)	Laser-based printing (Zopf et al., 2013); laser-based bioprinting (Keriquel et al., 2010); piezo-inkjet (Skardal et al., 2012); extrusion (pneumatic) (Ozbolat, 2015a)	EOS P 100 Formiga system (Zopf et al., 2013); HT-BioLP workstation (Keriquel et al., 2010); custom inkjet printer (Skardal et al., 2012); MABP (Ozbolat, 2015a)	Only transplantation of a splint (using a nonbioprinting technique) into a human and in situ bioprinting on animal models have been achieved in operating rooms

Cancer research	Ovarian cancer	Human ovarian cancer cells and MRC-5 fibroblasts (Xu et al., 2011)	Matrigel™ (substrate) (Xu et al., 2011)	Solenoid-valve ejection (Xu et al., 2011)	A custom dual-head bioprinter (Xu et al., 2011)	Only a technological platform has been demonstrated so far, but bioprinting of biomimetically developed ovarian cancer model is yet to be researched.
	Cervical cancer	HeLa (Zhao et al., 2014; Huang et al., 2014); 10 T1/2 fibroblasts (Huang et al., 2014)	Gelatin/alginate/fibrinogen (Zhao et al., 2014); PEGDA (Huang et al., 2014)	EBB (mechanical) (Zhao et al., 2014) and laser-based projection printing (Huang et al., 2014)	Cell assembly system I (Zhao et al., 2014); DMD-PP (Huang et al., 2014)	Only a very few attempts, at the basic research level, have been made for bioprinting of cervical cancer models.
	Breast cancer	MSC-differentiated adipose cells, mammary fibroblasts, and endothelial cells (King et al., 2014)	Cell pellet (King et al., 2014)	EBB (mechanical) (King et al., 2014)	NovoGen MMX Bioprinter™ (King et al., 2014)	Further substantial development is needed to use the bioprinted breast cancer model for cancer screening and drug testing.

EBB, Extrusion-based bioprinting; *GelMA*, gelatin-methacrylamide; *n-HA*, hydroxyapatite nanoparticle; *HUVEC*, human vascular endothelial cell; *LIFT*, laser-induced forward transfer; *MSC*, mesenchymal stem cell; *PEGDA*, polyethylene glycol diacrylate; *PEGDMA*, poly(ethylene glycol) dimethacrylate; *PU*, polyurethane.

tissue bioprinting attempts were mainly for the investigation of the science basis of stem cell differentiation toward osteogenic lineage within bioprinted tissue constructs (Kim et al., 2010). In vivo implantation has been performed for calvarium reconstruction or bone formation under subcutaneous tissue to assess in vivo performance and engraftment into the host (Bose et al., 2013); however, bioprinting of scale-up bone tissues for significant defects or substantial bone loss is still a challenge due to the lack of integration of blood vessels. In addition, most bioprinting approaches utilize soft materials such as hydrogels for bone tissue fabrication, which is not easy to implant into load-bearing sites of human body. Therefore, hydrogels should be reinforced with mechanically strong materials or integrated with supporting frames for large-size regeneration of bone tissue in vivo (Temple et al., 2014).

Bioprinting for cardiac tissue fabrication has been performed at cardiac patch level and successful regeneration of a cardiac patch in vivo has demonstrated so far, but bioprinting of the entire heart is still considered science fiction (Dababneh and Ozbolat, 2014). While bioprinting of hierarchical vascular network is the critical step toward fabrication of organs at the clinically relevant size, bioprinting of a whole-heart model vitally depends on the integration of vascular network as heart needs substantial vascularization due to its hectic metabolic activity. One of the major hurdles in cardiac tissue regeneration is that cardiomyocytes do not proliferate, and it is not trivial to obtain sufficient number of cardiomyocytes (Mollova et al., 2013); therefore, stem cell engineering for sufficient and practical derivation of stable cardiac cells will be the key factor in further advancements for cardiac tissue bioprinting.

Bioprinting for cartilage tissue fabrication has been well studied in the literature; however, bioprinting of zonally stratified articular cartilage has yet to be demonstrated. Articular cartilage is the lining on articulating surfaces of diarthroidal joints, and it functions as a shock absorber to distribute the load from weight and daily activities (Aydelottea et al., 1988). The superficial zone takes up to 20% of the total cartilage thickness and contains densely packed collagen fibers in parallel to the articulating surface, and cells in that zone secrete lubricants to minimize wear and tear to the joint. The deeper zones including middle zone, deep zone, and calcified zone are relatively less in cell density and have thicker collagen bundles, which are perpendicular to the articulating surface to resist compression force. This unique arrangement is formed due to the external loads over time, which is transmitted through the matrix of the tissue and converted into a biochemical signal, alerting cells to either produce more or catabolize existing ECM (Makris et al., 2014). Therefore, currently existing strategies are not sufficient in enabling controlled zonal differentiation for nativelike engineered articular cartilage tissues (Kock et al., 2012; Makris et al., 2014). Although not attempted yet, integration of bioprinted cartilage tissue with subchondral bone may be another challenge as it is a common problem in cartilage tissue repair (Makris et al., 2015).

Bioprinting for heart valve fabrication has been attempted by one research group so far, and different combinations of hydrogels, including alginate, PEGDA, gelatin, and Me-Gel, have been used for heart valve bioprinting (Jana and Lerman, 2015). Currently, there is no in vivo implantation demonstrated so far to test the efficacy and performance of the bioprinted cardiac valves. While only hydrogel-based materials have been used in the literature, long-term cultivation of bioprinted samples and their biological, mechanical, and functional characterization have not been reported so far. To transplant bioprinted heart valves, the constructs should possess sufficient mechanical properties to withstand the physiological blood flow pressure while providing an appropriate microenvironment to promote survival and growth of seeded cells.

Bioprinting for liver tissue fabrication has been primarily performed using human tumor–derived cell lines (i.e., HepG2) (Bertassoni, Cardoso, et al., 2014a; Tourlomousis and Chang, 2015). Compared to primary hepatocytes, HepG2s have reduced functional performance such as low level of ammonia removal, aminoacid metabolism, cytochrome P450s, and lack of a myriad of drug-metabolizing functions (Palakkan et al., 2013). Although no transplantation has been pursued with tumor-derived cell lines, these cells have potential to transmit the tumorigenic products or possible complications arising from their transmission (Knowles et al., 1980). Although primary hepatocytes are preferred, their limited availability and poor in vitro proliferation capability reduce their applicability in bioprinting research. In addition to cell source–related issues, bioprinting of scale-up liver tissue is still a challenge as there has not been any work reported yet. Transplantation of bioprinted liver tissue models has not been demonstrated yet, and long-term functionality and performance of such a tissue still remain elusive.

Bioprinting for lung tissue fabrication is still in its infancy, and there has been only a single work reported so far (Horváth et al., 2015). As lung is a highly complicated organ in its morphology comprising around half a billion alveoli to facilitate sufficient gas exchange. As the demonstrated multilayer pulmonary tissue model represents the air barrier mimicking the alveolus wall, bioprinting of an anatomically correct pulmonary tissue model with a highly dense capillary network is still a major cornerstone toward fabrication of a functional lung parenchyma (Nichols et al., 2009). Such a parenchymal tissue model should be mechanically stable; structurally strong and elastic enough to withstand air pressure; permeable enough to facilitate gas exchange across the tissue barrier; and vascularized enough to allow transfer of the gas from and to capillaries.

Bioprinting for nervous tissue fabrication is still in its infancy, and bioprinting for functional central nervous system components is yet far from the reality; however, recent work on peripheral nervous system by understanding neural stem growth through bioprinting (Lee et al., 2010) and fabricating heterocellular nerve grafts (Owens et al., 2013) for in vivo testing demonstrated the promise of bioprinting in this challenging field. A wide array of nerve grafts has been studied, including autologous, allogeneic, and xenogeneic neural tissues, naturally derived polymers (i.e., collagen, laminin, fibrin, fibronectin, hyaluronan), and polysaccharides (chitosan, alginate, and agarose); however, each of them has certain limitation such as but not limited to donor site morbidity, limited availability, mismatch in size, immunogenic issues, limited functionality, and degradation and associated by-products (Gu et al., 2014). Nerve conduits support generation of axon growth, but the regenerated tissue, beyond a certain length, does not imitate the native anatomy and functionality closely. Bioprinting thus has the ability to recapitulate the complex nerve anatomy, with conduits of nerve bundles along with blood vessels and other connective tissue, which can be further imitated with electrical or biochemical stimulation (Ghasemi-Mobarakeh et al., 2009).

Bioprinting for pancreatic tissue fabrication is relatively new, and a limited number of research have been done in this regard (Marchioli et al., 2015; Akkouch et al., 2015). Cells used in these studies were limited to mouse insulinoma cell, or islets of Langerhans were directly bioprinted as an alternative approach to manual islet encapsulation. As primary β-cells and islets of Langerhans are not stable in vitro, pancreatic regeneration work has been embodied to the extent where insulinoma cells or mouse cell lines used only, which is far from the human islet physiological conditions. In addition, pancreatic islets are comprised of multiple cells types (including α-cells, endothelial cells, δ-cells, and PP cells), which is highly crucial for islet biology and functionality (Migliorini et al., 2014), and current tissue engineering approaches do not enable successful derivation and aggregation of these cells as observed in islets of Langerhans.

Bioprinting for skin tissue fabrication has aimed at compartmentalization of dermal and epidermis layers by depositing fibroblasts and keratinocytes layer by layer in addition to a recent attempt in stimulating formation of microcapillaries by incorporating endothelial cells within layers (Yanez et al., 2014). Although bioprinting stratified zones has been demonstrated extensively, generating nativelike complete skin tissue with all components and appendages, such as hair follicles and sweat glands, and minimum wound contraction and scar formation, still remains elusive (Michael et al., 2013). Although recent regenerative medicine practices focus on understanding the regeneration of de nova hair follicles using human dermal papilla cells in 3D spheroid culture model (Higgins et al., 2013), incorporation of such a model has not been attempted in skin tissue bioprinting yet.

Bioprinting for vascular tissue fabrication has been well studied in the literature; several challenges are yet to be circumvented such as but not limited to the formation of physiologically relevant vascular grafts and their long-term evaluation in vivo (Ozbolat, 2015a). Although a recent effort demonstrated the functionality, suture retention and in vivo endothelialization of the vascular grafts on a murine model (Itoh et al., 2015), long-term functionality and durability, as one of the common problems in engineered vascular grafts (Kurobe et al., 2012), still remain elusive. For vascular network bioprinting in scale-up engineered tissues, bioprinting of multiscale hierarchical vascular networks from arteries and veins down to capillaries has not been demonstrated yet (Ozbolat, 2015b). Although integration of macroscale channels with the microcapillaries in fibrin has been demonstrated through gluing endothelial cells (Lee et al., 2014), generation of microcapillaries around free-standing macrovasculature still needs to be demonstrated toward bioprinting of scalable tissues and organs.

Bioprinting for composite tissue fabrication will be a highly influential step in regenerative medicine, but current attempts could be able to demonstrate very simple structures, not even close to their native counterparts. As significant amount of work has been done in the area of osteochondral tissue fabrication (Di Luca et al., 2015), bioprinting of such structures will be one of the first composite tissue models in the near horizon. Despite the great effort in inducing osteogenic and chondrogenic differentiation locally for knee replacement, biomimetic development of such anisotropy with gradual transition in mechanical, structural, and biological properties of osteochondral tissue models with well integration at the interface of cartilage and bone is still a challenge.

9.6.2 Limitations in Bioprinting for Transplantation and Clinics

Bioprinting for transplantation and clinics is a trending area of application, and a number of bioprinted tissue types have been tested in vivo; however, translation of bioprinting technology into clinics for human has yet to be succeeded as there are several impediments down the road. First of all, due to the lack of hierarchical vascular network, bioprinting of scale-up tissues is still a challenge (Ozbolat and Yu, 2013). Tissues at the clinically relevant sizes, except cartilage and skin, have not been reported yet (Ozbolat, 2015a). In the literature, bioprinted tissues have been implanted into vascularized sites on animal models such as subcutaneous tissue (Marchioli et al., 2015), but they need to be implanted into less immune-responsive sites and connected to blood stream as an intravascular device when bioprinted in larger sizes. Although a myriad of bioprinted tissue constructs have been demonstrated, one of the major issues is the cell source considering immunogenicity issues. Therefore, stem cell use in bioprinted tissues is a key factor in enabling translation of bioprinted tissues into clinical practices. There is no bioprinted product undergone FDA approval yet, and FDA has not taken any consideration on the classification of bioprinters and bioprinted tissues but as the technology evolves further through clinical trials, then the first product going through the FDA regulations will be exemplary for preceding ones.

9.6.3 Limitations in Bioprinting for Drug Screening and High-Throughput Assays

Bioprinting for drug screening and high-throughput assays is a highly powerful technology as 3D tissue models can be precisely formed in a high-throughput manner. Both extrusion- and inkjet-based bioprinting technologies can be used to create heterocellular tissue environment to predict drug toxicity (Feng et al., 2011). Currently employed techniques in liver fabrication employ HepG2 liver carcinoma cell line, which does not represent the human liver physiology closely (Palakkan et al., 2013). Although complex patterned structures have been successfully integrated within a perfusion system to assess drug toxicity in a control manner, the cell type used as well as the lack of other associated cell types reduces the reliability of the tissue model in predicting the performance of drugs (Chang et al., 2010). In this regard, Organovo's liver tissue model stands as a promising tool to represent a biomimetically developed liver tissue model for drug testing (Roskos et al., 2015). The employed scaffold-free technique comprising stem cell–derived hepatocytes as well as hepatic satellite cells and endothelial cells facilitates physiologically relevant liver tissue, and further progress is needed to create a standardized bioprinted liver tissue model for pharmaceutical industry. In addition to liver tissue models, cells can be bioprinted in a high-throughput manner to study their behavior as well as bacterial cells can be bioprinted along with drugs to understand the interactions between applied drugs and bioprinted different bacterial strains (Rodríguez-Dévora et al., 2012). Different dosages can be bioprinted in high-throughput manner to effectively analyze the influence of different antibiotics on bacterial cells; however, a translational effort is yet to be demonstrated for the pharmaceutical industry.

9.6.4 Limitations in Bioprinting for Cancer Research

Bioprinting for cancer research is relatively new, and there are only a few efforts in fabrication of tumor models (i.e., ovarian, cervical, and breast tissue models) (Knowlton et al., 2015). To study cancer pathogenesis, inkjet-based bioprinting stands as a promising tool in generating 3D tumor models with multiple cell types in controlled composition; however, there is no well-established model in abovementioned tumor types that can be used in pharmaceutics industry yet. Formation of larger tissues as an in vitro cancer tissue model for exploration of cancer metastasis has not been attempted using bioprinting yet; however, there are various microfluidics-based platforms with closely recapitulated cancer microenvironment for cancer metastasis research (Jeon et al., 2015; Zervantonakis et al., 2012). These platforms lack precise placement of multiple cell types in a localized manner. Bioprinting has the capability of patterning the cellular microenvironment, but further research is required in angiogenesis work in bioprinting to establish standard cancer tissue models for cancer metastasis research.

9.7 Future Directions

Currently, there are around 15 different tissue types attempted in bioprinting field; however, there exist a number of other tissues in human body that have not been investigated yet. In this regard, diverging the focus into other tissue and organ models, which are challenging but can revolutionize the medicine, is necessary in the near horizon. This also depends on the advancements in tissue engineering field as bioprinting research vitally depends on our understanding of unexplored tissue types. In addition, bioprinting of new types of organs, such as bionic organs or organs that do not exist in nature, will be one of the new directions in bioprinting.

Majority of bioprinting research has evolved around homocellular tissue construct using a single cell type; however, native tissues have a heterocellular nature with multiple cell type patterned in a highly complex anatomy. Although bioprinting-simplified tissue models are relatively acceptable in basic research, functional tissue fabrication for clinics or pharmaceutics necessitates inclusion of multiple cell types as some of the functionality of cells can be enabled or further boosted by cell–cell interactions. Bioprinting multiple cell types requires further understanding of the optimum culture conditions including the right medium and cocktail to support growth and behaviors of multiple cell types.

Current efforts in translation of bioprinting into transplantation are mainly limited to murine models. As murine models are highly small and their physiological conditions are not closely relevant to that of humans. For example, a small representative pancreatic model with bioprinted pancreatic islets can be implanted into a diabetic murine model and can regulate insulin secretion, but average volume of mouse model is approximately 100,000 smaller than that of human model (Bock et al., 2003; Ionescu-Tirgoviste et al., 2015). Therefore, bioprinting of scale-up tissues and organs is highly important in fabricating tissues in clinically relevant dimensions. Larger animals such as a pig model can be a transitional step toward trials on humans as these models represent human physiology closer than small animals (Meurens et al., 2012). To scale-up bioprinted organs, bioprinting of hierarchical vascular network is vital as detailed out in Chapter 8. To generate clinically relevant tissue and organ models, mechanical strength and elasticity as well as long-term structural stability is highly important. In addition, integration of nerve tissues and establishing innervation is a vital step toward functional tissue and organ fabrication as tissues such as cardiac, muscle, and skin need innervation, which is currently a challenge in bioprinting. Majority of the bioprinting research entails the use of hydrogel-based bioink due to their favorable environment for 3D growth of cells; however, hydrogels are highly weak in mechanical properties when they are used at a concentration compatible with cell proliferation. In addition, biodegradable materials such as thermoplastics can be used as a supporting frame for the scale-up tissues and organs. Current biomaterials using synthetic polymers are highly strong, but their degradation takes prolonged times and does not synchronize with the tissue regeneration process. Therefore, new biomaterial development is highly crucial for the advancement in bioprinting of tissues and organs for clinical use. In addition to biomaterials, selection of the right cell source is also a critical factor in translation of bioprinting technologies into clinics and pharmaceutics. For personalized medicine, as it is highly challenging to acquire different primary cell types. Stem cell stands as a promising source of cells, and further advances are needed to establish highly standard protocols for differentiation of stem cells into various stable and functional cell lineages.

In addition, bioprinting for cancer research needs further advancement to enable philologically relevant microenvironment for cancer pathology and metastasis. There exist 3D tumor models that need to be integrated with vascular network and the rest of the parenchymal tissue using bioprinting. Tumor tissue models should be precisely placed within bioprinted vascularized parenchymal tissues to study tumor growth and tumor cell intravasation and extravasation. Physiologically relevant cancer microenvironment has been well established in microfluidics-based organ-on-chip-models, but bioprinting can bring precise control on positioning tumor spheroids and cells as well as tight control on the formation of microvascular network.

9.8 Summary

This chapter presented a detailed discussion on the application areas of 3D bioprinting technology. The noble effort by Klebe in cytoscribing cells has opened up great avenues in bioprinting of living tissue and organ constructs, which has been adopted into various fields including basic research in tissue engineering, regenerative medicine and cancer pathogenesis, tissue printing for transplantation and clinics, and some recent efforts in beginning translational technologies in pharmaceutics for drug testing and high-throughput screening. With the current advancements in various bioprinting technologies as well as progress in cell and biomaterial research, fabrication of physiologically relevant scalable tissues is expected to be feasible in the near future.

References

Akkouch, A., Yu, Y., Ozbolat, I.T., 2015. Microfabrication of scaffold-free tissue strands for three-dimensional tissue engineering. Biofabrication 7 (3), 31002.

Aydelottea, M., Greenhilla, R., Kuettnerab, K., 1988. Differences between sub-populations of cultured bovine articular chondrocytes. II. Proteoglycan metabolism. Connective Tissue Research 18 (3), 223–234.

Bertassoni, L.E., Cardoso, J.C., et al., 2014a. Direct-write bioprinting of cell-laden methacrylated gelatin hydrogels. Biofabrication 6 (2), 024105.

Bertassoni, L.E., Cecconi, M., et al., 2014b. Hydrogel bioprinted microchannel networks for vascularization of tissue engineering constructs. Lab on a Chip 14 (13), 2202–2211.

Bhise, N.S., et al., 2016. A liver-on-a-chip platform with bioprinted hepatic spheroids. Biofabrication 8 (1). http://dx.doi.org/10.1088/1758-5090/8/1/014101.

Blaeser, A., et al., 2013. Biofabrication under fluorocarbon: a novel freeform fabrication technique to generate high aspect ratio tissue-engineered constructs. BioResearch Open Access 2 (5), 374–384.

Bock, T., Pakkenberg, B., Buschard, K., 2003. Increased islet volume but unchanged islet number in ob/ob mice. Diabetes 52 (7), 1716–1722.

Bose, S., Vahabzadeh, S., Bandyopadhyay, A., 2013. Bone tissue engineering using 3D printing. Materials Today 16 (12), 496–504.

Chang, R., et al., 2010. Biofabrication of a three-dimensional liver micro-organ as an in vitro drug metabolism model. Biofabrication 2 (4), 45004.

Chang, R., Nam, J., Sun, W., 2008. Direct cell writing of 3D microorgan for in vitro pharmacokinetic model. Tissue Engineering Part C: Methods 14 (2), 157–166.

Christensen, K., et al., 2015. Freeform inkjet printing of cellular structures with bifurcations. Biotechnology and Bioengineering 112 (5), 1047–1055.

Cohen, D.L., et al., 2010. Increased mixing improves hydrogel homogeneity and quality of three-dimensional printed constructs. Tissue Engineering Part C: Methods 17 (2), 239–248.

Coruh, A., Yontar, Y., 2012. Application of split-thickness dermal grafts in deep partial- and full-thickness burns: a new source of auto-skin grafting. Journal of Burn Care and Research 33 (3).

Cui, X., Breitenkamp, K., Finn, M.G., et al., 2012a. Direct human cartilage repair using three-dimensional bioprinting technology. Tissue Engineering Part A 18 (11–12), 1304–1312.

Cui, X., Breitenkamp, K., Lotz, M., et al., 2012b. Synergistic action of fibroblast growth factor-2 and transforming growth factor-beta1 enhances bioprinted human neocartilage formation. Biotechnology and Bioengineering 109 (9), 2357–2368.

Dababneh, A.B., Ozbolat, I.T., 2014. Bioprinting technology: a current state-of-the-art review. Journal of Manufacturing Science and Engineering 136 (6), 061016.

Demirci, U., Montesano, G., 2007. Single cell epitaxy by acoustic picolitre droplets. Lab on a Chip 7 (9), 1139–1145.

Dolati, F., et al., 2014. In vitro evaluation of carbon-nanotube-reinforced bioprintable vascular conduits. Nanotechnology 25 (14), 145101.

Duan, B., et al., 2013. 3D Bioprinting of heterogeneous aortic valve conduits with alginate/gelatin hydrogels. Journal of Biomedical Materials Research Part A 101A (5), 1255–1264.

Duan, B., et al., 2014. Three-dimensional printed trileaflet valve conduits using biological hydrogels and human valve interstitial cells. Acta Biomaterialia 10 (5), 1836–1846.

Eulalio, A., et al., 2012. Functional screening identifies miRNAs inducing cardiac regeneration. Nature 492 (7429), 376–381.

Faulkner-Jones, A., et al., 2015. Bioprinting of human pluripotent stem cells and their directed differentiation into hepatocyte-like cells for the generation of mini-livers in 3D. Biofabrication 7 (4), 44102.

Fedorovich, N.E., et al., 2011. Biofabrication of osteochondral tissue equivalents by printing topologically defined, cell-laden hydrogel scaffolds. Tissue Engineering Part C: Methods 18 (1), 33–44.

Fedorovich, N.E., et al., 2008. Three-dimensional fiber deposition of cell-laden, viable, patterned constructs for bone tissue printing. Tissue Engineering Part A 14 (1), 127–133.

Feng, X., et al., 2011. Microengineering methods for cell-based microarrays and high-throughput drug-screening applications. Biofabrication 3 (3), 34101.

Gaebel, R., et al., 2011. Patterning human stem cells and endothelial cells with laser printing for cardiac regeneration. Biomaterials 32 (35), 9218–9230.

Gaetani, R., et al., 2012. Cardiac tissue engineering using tissue printing technology and human cardiac progenitor cells. Biomaterials 33 (6), 1782–1790.

Gao, G., et al., 2014. Bioactive nanoparticles stimulate bone tissue formation in bioprinted three-dimensional scaffold and human mesenchymal stem cells. Biotechnology Journal 9 (10), 1304–1311.

Ghasemi-Mobarakeh, L., et al., 2009. Electrical stimulation of nerve cells using conductive nanofibrous scaffolds for nerve tissue engineering. Tissue Engineering Part A 15 (11), 3605–3619.

Gruene, M., et al., 2010. Laser printing of stem cells for biofabrication of scaffold-free autologous grafts. Tissue Engineering Part C: Methods 17 (1), 79–87.

Gu, X., Ding, F., Williams, D.F., 2014. Neural tissue engineering options for peripheral nerve regeneration. Biomaterials 35 (24), 6143–6156.

Gudapati, H., Dey, M., Ozbolat, I., 2016. A comprehensive review on droplet-based bioprinting: past, present and future. Biomaterials 102, 20–42.

Gurkan, U.A., et al., 2014. Engineering anisotropic biomimetic fibrocartilage microenvironment by bioprinting mesenchymal stem cells in nanoliter gel droplets. Molecular Pharmaceutics 11 (7), 2151–2159.

Higgins, C.A., et al., 2013. Microenvironmental reprogramming by three-dimensional culture enables dermal papilla cells to induce de novo human hair-follicle growth. Proceedings of the National Academy of Sciences 110 (49), 19679–19688.

Hirt, M.N., Hansen, A., Eschenhagen, T., 2014. Cardiac tissue engineering: state of the art. Circulation Research 114 (2), 354–367.

Hockaday, L.A., et al., 2014. 3D-Printed hydrogel technologies for tissue-engineered heart valves. 3D Printing and Additive Manufacturing 1 (3), 122–136.

Hockaday, L.A., et al., 2012. Rapid 3D printing of anatomically accurate and mechanically heterogeneous aortic valve hydrogel scaffolds. Biofabrication 4 (3), 35005.

Horváth, L., et al., 2015. Engineering an in vitro air-blood barrier by 3D bioprinting. Scientific Reports 5, 7974.

Hsieh, F.-Y., Lin, H.-H., Hsu, S.-H., 2015. 3D bioprinting of neural stem cell-laden thermoresponsive biodegradable polyurethane hydrogel and potential in central nervous system repair. Biomaterials 71, 48–57.

Huang, T., et al., 2014. 3D printing of biomimetic microstructures for cancer cell migration. Biomedical Microdevices 16 (1), 127–132.

Ionescu-Tirgoviste, C., et al., 2015. A 3D map of the islet routes throughout the healthy human pancreas. Scientific Reports 5, 14634.

Itoh, M., et al., 2015. Scaffold-free tubular tissues created by a Bio-3D printer undergo remodeling and endothelialization when implanted in rat aortae. PLoS One 10 (9), e0136681.

Jakab, K., et al., 2010. Tissue engineering by self-assembly and bio-printing of living cells. Biofabrication 2 (2), 22001.

Jakab, K., et al., 2008. Tissue engineering by self-assembly of cells printed into topologically defined structures. Tissue Engineering Part A 14 (3), 413–421.

Jana, S., Lerman, A., 2015. Bioprinting a cardiac valve. Biotechnology Advances 33 (8), 1503–1521.

Jeon, J.S., et al., 2015. Human 3D vascularized organotypic microfluidic assays to study breast cancer cell extravasation. Proceedings of the National Academy of Sciences 112 (1), 214–219.

Keriquel, V., et al., 2010. In vivo bioprinting for computer- and robotic-assisted medical intervention: preliminary study in mice. Biofabrication 2 (1), 14101.

Kesti, M., et al., 2015. A versatile bioink for three-dimensional printing of cellular scaffolds based on thermally and photo-triggered tandem gelation. Acta Biomaterialia 11, 162–172.

Kim, K., et al., 2010. Stereolithographic bone scaffold design parameters: osteogenic differentiation and signal expression. Tissue Engineering Part B: Reviews 16 (5), 523–539.

King, S.M., Presnell, S.C., Nguyen, D.G., 2014. Abstract 2034: development of 3D bioprinted human breast cancer for in vitro drug screening. Cancer Research 74 (Suppl. 19), 2034.

Knowles, B.B., Howe, C.C., Aden, D.P., 1980. Human hepatocellular carcinoma cell lines secrete the major plasma proteins and hepatitis B surface antigen. Science 209 (4455), 497–499.

Knowlton, S., et al., 2016. Advancing cancer research using bioprinting for tumor-on-a-chip platforms. International Journal of Bioprinting 2 (2), 3–8.

Knowlton, S., et al., 2015. Bioprinting for cancer research. Trends in Biotechnology 33 (9), 504–513.

Koch, L., et al., 2012. Skin tissue generation by laser cell printing. Biotechnology and Bioengineering 109 (7), 1855–1863.

Kock, L., van Donkelaar, C.C., Ito, K., 2012. Tissue engineering of functional articular cartilage: the current status. Cell and Tissue Research 347 (3), 613–627.

Kurobe, H., et al., 2012. Concise review: tissue-engineered vascular grafts for cardiac surgery: past, present, and future. Stem Cells Translational Medicine 1 (7), 566–571.

Lee, V., et al., 2013. Design and fabrication of human skin by three-dimensional bioprinting. Tissue Engineering Part C: Methods 20 (6), 473–484.

Lee, V., et al., 2014. Generation of multi-scale vascular network system within 3D hydrogel using 3D bio-printing technology. Cellular and Molecular Bioengineering 7 (3), 460–472.

Lee, Y.-B., et al., 2010. Bio-printing of collagen and VEGF-releasing fibrin gel scaffolds for neural stem cell culture. Experimental Neurology 223 (2), 645–652.

Leon-Villapalos, J., Eldardiri, M., Dziewulski, P., 2010. The use of human deceased donor skin allograft in burn care. Cell and Tissue Banking 11 (1), 99–104.

Lorber, B., et al., 2014. Adult rat retinal ganglion cells and glia can be printed by piezoelectric inkjet printing. Biofabrication 6 (1), 15001.

Lozano, R., et al., 2015. 3D printing of layered brain-like structures using peptide modified gellan gum substrates. Biomaterials 67, 264–273.

Di Luca, A., Van Blitterswijk, C., Moroni, L., 2015. The osteochondral interface as a gradient tissue: from development to the fabrication of gradient scaffolds for regenerative medicine. Birth Defects Research Part C: Embryo Today: Reviews 105 (1), 34–52.

Makris, E.A., MacBarb, R.F., Paschos, N.K., Hu, J.C., Athanasiou, K.A., 2014. Combined use of chondroitinase-ABC, TGF-Beta1, and collagen crosslinking agent lysyl oxidase to engineer functional neotissues for fibrocartilage repair. Biomaterials 35 (25), 6787–6796.

Makris, E.A., et al., 2015. Repair and tissue engineering techniques for articular cartilage. Nature Reviews Rheumatology 11 (1), 21–34.

Malone, E., Lipson, H., 2007. Fab@Home: the personal desktop fabricator kitnull. Rapid Prototyping Journal 13 (4), 245–255.

Mannoor, M.S., et al., 2013. 3D printed bionic ears. Nano Letters 13 (6), 2634–2639.

Marchioli, G., et al., 2015. Fabrication of three-dimensional bioplotted hydrogel scaffolds for islets of Langerhans transplantation. Biofabrication 7 (2), 25009.

Markstedt, K., et al., 2015. 3D bioprinting human chondrocytes with nanocellulose–alginate bioink for cartilage tissue engineering applications. Biomacromolecules 16 (5), 1489–1496.

Merceron, T.K., et al., 2015. A 3D bioprinted complex structure for engineering the muscle–tendon unit. Biofabrication 7 (3), 35003.

Metcalfe, A.D., Ferguson, M.W.J., 2007. Tissue engineering of replacement skin: the crossroads of biomaterials, wound healing, embryonic development, stem cells and regeneration. Journal of the Royal Society Interface 4 (14), 413–437.

Meurens, F., et al., 2012. The pig: a model for human infectious diseases. Trends in Microbiology 20 (1), 50–57.

Michael, S., et al., 2013. Tissue engineered skin substitutes created by laser-assisted bioprinting form skin-like structures in the dorsal skin fold chamber in mice. PLoS One 8 (3), e57741.

Migliorini, A., Bader, E., Lickert, H., 2014. Islet cell plasticity and regeneration. Molecular Metabolism 3 (3), 268–274.

Miller, J.S., et al., 2012. Rapid casting of patterned vascular networks for perfusable engineered three-dimensional tissues. Nature Materials 11 (9), 768–774.

Mollova, M., et al., 2013. Cardiomyocyte proliferation contributes to heart growth in young humans. Proceedings of the National Academy of Sciences 110 (4), 1446–1451.

Moroni, L., De Wijn, J.R., Van Blitterswijk, C.A., 2006. 3D fiber-deposited scaffolds for tissue engineering: influence of pores geometry and architecture on dynamic mechanical properties. Biomaterials 27, 974–985.

Nam, K.-H., et al., 2015. Biomimetic 3D tissue models for advanced high-throughput drug screening. Journal of Laboratory Automation 20 (3), 201–215.

Nelson, B., 2015. 3-dimensional bioprinting makes its mark: new tissue and organ printing methods are yielding critical new tools for the laboratory and clinic. Cancer Cytopathology 123 (4), 203–204.

Nichols, J.E., Niles, J.A., Cortiella, J., 2009. Design and development of tissue engineered lung: progress and challenges. Organogenesis 5 (2), 57–61.

Nishiyama, Y., et al., 2008. Development of a three-dimensional bioprinter: construction of cell supporting structures using hydrogel and state-of-the-art inkjet technology. Journal of Biomechanical Engineering 131 (3), 35001.

Norotte, C., et al., 2009. Scaffold-free vascular tissue engineering using bioprinting. Biomaterials 30 (30), 5910–5917.

Ott, H.C., et al., 2008. Perfusion-decellularized matrix: using nature's platform to engineer a bioartificial heart. Nature Medicine 14 (2), 213–221.

Owens, C.M., et al., 2013. Biofabrication and testing of a fully cellular nerve graft. Biofabrication 5 (4), 45007.

Ozbolat, I.T., 2015a. Bioprinting scale-up tissue and organ constructs for transplantation. Trends in Biotechnology 33 (7), 395–400. Available at: http://www.ncbi.nlm.nih.gov/pubmed/25978871.

Ozbolat, I.T., 2015b. Scaffold-based or scaffold-free bioprinting: competing or complementing approaches? Journal of Nanotechnology in Engineering and Medicine 6 (2), 24701.

Ozbolat, I.T., Chen, H., Yu, Y., 2014. Development of "Multi-arm Bioprinter" for hybrid biofabrication of tissue engineering constructs. Robotics and Computer-Integrated Manufacturing 30 (3), 295–304.

Ozbolat, I.T., Hospodiuk, M., 2016. Current advances and future perspectives in extrusion-based bioprinting. Biomaterials 76, 321–343.

Ozbolat, I.T., Yu, Y., 2013. Bioprinting toward organ fabrication: challenges and future trends. IEEE Transactions on Bio-Medical Engineering 60 (3), 691–699.

Pagliuca, F.W., et al., 2015. Generation of functional human pancreatic β cells in vitro. Cell 159 (2), 428–439.

Pagliuca, F.W., Melton, D.A., 2013. How to make a functional β-cell. Development 140 (12), 2472–2483.

Palakkan, A.A., et al., 2013. Liver tissue engineering and cell sources: issues and challenges. Liver International 33 (5), 666–676.

Park, J.Y., et al., 2014. A comparative study on collagen type I and hyaluronic acid dependent cell behavior for osteochondral tissue bioprinting. Biofabrication 6 (3), 35004.

Pati, F., et al., 2014. Printing three-dimensional tissue analogues with decellularized extracellular matrix bioink. Nature Communications 5, 3935.

Peng, W., Unutmaz, D., Ozbolat, I.T., September 2016. Bioprinting towards physiologically relevant tissue models for pharmaceutics. Trends in Biotechnology 34 (9), 722–732. http://dx.doi.org/10.1016/j.tibtech.2016.05.013.

Perkins, J.D., 2007. Are we reporting the same thing?: comments. Liver Transplantation 13, 465–466.

Phillippi, J.A., et al., 2008. Microenvironments engineered by inkjet bioprinting spatially direct adult stem cells toward muscle- and bone-like subpopulations. Stem Cells 26 (1), 127–134.

Proks, P., Ashcroft, F.M., 1995. Effects of divalent cations on exocytosis and endocytosis from single mouse pancreatic beta-cells. The Journal of Physiology 487 (2), 465–477.

Quint, C., et al., 2011. Decellularized tissue-engineered blood vessel as an arterial conduit. Proceedings of the National Academy of Sciences 108 (22), 9214–9219.

Raikwar, S.P., et al., 2015. Human iPS cell-derived insulin producing cells form vascularized organoids under the kidney capsules of diabetic mice. PLoS ONE 10 (1), e0116582.

Rodríguez-Dévora, J.I., et al., 2012. High throughput miniature drug-screening platform using bioprinting technology. Biofabrication 4 (3), 35001.

Roskos, K., et al., 2015. Essentials of 3D Biofabrication and Translation. Elsevier.

Saunders, R., Derby, B., 2014. Inkjet printing biomaterials for tissue engineering: bioprinting. International Materials Review 59 (8), 430–448.

Shim, J.-H., et al., 2012. Bioprinting of a mechanically enhanced three-dimensional dual cell-laden construct for osteochondral tissue engineering using a multi-head tissue/organ building system. Journal of Micromechanics and Microengineering 22 (8), 85014.

Skardal, A., et al., 2012. Bioprinted amniotic fluid-derived stem cells accelerate healing of large skin wounds. Stem Cells Translational Medicine 1 (11), 792–802.

Snyder, J.E., et al., 2011. Bioprinting cell-laden matrigel for radioprotection study of liver by pro-drug conversion in a dual-tissue microfluidic chip. Biofabrication 3, 034112.

Temple, J.P., et al., 2014. Engineering anatomically shaped vascularized bone grafts with hASCs and 3D-printed PCL scaffolds. Journal of Biomedical Materials Research Part A 102 (12), 4317–4325.

Tourlomousis, F., Chang, R.C., 2015. Numerical investigation of dynamic microorgan devices as drug screening platforms. Part I: Macroscale modeling approach & validation. Biotechnology and Bioengineering 113 (3), 612–622.

Vaidya, M., 2015. Startups tout commercially 3D-printed tissue for drug screening. Nature Medicine 21 (1), 2.

Wu, W., DeConinck, A., Lewis, J.A., 2011. Omnidirectional printing of 3D Microvascular networks. Advanced Materials 23 (24), H178–H183.

Xiong, R., Zhang, Z., Chai, W., et al., 2015a. Freeform drop-on-demand laser printing of 3D alginate and cellular constructs. Biofabrication 7 (4), 45011.

Xiong, R., Zhang, Z., Huang, Y., 2015b. Identification of optimal printing conditions for laser printing of alginate tubular constructs. Journal of Manufacturing Processes 20, 450–455.

Xu, F., Moon, S., Emre, A., Lien, C., Turali, E., Demicri, U., 2009a. Cell bioprinting as a potential high-throughput method for fabricating cell-based biosensors (CBBs). IEEE Sensors 387–391.

Xu, C., et al., 2012. Scaffold-free inkjet printing of three-dimensional zigzag cellular tubes. Biotechnology and Bioengineering 109 (12), 3152–3160.

Xu, F., et al., 2011. A three-dimensional in vitro ovarian cancer coculture model using a high-throughput cell patterning platform. Biotechnology Journal 6 (2), 204–212.

Xu, T., et al., 2009b. Fabrication and characterization of bio-engineered cardiac pseudo tissues. Biofabrication 1 (3), 35001.

Xu, T., et al., 2013. Hybrid printing of mechanically and biologically improved constructs for cartilage tissue engineering applications. Biofabrication 5 (1), 15001.

Yanez, M., et al., 2014. Vivo assessment of printed microvasculature in a bilayer skin graft to treat full-thickness wounds. Tissue Engineering Part A 21 (1–2), 224–233.

Yu, Y., Ozbolat, I.T., 2014. Tissue strands as "bioink" for scale-up organ printing. In: Conference Proceedings: Annual International Conference of the IEEE Engineering in Medicine and Biology Society. IEEE Engineering in Medicine and Biology Society. Annual Conference, pp. 1428–1431.

Yoon No, D., et al., 2015. 3D liver models on a microplatform: well-defined culture, engineering of liver tissue and liver-on-a-chip. Lab on a Chip 15 (19), 3822–3837.

Yoshida, Y., Yamanaka, S., 2010. Recent stem cell advances: induced pluripotent stem cells for disease modeling and stem cell–based regeneration. Circulation 122 (1), 80–87.

Yu, Y., et al., 2013. Evaluation of cell viability and functionality in vessel-like bioprintable cell-laden tubular channels. Journal of Biomechanical Engineering 135 (9), 91011.

Yu, Y., et al., 2016. Three-dimensional bioprinting using self-assembling scalable scaffold-free "tissue strands" as a new bioink. Scientific Reports 6, 28714.

Yu, Y., Zhang, Y., Ozbolat, I.T., 2014. A hybrid bioprinting approach for scale-up tissue fabrication. Journal of Manufacturing Science and Engineering 136 (6), 61013.

Zervantonakis, I.K., et al., 2012. Three-dimensional microfluidic model for tumor cell intravasation and endothelial barrier function. Proceedings of the National Academy of Sciences 109 (34), 13515–13520.

Zhang, Y., Yu, Y., Chen, H., et al., 2013a. Characterization of printable cellular micro-fluidic channels for tissue engineering. Biofabrication 5 (2), 025004.

Zhang, Y., et al., 2015. In vitro study of directly bioprinted perfusable vasculature conduits. Biomaterials Science 3 (1), 134–143.

Zhang, Y., Yu, Y., Ozbolat, I.T., 2013b. Direct bioprinting of vessel-like tubular microfluidic channels. Journal of Nanotechnology in Engineering and Medicine 4, 020902.

Zhao, L., et al., 2012. The integration of 3-D cell printing and mesoscopic fluorescence molecular tomography of vascular constructs within thick hydrogel scaffolds. Biomaterials 33 (21), 5325–5332.

Zhao, Y., et al., 2014. Three-dimensional printing of Hela cells for cervical tumor model in vitro. Biofabrication 6 (3), 35001.

Zopf, D.A., et al., 2013. Bioresorbable airway splint created with a three-dimensional printer. New England Journal of Medicine 368 (21), 2043–2045.

10

Future Trends

CHAPTER OUTLINE

Let the future tell the truth, and evaluate each one according to his work and accomplishments. The present is theirs; the future, for which I have really worked, is mine

Nikola Tesla

10.1 Introduction

Due to its great benefit in spatial arrangements of multiple cell types to recapitulate tissue biology, bioprinting has assumed a game-changer role in the rapid development of tissue constructs and has gained enormous attention (Dababneh and Ozbolat, 2014). Despite the great progress made in the last decade, bioprinting still faces several challenges associated with biology, biotechnology, biomaterials, and medicine. New technologies and trends are needed to advance the bioprinting technology in multiple aspects. Therefore, this chapter highlights trends in bioprinting technology with new prospects in a wide variety of aspects of bioprinting.

This chapter first discusses general needs for advancement in bioprinting technology and its major components, including bioprinters, bioink materials, bioprinting processes, and pre- and postprocesses. Although a number of bioprinters, bioink materials, and bioprinting processes are available both noncommercially and commercially, bioprinting technology is still in its infancy, and further research, development, and advancements are needed in all aspects of bioprinting to generate viable end products for use in tissue engineering, medicine, pharmacies, and clinics.

The chapter then focuses on four-dimensional (4D) bioprinting, which can be considered a promising direction in the fabrication of living tissues in a shorter period of culture time in vitro. With the rapid fusion, folding, and remodeling capabilities of the new bioink materials, tissues can be generated quickly, enabling bioprinting in the fourth dimension, "time." This will be a groundbreaking technology that will enable mass fabrication of living tissues for pharmaceutics in the short-term and create an alternative strategy for future organ-printing technologies.

Functional organ bioprinting in clinically relevant volumes holds great promise. Bioprinting "mini-organs" that mimic the functionality of their natural counterparts with relatively simple vascular networks seems to be the transitional step toward bioprinting scale-up organs. This chapter outlines a systematic approach to bioprinting scale-up tissues and organs using a new bottom-up concept, "from vascular network to full organs." This will enable the generation of perfusable tissues and organs with hierarchical blood vessel networks and will truly revolutionize organ-fabrication technology in the near future.

Next, the chapter highlights in-situ bioprinting technology, which has rarely been attempted due to limitations such as the need for a highly effective printable bioink enabling instant solidification in a living body, the need for a biologically appealing ink for enhanced tissue formation, and regulatory issues related to living models necessitating safe and sterile delivery of the tissue construct in minimum time under anesthesia. However, overcoming these issues will be a very critical milestone toward using bioprinters in clinical settings. The chapter provides an extensive discussion on the current state of the art in in situ bioprinting as well as possibilities and approaches for in situ bioprinting of various tissues and organs to overcome the existing grand challenges. Strategies to translate the technology from bench to bedside are presented because in situ bioprinting has great promise in operating rooms in the near future.

In addition, this chapter highlights gene therapy and its potentials in bioprinting, particularly in recapitulating tissue biology, where gene therapy can enable differentiation of bioprinted stem cells into multiple lineages spatially. With bioprinting-mediated gene therapy, one can engineer a release profile for genes, resulting in sustained release of genes spatially and temporally for an advanced tissue-regeneration process. Bioprinting-mediated gene therapy can be applied in vitro and in vivo by creating hybrid tissue constructs in petri dishes and inside lesions, respectively.

Although the majority of current and past research attempts have investigated the possibility of mimicking natural organs for various applications, including transplantation and in-vitro testing, bioprinting of new types of organs that do not exist in nature unveils a great future for medicine. With such possibilities in the near future, scientists can achieve organs that are completely biological or in the form of cyborg organs enhancing the physiology of the human body beyond its ordinary capabilities.

Finally, this chapter discusses regulatory concerns, which will be crucial in translating research and development capabilities into products for transplantation or human use. Bioprinting technology, including bioprinters, bioinks, and bioprinted tissue and organ constructs, should go through Food and Drug Administration (FDA) regulations in addition to overcoming potential issues with ethical and religious barriers.

10.2 Innovative Developments in Bioprinting Technology and Its Components

Despite the great progress and many breakthroughs of the last decade, bioprinting technology is still in its infancy and has met several challenges and limitations associated with bioprinters, bioink materials, and bioprinting processes, as well as advancements in other fields such as biology, tissue engineering, and regenerative medicine (Ozbolat and Yin, 2013). In addition to bioprinting, advancements in processes associated with prebioprinting are also essential, such as new stem cell technologies enabling successful and efficient generation of tissue- and organ-specific cells from autologous cells, rapid and cost-effective expansion of cells into desired numbers comparable to the high cell numbers in native organs, such as 1.3×10^8 cells per gram in liver (Marcos et al., 2006), and more robust and automated approaches for blueprint modeling. Unless other associated fields can make great strides in advancement, bioprinting will be bottlenecked and limited in its potential. Fig. 10.1 demonstrates the need for advancements in different stages and related components of bioprinting, including (1) prebioprinting, (2) bioprinting (bioink, bioprinters, and bioprinting processes), and (3) postbioprinting.

Although great progress has been made with novel biomaterials and biomaterial processing techniques, the development of bioink materials that are well suited to bioprinting and allow one to coax cells into their native tissue-like functional structures is a great need. Particularly, new biomaterials with very quick gelation or solidification capabilities providing a mild environment for cells would be highly desirable. Despite the great success in developing new hydrogels for tissue engineering, unfortunately not all of them have been adopted to bioprinting (Malda et al., 2013). Thus a new field of study, such as "bioprintable biomaterials," potentially under the biomaterials and biofabrication fields could be a great leap to promote research in this direction. In general, highly novel bioink materials that possess the following characteristics should be developed: promotion of cell adhesion, proliferation, aggregation, and differentiation toward multiple lineages; exhibition of high mechanical integrity and structural stability without dissolving after bioprinting; facilitation of engraftment with endogenous tissue without generating immune response; bioprintability with ease of shear thinning, rapid solidification, and formability; and affordability, abundance, and commercial availability with appropriate regulations for clinical use.

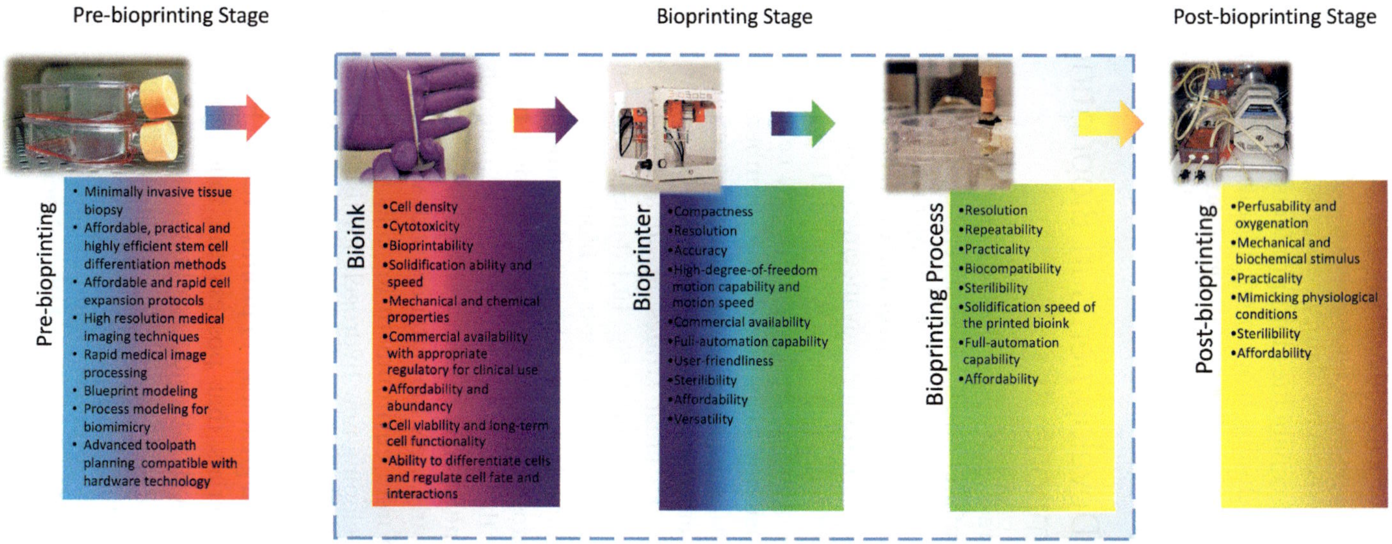

FIGURE 10.1 Components of bioprinting technology and the need for advancement in various dimensions. *(Bioprinter image, image courtesy of Biobots; bioreactor culture, reproduced/adapted with permission from Norotte et al. (2009)).*

In addition to new bioink development, there is also a great need for progress in bioprinting technologies. To fabricate scalable tissues and organs, a bioprinter needs to run for several hours because the resolution of the system is in microscale. During this prolonged fabrication time, it should deliver biological substances through a micro-nozzle or other means without clogging problems or collision issues between the nozzle tip and the printed structure. For future bioprinters, multiaxis bioprinters (for printing on nonplanar surfaces) with multiple arms (for printing hybrid constructs rapidly and more precisely (Ozbolat et al., 2014)) can be considered for bioprinting hybrid tissues both in vitro and in vivo. Therefore, bioprinters should be compact enough to fit into biosafety cabinets; easy to sterilize to facilitate aseptic conditions; have high resolution to accurately place cells; have a high-degree-of-freedom motion capability and motion speed to bioprint large constructs into lesions directly and rapidly; have full automation capabilities without any user intervention from blueprint model to posttissue maturation stage; be user-friendly, enabling ease of operation; be versatile enough to support various bioink materials and bioprinting processes; and be affordable and commercially accessible to promote further research and investigations.

In addition to advances in bioprinters and bioink materials, there is also a great need for innovative bioprinting processes that exhibit characteristics such as high-resolution capability enabling bioprinting at a single-cell-scale at high precision and repeatability. For example, a bioprinting process with the capability to print a single cell with controlled orientation and rotation in three-dimensional (3D) will have great benefits for engineering a native milieu tissue microenvironment. Moreover, the process should be practical enough to be used and advanced by fellow scientists. Most importantly, it should be biocompatible in the sense that cells should be delivered to the printing stage safe and alive with minimal or no damage, which necessitates ease of sterility for the process as well. The process should facilitate solidification of the bioink as soon as it is deposited onto the printing stage so that structural integrity can be preserved. Lastly, the process should be fully automated with in situ monitoring and self-healing capabilities, enabling detection of faulty bioprinted constructs and repairing them directly in place immediately.

The postbioprinting process is also crucial and entails physical (i.e., mechanical and electrical stimulation) and molecular (i.e., biochemical stimulation including biochemical concentration and gradient) cues and signaling to regulate tissue remodeling and growth, with rapid and accelerated tissue or organ maturation process toward a solid construct that is mechanically and structurally rigid, functional, and innervated for transplantation. Biochemical cues that accelerate tissue maturation are defined as "maturogens" (Hajdu et al., 2010), and they play an essential role in tissue and organ fabrication. Maturogens such as transforming growth factor beta-1 (TGFβ-1), serotonin, and periostin are effective in collagen accumulation, fibrogenic activity, and collagen fibrillogenesis, respectively. This makes the tissue cohesive and rapidly facilitates tissue maturation. After the bioprinting process, the fabricated constructs need to be transferred to a bioreactor, which is an important part of the tissue- and organ-fabrication process. A bioreactor is a device for tissue cultivation that facilitates efficient perfusion and oxygenation of the tissue constructs during the maturation period. Although a number of bioreactors are available for culturing various tissues and organs (Bhumiratana et al., 2014), there is a great need for new developments in bioreactor technologies that provide an optimum environment to mimic physiological conditions and better cultivate tissues and organs. The transfer of bioprinted tissues and organs to a bioreactor should be performed gently without inducing any damage that can induce disintegration and degeneration of immature and fragile tissue constructs. Therefore, future bioprinter systems can be compact enough to be enclosed in a bioreactor system, or they can be seamlessly integrated in a biofabrication line (Mironov et al., 2011) that will allow rapid and direct transfer of the bioprinted construct into a bioreactor enclosure, automatically allowing cultivation of the tissue construct under controlled aseptic conditions with high reproducibility and efficiency. This will ultimately enable biofabrication of consistently high-quality products complying with future regulations for transplantation and human use.

10.3 Toward Four-Dimensional Bioprinting

Bioprinting of scaffold-free tissues, pioneered by Mironov et al. (2009), has been a highly impressive way of fabricating tissues in vitro in a reasonably short time. Using cell aggregates in spheroid form (also known as "tissue spheroids") and their rapid self-assembly capabilities, it has already been demonstrated that tissue types that are hollow or thin in morphology can be biomimetically fabricated; these include nerve grafts and blood vessels (Owens et al., 2013; Norotte et al., 2009). Although integration of a vascular network, as discussed in Chapter 8, is the main impediment toward the ambitious idea of whole-organ printing, the self-assembling capabilities of cell aggregates and their ability to fuse into a larger-scale fully biological tissue are very promising in a sense that scaffold-based approaches cannot avail. Currently, the fusion timing capabilities are on the order of 12 h to a few days; however, technologies should be developed for more expedited fusion to enable bioprinting without the need for cell adhesion–inert molds to keep the cell aggregates in contact and make them fuse to each other. Thus 4D bioprinting can be considered a promising direction in the fabrication of living tissues in a shorter period of in vitro culture without the need for extensive casting in molds that prevent fabrication of larger tissues or their integration with vascular networks. With the rapid fusion, folding, and remodeling capabilities of cell-aggregate–based bioink materials, tissues can be generated in relatively shorter times, enabling bioprinting in the fourth dimension, "time." Printed cell aggregates need to fold and fuse to each other to create larger-scale tissues within hours to enable scale-up tissue printing technologies. This period depends on several factors, including cell phenotype, cell-to-cell interactions, cell–matrix interactions, applied maturogens, optimized media conditions for cocultured systems (i.e., medium and growth factors), culture conditions (i.e., static or dynamic), and applied cell aggregation methods. Although short fusion time after bioprinting is highly desirable, cell aggregates do not possess sufficient mechanical integrity; thus rapid deposition or exogenous reinforcement of connective tissue proteins of stroma (such as collagen and elastin) is required. The latter, however, can diminish the fusion, folding, and contraction capabilities of cell aggregates (Olsen et al., 2015). To expedite the tissue assembly process, three approaches have been recently investigated: maturogens, lockyball structures, and magnetic nanoparticles. As discussed in the previous section, maturogens such as TGFβ-1, serotonin, and periostin are biochemical molecules that accelerate the tissue fusion and maturation process as demonstrated using in vitro screening assays (Hajdu et al., 2010). Lockyball is a 3D-printed frame structure or a carrier to encage tissue spheroids, where protruding Velcro-like hooks enable interlocking of neighboring spheroids. Although this approach has been proposed for in situ tissue repair (Rezende et al., 2012), bioprinting of lockyballs has not been demonstrated yet. In the second approach, magnetic nanoparticles can be loaded in cells before the cell aggregate fabrication process; cells under magnetic forces stay in physical contact that improves their interaction. In addition to assembling prefabricated cell aggregates using magnetic forces, the entire large cell-aggregate construct can be generated using magnetic forces as well. A recently published work (Du et al., 2015) demonstrated rodlike cell aggregates under miniature magnetic forces. Upon releasing the magnetic forces, cell aggregates first form self-fold in 3 h and then bend into snaillike tissues in 13 h demonstrating a time-based transformation of tissues in 4D (see Fig. 10.2A–E). Although the presented study was not performed using bioprinting, bioprinting would ultimately bring more capabilities. With the great benefit of magnetic forces, in a few hours cells can be clustered into complex shapes, which can fold and transform into various different tissue shapes. For example, cell pellet can be printed into a sheet form in multiple layers using different cells such as smooth muscle cells and fibroblasts to generate smooth muscle and adventitia layers of a vascular tissue, respectively (see Fig. 10.2F). Upon being exposed to an engineered magnetic field, cells aggregate and form a multilayer sheet of tissue in a short period of time. After releasing the magnetic field, tissue in sheet form self-bends into a tubular form, generating a vascular tube upon fusion of both ends of the tissue. This can eliminate the need for printing a complex mold structure for vascular tissue bioprinting. In addition, cells can be used as building blocks rather than cell aggregates, which are labor-intensive and expensive to make (Ozbolat, 2015a). Further, complex tissues can be bioprinted and fabricated using magnetic engineering of cells in 4D space.

Although advancements are needed in the content of bioink materials, further development is absolutely necessary in bioprinting technologies as well as the bioprinting processes so that cell-aggregate–based bioink in near-solid state can be delivered to the printing stage without inclusion or with minimum inclusion of a delivering medium. In such cases, highly efficient cartridge systems should be designed to enable loading and extrusion of cell aggregates with minimum damage. Once established, 4D

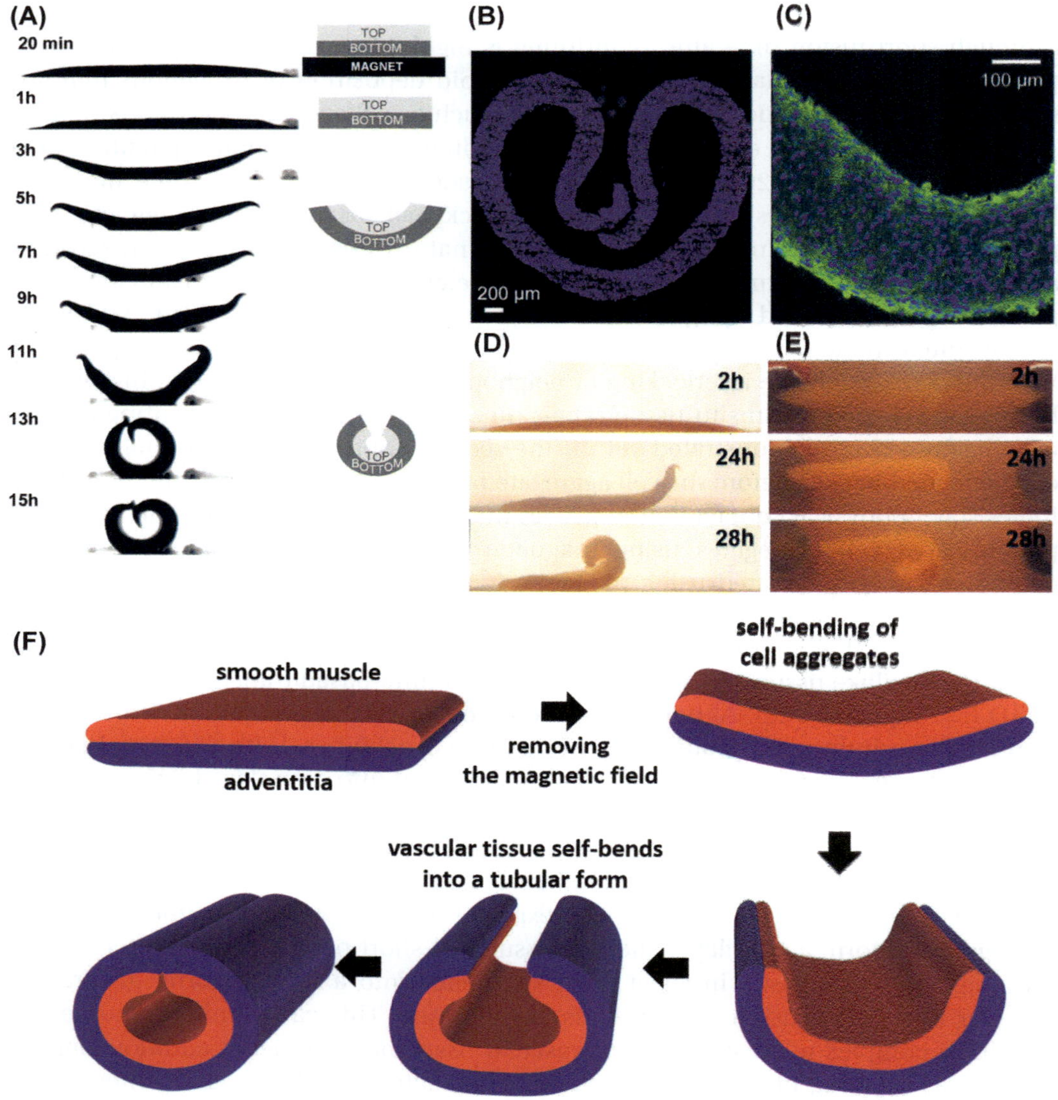

FIGURE 10.2 (A) The rod-shaped aggregate bends and folds, eventually forming a snaillike shape. The image sequences start at 20 min (immediately after turning off the magnetic field) and continue every 2 h from 1 h until 15 h. (B) A cryosection of a rod fixed 15 h after its formation (4× magnification) where *blue staining* [4′,6-diamidino-2-phenylindole (DAPI)] shows cell nucleus and (C) a cryosection of a rod fixed 15 h after its formation (20× magnification) where *blue* and *green staining* shows DAPI and E-Cadherin, respectively. (D–E) With one magnet at each end of the rod, the force was not enough to prevent bending, which occurred 24 h after rod formation *(Images from (A) to (E) are adapted/reproduced with permission from Du et al. (2015))*. (F) A conceptual image of self-bending of bioprinted cell aggregates in sheet form into a tubular form after removal of the magnetic field.

bioprinting technologies will be a highly efficient in enabling mass fabrication of living tissues for pharmaceutics in the short run.

10.4 Toward Functional Organ Fabrication

Organ bioprinting holds great promise for the future; however, whole-organ fabrication technology via bioprinting has remained elusive due to limitations associated with the integration of the vascular hierarchical network from arteries and veins down to capillaries. The field is moving forward, though, and giving the hope that shortages in tissue grafts and organ transplantation will be mitigated to some extent in the future (Dababneh and Ozbolat, 2014). Currently, the technology allows development of organs or tissues that are not metabolically highly active or that do not require vascularization, as well as mini-tissue models mimicking the biology of natural counterparts for pharmaceutical testing or cancer studies (Peng et al., 2016).

10.4.1 Bioprinting Mini-Organs

Miniature organs with neovascularization are considered an intermediate stage on the way to functional whole organs. Miniature organs can be built on a smaller scale than their natural counterparts because they do not need vascularization. In addition, they closely perform the most vital function of the associated natural organ, such as a glucose-sensitive pancreatic organ, very rich in islet density, which can produce and secrete insulin in substantial amounts to regulate the glucose level to normoglycemia, or a liver tissue closely performing the essential metabolic activities of liver (Takebe et al., 2013; Greggio et al., 2013; see Fig. 10.3). Although mini-organs or organoids are too small to restore the functionality of whole organs that are in clinically relevant volumes, they can recapitulate the tissue biology very closely and reflect the tissue physiology accurately, which has great potential in drug screening assays in vitro and can be used in cancer research.

10.4.2 Bioprinting Scale-Up Tissues and Organs

Although several studies have been performed in bioprinting of tissue constructs, fabrication of vascularized metabolically highly active thick tissues such as cardiac, pancreas, lung, or liver tissue is still a challenge. Both the general public and academics in the fields of medicine and biology have a great perception of bioprinting of fully functional whole organs as demonstrated in Fig. 10.4, where cells can be bioprinted very accurately and coaxed and self-organized into organ biomimicry that can be readily available for transplantation. In the author's opinion, the science and technology will not be at that point even in the very far future; however, that may not be absolutely essential because tissue and organ analogues that are sufficient to restore and partially replace the functionality of diseased or damaged counterparts is a more realistic vision. To bioprint

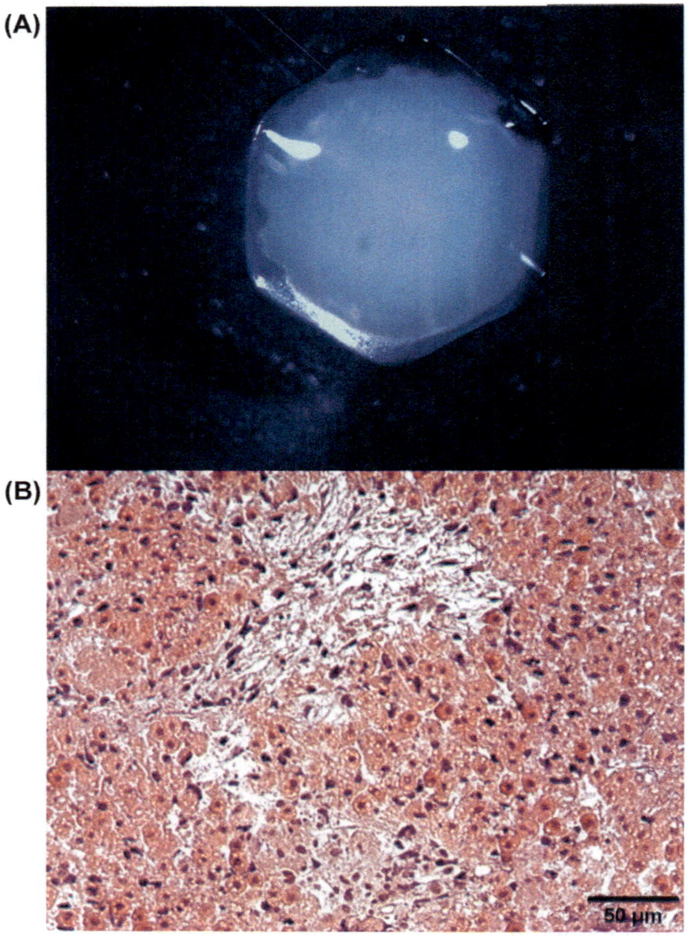

FIGURE 10.3 (A) Bioprinted mini-liver tissue for pharmaceutics using a scaffold-free bioprinting approach (3 mm × 3 mm), where (B) hepatocytes, satellite cells, and endothelial cells self-organize into liverlike constructs recapitulating liver functionality *(Image courtesy of Organovo Holdings, Inc.)*.

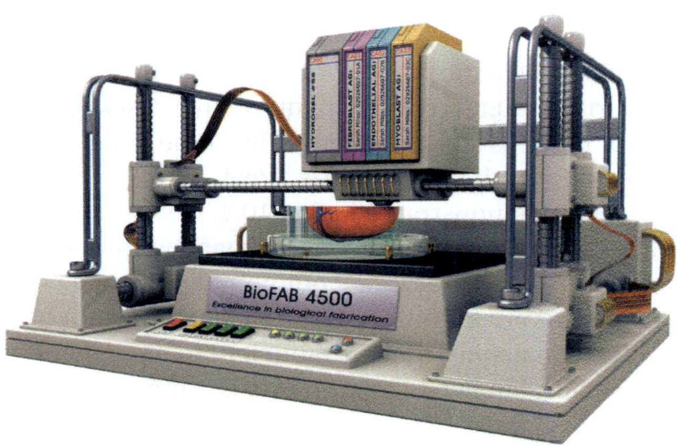

FIGURE 10.4 Futuristic organ printing concept demonstrating fabrication of organs readily available for transplantation *(Image courtesy of Christopher Barnatt, www.explainingthefuture.com.)*. Can we ever reach it?

vascularized thick tissues, robust technologies and protocols should be developed in logical steps toward this ambitious goal. Since it is very difficult to print capillaries at the submicron scale using current technology, one alternative can be bioprinting the macrovasculature and having the capillaries created by nature. However, generation of capillaries does not take place in the same timeframe as tissue formation because angiogenesis takes from 10 days to 2 weeks. Therefore, mass transport to cells in parenchyma is very limited during the time course of angiogenesis. In addition, hypoxia supports angiogenesis (Krock et al., 2011); however, it brings considerable apoptosis in parenchymal tissues. Therefore, a bottom-up strategy, building vascular network in multiple scales followed by integrating parenchyma thereafter, is preferred. Although a hierarchical vascular network in multiple scales using currently available bioprinting technology seems to be far-fetched, this can be achieved using an alternative approach. For example, a temporary supporting structure (such as fugitive wax in the investment casting process) can be printed using a biocompatible material, mimicking a vascular network in 3D. This structure should possess the capability to attract cells to gather around it and facilitate the aggregation of cells around it; however, it should be inert to cell adhesion, such as nonmodified alginate, allowing cells to attach only to each other rather than attaching to alginate. In this way, cells can aggregate with each other around a support structure, generating a tubular vascular tissue. This attraction can be achieved by hydrogels enclosing free radicals in their boundaries (Tasoglu et al., 2014), which are paramagnetic enough to attract cells infused with magnetic nanoparticles (Du et al., 2015). With this approach, vascular network can be built by assembling different layers of cell types sequentially around the temporary support, followed by degrading or decrosslinking the support structure that generates the luminal cavity and makes it ready for intravascular perfusion. Later, cells in suspension, or in aggregate or mini-tissue form, can be integrated using various means, such as assembling parenchymal and stromal cells around the vascular network by perfusing and attaching them, spraying them (Gerlach et al., 2011), or using robotic-assisted placement of mini-tissues via bioprinting, where further vascularization can be achieved via capillary sprouting to the parenchyma part of the organ construct. In this way, large-scale tissues and organs can be built with vascularization in multiple scales.

10.5 From In Vitro to In Situ: Translation of Bioprinting Technologies Into Operating Rooms

Bioprinting living tissue constructs or cell-laden scaffolds in vitro have been well studied in the literature. Success has been achieved with growing tissues such as thin tissues or tissues that do not need vascularization, including skin, cartilage, and blood vessels (Murphy and Atala, 2014), in laboratory settings. In situ bioprinting, on the other hand, can enable the growth of thick tissues in critical defects with the help of vascularization driven by nature in lesions. Therefore, in situ bioprinting stands as a promising direction for the bioprinting of porous tissue analogues that can engraft with the endogenous tissue and generate new tissue along with vascularization through recruitment of endothelial cells from the host and sprouting of capillaries from the endogenous tissue.

The idea of in-situ bioprinting was first proposed by Campbell and Weiss (2007) using inkjet technology; however, the potential of translating the bioprinters into operating rooms was considered very challenging due to the perception that surgeons can be considered artists and like off-the-shelf solutions such as using prefabricated tissue constructs and cutting or carving them into a form to be implanted into the defect site. Very limited research has been performed on in situ bioprinting since then. Only inkjet-based bioprinting has been tested for printing skin cells in the form of a thin film for burn wound healing (Skardal et al., 2012); laser-assisted bioprinting has been performed as a preliminary study to test the feasibility of printing nano-hydroxyapatite (n-HA) particles on a mouse model (Keriquel et al., 2010).

The technology for in situ bioprinting of skin tissue developed at Wake Forest Regenerative Medicine Institute was a laser scanner–integrated inkjet-based bioprinting platform enabling scanning burn wounds on pigs and processing the scanned data to obtain the wound periphery (Skardal et al., 2012). First, the geometry was postprocessed for bioprinting using custom-made software to identify the path plan, and the bioprinter heads, loaded with fibroblasts and keratinocytes, deposit cells in collagen droplets spatially. Fibroblasts were printed first, creating the first layer of the skin graft, and then keratinocytes were printed on the second layer to create the epidermis layer. The bioink made of collagen in that study has several advantages. First of all, it is the main component of the skin that gives comparable properties to the native skin properties and it enabled fibroblasts and keratinocytes to grow and proliferate efficiently. Secondly, collagen is in liquid state when loaded in a cold chamber and gels quickly when it is printed in small droplets into the body at 37°C. The bioprinted skin graft healed the wound in 3 weeks and resulted in better healing and less scar formation compared to the control groups, which used manual injection of a random mix of the aforementioned two cell types. The technology was intended for use by the United States Armed Forces for treatment for wounded soldiers in the battlefield, which would enable rapid healing of the burn wounds. In addition to inkjet-based bioprinting, attempts have been made with laser-based systems to deposit n-HA into mouse calvarial defects as a framework study (Keriquel et al., 2010). First, the effect of laser irritation on inflammation in the dura site was determined by means of magnetic resonance imaging. Then, the preliminary results obtained using decalcified sections and microtomography demonstrated the possibility and promise of in situ printing of n-HA particles. Although the ink in the demonstrated work did not comprise any biologics, it unveiled the application of a laser-based printing system in operating rooms. In addition, the recently commercialized bioprinting pen technology has been an exemplary approach in the clinical settings (O'Connell et al., 2016); the bioprinting pen can dispense cells in hydrogels into a lesion and fill the defect. Although the bioprinting pen is manually used rather than computer-controlled, the new technology has given rise to hope that translating in-situ bioprinting technology into operating rooms will be highly useful.

In situ bioprinting for deep and major defects with tunable biological, mechanical, gene delivery, and anatomical properties such as a porous tissue analog enabling enhanced and rapid tissue formation is one of the trends in bioprinting. Although droplet- or laser-based bioprinting has been used in printing nonporous bulk scaffolds, it cannot be used in printing porous architecture due to the intrinsic limitations of these bioprinting modalities to enable continuous fibers (Gudapati et al., 2016). In situ bioprinting using extrusion-based bioprinting has been recently attempted by the author's laboratory (Ozbolat, 2015b). In general, extrusion-based bioprinting has several major challenges associated with biological, biomaterial, and engineering aspects, such as printing difficulties on nonplanar or nonhorizontal surfaces, the need for a highly effective extrudable bioink enabling instant solidification [without need for an external solidifier such as ultraviolet (UV) light (Hockaday et al., 2012) or a chemical crosslinker (Zhang et al., 2013)] in a living body, the need for a biologically appealing ink for enhanced tissue formation, and regulatory issues related to animals necessitating safe and sterile delivery of the tissue construct in minimum time under anesthesia (Khatiwala et al., 2012). The author's laboratory recently developed a technology to print multiple tissue constructs into calvarial defects for bone tissue regeneration. In that approach, the Multi-Arm BioPrinter (discussed in Chapter 7) was used to print multiple tissue analogues with tunable bioink properties with controlled plasmid-deoxyribonucleic acid (pDNA) delivery using gene-activated matrices.

In general, in situ bioprinting is not trivial, and there are several major challenges associated with biological, biomaterial, and engineering limitations. Further systematic research is required to take the bioprinting technology into a robust state in situ. In this regard, bioprinting ex vivo on explants can be considered as a transitional stage (see Fig. 10.5A), where explants can be harvested from the animal model, and the tissue construct can be built and engineered inside the defect. When the defect model is still alive with living cells inside, it allows cells of native tissue to migrate and grow through the printed tissue construct or vice versa, depending on the tissue type. Although bioprinting into the explant model has been performed using inkjet-based bioprinting only (Cui et al., 2012), it has not been attempted using other bioprinting means so far, except for a preliminary effort on extrusion-based printing into a defect on a nonliving femur model placed on a fixture (Cohen et al., 2010), which was then filled with precrosslinked sodium alginate. Printing ex vivo into a defect model using bioprinting has some advantages and disadvantages compared to bioprinting in vitro. First of all, the success of tissue generation is higher compared to bioprinting in vitro because cells from native tissue can migrate into the printed tissue analogues, which will further promote tissue formation in ex vivo organ culture. Similar attempts, not using bioprinting but rather manual injection, have been demonstrated in the literature for cartilage defects (Yu et al., 2015). The major advantage of bioprinting compared to injection is that bioprinting

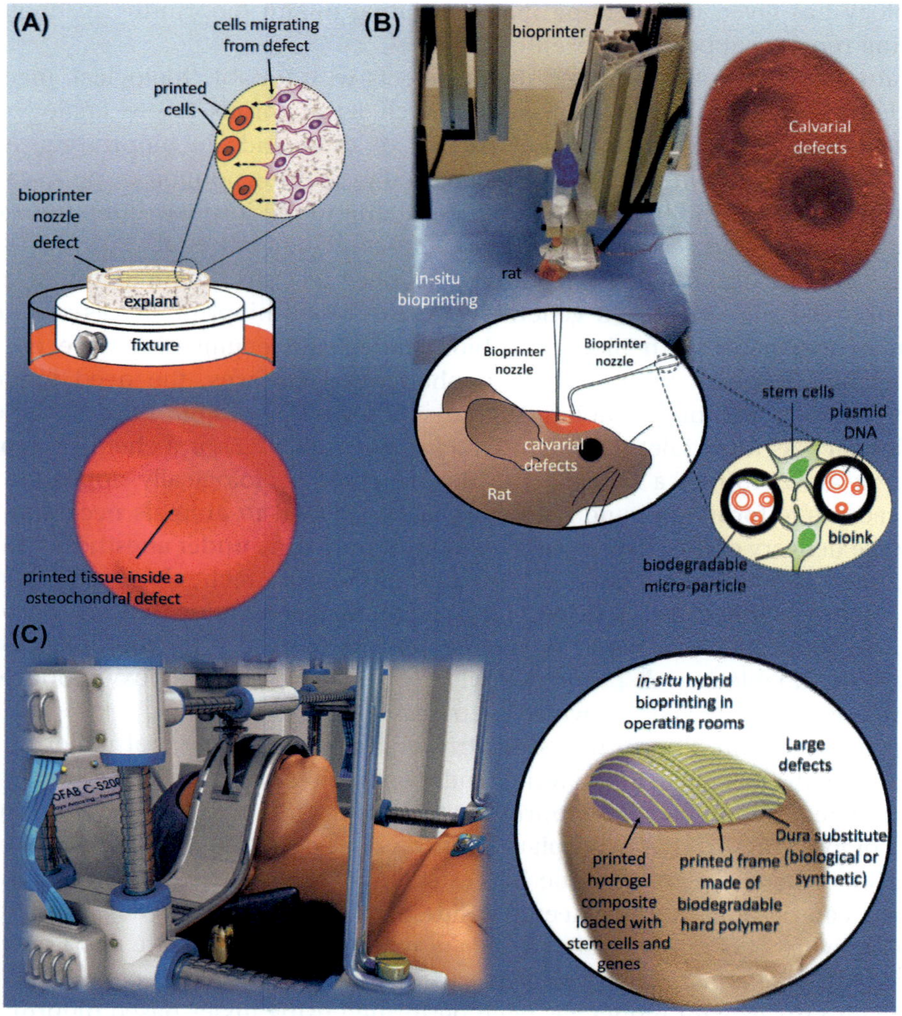

FIGURE 10.5 In situ bioprinting. (A) Bioprinting cells into explants in situ can be considered an intermediate step toward (B) bioprinting tissue constructs directly into animal models, where DNA can also be deposited for bioprinting-mediated gene therapy to transfect and differentiates printed stem cells into multiple lineages. This will have a great impact on (C) transitioning in situ bioprinting technology into operating rooms for humans in the near future *(Image courtesy of Christopher Barnatt)*. For example, large and deep calvarial defects can be regenerated on a synthetic or biological dura substitute, where a hard polymeric biodegradable frame can be printed along with stem cells and genes loaded in hydrogels to generate the vascularized bone tissues.

enables locating different cell types spatially, such as zonally controlled stratified cartilage, that allows one to biomimetically engineer the printed tissues. In addition, creating a bulk tissue construct (nonporous) is very straightforward because the bioink can be printed into the confined shape without any consideration for internal architecture design. Bioprinting a porous construct into an ex vivo defect, on the other hand, is more challenging than bioprinting in vitro because the defect models confine the motion of the nozzle tip. Therefore, very small nozzle tips are preferable, and advanced toolpath algorithms such as spiral paths should be developed to overcome issues with the nozzle interfering with the defect periphery. In general, zigzag printing can increase the chance of nozzle collision and creates significant overdeposition on the periphery of the defect. In addition, there will be challenges with attachment of the printed tissue construct on the bottom surface of the defect; thus surface modifications can be performed on the explant model to enhance the adherence capabilities of printed tissue constructs. The major advantage of printing into ex vivo defect models is that it provides a translational step toward in situ bioprinting on a live animal model, which will one day bring the bioprinter technologies from benchside to bedside. For naturally forming defects resulting from trauma, surgical excision or other issues are random in morphology and shape, and integrated laser- or image-based can be considered to automatically capture the shape and generate a path plan for in situ bioprinting.

In situ bioprinting can be considered very promising for developing tissue analogues directly on the defect model in the operating rooms (see Fig. 10.5B), which would pave the way to developing associated enabling technologies for humans in the future. It can be envisioned that in situ bioprinting into the defect on live models can have several advantages, as listed in Box 10.1. Because of these advantages, in-situ bioprinting of tissue analogues can be applied to various sites on the body, such as deep dermal or extreme injuries, calvarial or craniofacial defects during maxillofacial or neurosurgeries, and plastic surgeries for facial reconstructions.

For long-term future directions, in situ bioprinting technology can be considered for reasonably large defects in humans (see Fig. 10.5C). To fix such large defects that need a great deal of vascularization along with structural support, one can envision bioprinting a framework in tandem with stem cells (i.e., bone marrow or adipose-derived stem cells) to be differentiated toward multiple lineages, including osteoblasts and endothelial cells for bone generation and vascularization, respectively. To this end, two 6-axis bioprinter arms are required to bioprint the framework using hard polymers that can be extruded at or below human body temperature (i.e., a newly discovered protein obtained from squid ring teeth (Pena-Francesch et al., 2014)) and the stem cells using hydrogels (i.e., blend of collagen and fibrin) that can support bone matrix deposition and angiogenesis (Temple et al., 2014). In situ bioprinting of porcine aortic endothelial cells in fibrin gel has already demonstrated vascularization in the subcutaneous tissue of mice one week after implantation (Xu et al., 2008). In another long-term future application, in situ bioprinting can assist placement of different cell types in different compartments in very deep and large defects for composite tissue regeneration, where manual surgical interventions are required for suturing supplemental blood vessels and nerves. In that case, bioprinting can be performed with a deposition head mounted on a 6-axis robotic arm controlled by the surgeon. The printed bioink should have a highly porous microstructure or can be mixed with a sacrificial (quickly bioresorbable) biomaterial leaving porosity upon

BOX 10.1 CHALLENGES IN IN SITU BIOPRINTING AND FORESEEABLE ADVANTAGES WHEN THE TECHNOLOGY EVOLVES INTO A ROBUST STATE

In situ bioprinting is not trivial, and there are several major challenges associated with its biological, biomaterial, and engineering aspects, such as printing difficulties on non-horizontal surfaces, the need for highly advanced robotics bioprinting technologies, the requirement for a highly effective extrudable bioink enabling instant solidification in a living body (without need for an external solidifier such as a UV light or a chemical crosslinker), the need for a biologically appealing ink for enhanced tissue formation, and regulatory issues related to animals or humans necessitating safe and sterile delivery of the tissue construct under anesthesia (Khatiwala et al., 2012).

When the technology is translated into clinics, it will have several advantages, including the following:

- Direct bioprinting of tissue constructs into defects can eliminate the need for preshaping or reshaping the scaffold based on the defect geometry. This can surpass the laborious nature of scaffold preparation and overcome the risks associated with contamination and limited activity of cells in vitro.
- For bioprinting of cell-laden tissue constructs for critical- or large-size defects, in situ bioprinting can eliminate the need for differentiation of stem or progenitor cells in vitro, which might be expensive and time-consuming. When bioprinting stem or progenitor cells in situ, cells are exposed to the natural environment with growth factors that can induce their differentiation into the desired lineages.
- In situ bioprinting can enable very precise deposition of cells, genes, or cytokines inside the defect, unlike manual interventions such as prefabricated scaffolds, in which the shape can alter due to swelling, contraction, or deformations. Localized control via bioprinting, such as printing different cytokines at different layers, is an asset for future bioprinting research.
- Standard defects made by surgery tools are easily addressed by manipulation and bioprinting of tissue analogues. However, naturally occurring defects resulting from trauma, surgical excision, or other issues are random in morphology and geometry and need to be captured precisely; laser- or image-based scanning systems can overcome this challenge. In situ bioprinting can eliminate the need for multiple operations because the tissue constructs can be bioprinted into the defect right away.
- Twisting multiaxis robotic arms can enable angled deposition and printing of the bioink into nonhorizontally oriented defects. Defects on the live model can be at random locations, and it is not convenient for the surgeon to change the position of the anesthetized model during bioprinting.

transplantation, which will enable diffusion and interstitial flow of blood for survivability of cells until neovascularization is completed. A major challenge is lack of growth factors far from the defect periphery, which are needed to induce differentiation of printed stem cells or progenitor cells recruited from the host. This can be overcome with gene therapy, where gene delivery can be sustained and controlled using gene-activated matrices (GAMs), such as microparticles loaded with genes, for long-term release of genes for transduction and differentiation of autologous cells into multiple lineages (Evans, 2012). Printing nonviral vectors in GAMs is safe and efficient for transfecting target cells and surpasses the benefits of direct delivery of growth factors during in situ bioprinting.

It is hoped that these highly transformative recent efforts in in situ bioprinting will pioneer the translation of robotics bioprinting technology into operating rooms and will be used for printing body parts in humans after going through very strict FDA procedures. This will pave the road to the future of medicine with automated technologies to build engineered tissue and body parts on humans.

10.6 Bioprinting New Types of Organs

In addition to bioprinting tissues and organs to replace their existing counterparts, the author also envisions bioprinting of new types of organs that do not exist in nature but can be engineered to perform specific and useful functions when transplanted, such as treating diseases or enhancing the physiology of the human body beyond its ordinary capabilities. Such an organ can be either fully biological or in the form of cyborg organs interweaving electronics and biology. A recently published study demonstrated a proof of concept of such a cyborg organ example, where bionic ears were printed using a hybrid approach via integration of bioprinting chondrocytes in sodium alginate matrix along with printed silver nanoparticles in the form of an inductive coil antenna (Mannoor et al., 2013). The cultured cyborg organ model was then tested and was found to exhibit enhanced auditory sensing for radio frequency reception (see Fig. 10.6). 3D printing in that study demonstrated the proof of concept for cyborg ears, promising a seamless integration of electronics and biology for future off-the-shelf cyborg organs.

These organs can also be constructed fully biologically and even generate functions that power systems do in daily life, such as producing electricity. With recent advances in understanding the genomic basis of electric organs (EOs) (Gallant et al., 2014), which exist in electric eels and produce electricity for communication, sensing, navigation, predation ,and defense, the possibility of reconstructing similar models of EOs through additive manufacturing has been considered. Electric organs are constructed from cells called electrocytes, which have cation-specific ion channels on an innervated surface and an invaginated plasma membrane enriched in sodium pumps on the opposite surface (Gallant et al., 2014). Due to the asymmetric functionality of their anatomy and their spatial arrangements in series configuration in an EO, electrocytes produce a significant amount of electricity. This unique spatial arrangement can be enabled by 3D bioprinting (particularly with a laser- or droplet-based bioprinting system), allowing one to aggregate and collect the voltage produced by electrocytes. One can envision differentiating stem cells or muscle cells to produce such a cell source for a human-specific organ type for future attempts in using such an organ for transplantation or for

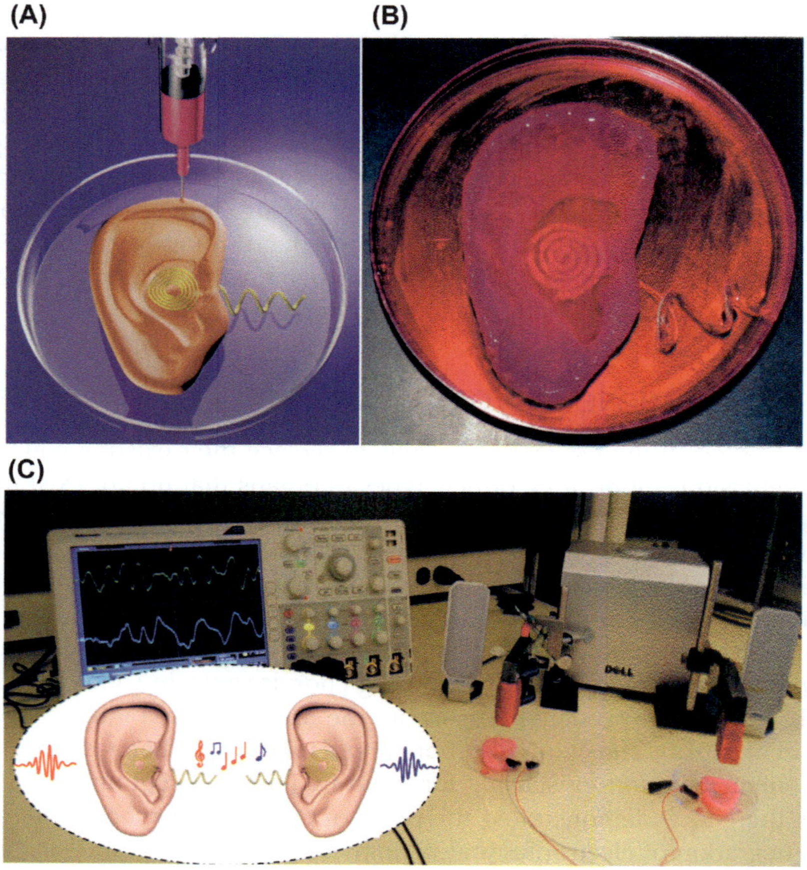

FIGURE 10.6 Three-dimensional (3D)-printed cyborg ears. (A) Bioprinting of anatomically correct cartilage scaffold loaded with chondrocytes along with printing of coil antenna. (B) Scaffolds were cultured 10 weeks, resulting in neocartilaginous tissue in alginate matrix. (C) 3D-printed complementary ears (right and left) demonstrated the ability to listen to stereophonic audio music *(Reprinted (adapted) with permission from Mannoor et al. (2013). Copyright (2013) American Chemical Society).*

replacing batteries for pacemakers (Ozbolat and Yu, 2013) or cochlear implants (Fritzsch, 2014) or powering the human body.

Another exciting direction in bioprinting is to fabricate biological robots or human–machine interfaces such as biologically made electromechanical circuits. A recent study (Cvetkovic et al., 2014) demonstrated the great potential of 3D printing in generating untethered biological machines through stereolithography-based fabrication of a device, called a biobot, composed of two stiff pillars connected by a beam made of poly(ethylene glycol) diacrylate hydrogel followed by seeding of mouse skeletal muscle myoblast cells with the assistance of extracellular matrix proteins, resulting in muscle strips. By exciting the fabricating structure using electrical stimulation, cells in the muscle strip contracted and resulted in locomotion of the biobot with a maximum velocity of 156 μm/s. Although bioprinting was not applied in this study, it has great potential to make more advanced versions of such a biological machine due to its accuracy in placements of multiple cell types spatially.

10.7 Bioprinting Deoxyribonucleic Acid for Controlled Gene Therapy

To date, both in vivo and ex vivo gene therapy have been used in tissue repair (Kay, 2011); however, limited attempts have been made to bioprint genes (Loozen et al., 2013). While differentiating stem cells into multiple lineages is crucial to recapitulate the tissue nature, bioprinting genes spatially could be a solution to overcome this limitation and could allow transduction and differentiation of autologous cells into multiple lineages per demand spatially. In addition to bioprinting-mediated ex vivo gene therapy, bioprinting-mediated in vivo gene therapy can also be used and is very appealing because it is technically feasible and will be highly effective in operating rooms, as discussed earlier. Bioprinting genes for locally controlled gene therapy can surpass the limitations of currently available methods, including direct injection or gene-activated matrices such as potential spreading of genes to nontarget sites (Evans et al., 2009).

Although naked pDNA can be applied for gene delivery, it typically results in low-transfection efficiency and high toxicity (Elangovan et al., 2014). Therefore, loading pDNA in biodegradable microparticles has recently generated promising results for controlled gene delivery. In this regard, bioprinting will not only allow spatial control over gene therapy but also enable slow release of the gene vector to the surrounding cells or tissues. By bioprinting tissue constructs ex vivo or in vivo, one can engineer the gene therapy through the sustained and controlled release of genes loaded in microparticles. This way, new delivery systems can be developed with controlled, localized, and sustained release of genes with high efficiency and low toxicity, and the release profile can be mediated by altering bioprinting parameters and releasing multiple genes sequentially and spatiotemporally. This is particularly important for tissue systems with functionality-graded tissue heterogeneity, such as osteochondral tissues with multiple osteal and chondral regions interfacing at a unique zone with extremely unique tissue anatomy. Thus gene release systems can efficiently generate such zonal differentiation gradually. Fig. 10.7 demonstrates bioprinting of hybrid tissue constructs where multiple types of genes are located spatially to transfect the stem cells in a way to trigger them to secrete growth factors A and B, which will differentiate stem cells into multiple lineages such as BMP-2 and VEGF. In this way, bone tissue can be fabricated with more bony tissue in the outer regions and more vascularized tissue in the core sections. There exist several parameters that will determine the release profile and kinetics of genes, including tissue construct properties (i.e., composition and porosity), bioink properties (i.e., biomaterial type and concentration), gene loading conditions (i.e., gene types and

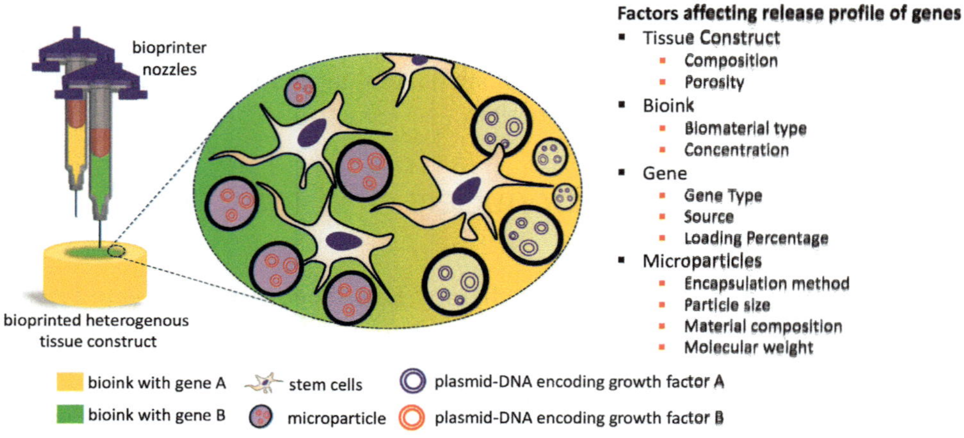

FIGURE 10.7 Bioprinting-mediated gene therapy where multiple genes can be used to transfect stem cells spatially to differentiate them into multiple lineages to recapitulate heterocellular tissue biology. The spatiotemporal control of gene delivery can be regulated by controlling several factors, including tissue construct material and morphology, gene type and loading rates, and microparticle characteristics.

sources, and loading percentages), and microparticle properties (i.e., encapsulation method, particle size, and encapsulating material properties).

10.8 Regulatory Issues

Although several attempts have been made to advance bioprinting technology, regulatory issues seem to be imminent as the technology transforms into products for transplantation and human-use purposes. Currently, no regulations have been set for bioprinting, including bioink, bioprinters, and bioprinted products such as tissues, and the FDA has not imposed any regulatory restrictions on bioprinting technology yet. Cutting-edge technologies such as bioprinting cannot be easily categorized for regulatory purposes because they do not fit into the general classifications of "device," "drug," or "biologic" under FDA regulations. The Office of Combination Products (OCP) formed by the FDA can handle this situation; "combination product" is defined in 21 CFR §3.2(e) as "A product comprised of two or more regulated components, i.e., drug/device, biologic/device, drug/biologic or drug/device/biologic, that are physically, chemically, or otherwise combined or mixed and produced as a single entity" (Hellman, 2008). The OCP does not conduct product reviews but assigns combination products to the appropriate FDA center (i.e., the Center for Drug Evaluation and Research , The Center for Biologics Evaluation and Research , or the Center for Devices and Radiological Health), ensures timely and effective premarket review and appropriate postmarket regulations, and serves as a resource to industry and the FDA center's review staff (Hellman, 2008). The OCP determines jurisdiction and classification assignments for medical products. Ultimately, both the bioprinted tissues and the 3D bioprinter itself could be classified as combination products. The bioprinter is classifiable as a medical device as it is used for treating humans and is intended to affect the structure and function of the human body. For it to function, the bioprinter should be loaded with a bioink, which is composed of cells and other biologics that can be classified as biologics (cells) or drugs (genes, growth factors, etc.). The tissues printed by the bioprinter could be classified as a biologic. Currently, there are only few companies in the world (Root Analysis Private Ltd., 2014) working in this area; however, with the increasing global interest and needs, more businesses will be established in the growing bioprinting market. The success of the first technology going through FDA regulations will be exemplary for subsequent technologies and products.

In addition to regulatory concerns with bioprinting, ethical concerns will also need to be considered for future attempts. Although the majority of the trials have been on animals, ethical concerns will arise when printing tissues or organs for transplant to humans. Patients' own stem cells will be required to overcome rejection issues, and patients may not be willing to allow their cells to go through several procedures, such as mixing their cells with biomaterials obtained from animals, to 3D bioprint an organ. New types of organs can also be manipulated. One example is organs for superior functionalities, which can mutate the human body or make it superior, such as energy-generating organs or muscles that do not produce lactic acid, providing the body with extra stamina and making athletes extra competitive. This is not ethical and is not likely to be accepted in the future. Religious and cultural norms will also play an important role in ethical concerns; transplantation of a patient's own cells within a scaffold made from animal proteins will not be acceptable for some religious and cultural rules. Although these seem to be speculations at this point, the future of bioprinting will certainly encounter some constraints and impediments.

10.9 Summary

This chapter presents future perspectives in bioprinting science and technology over the next few decades. The future trends include advancements in bioprinting and its components; 4D bioprinting to expedite the tissue fusion and maturation process for in vitro tissue fabrication processes; in situ bioprinting to translate the technology into operating rooms and enable printing body parts on humans in the future; a systematic step-by-step approach to generate enabling technologies for vascularized scale-up organ fabrication; bioprinting of new types of organs to generate advanced capabilities for humans beyond their ordinary physiology; sustained gene therapy to develop complex heterocellular tissues mimicking natural tissues; and prospects of regulatory barriers. Although the future trends demonstrate some promising concepts, there is still a need for great progress in several components of bioprinting. One such area is stem cell technology, particularly in the differentiation capability of current stem cell sources or the invention of new stem cell sources and methods to mimic the evolutionary development of tissues and organs.

References

Bhumiratana, S., Bernhard, J., Cimetta, E., Vunjak-Novakovic, G., 2014. Chapter 14-principles of bioreactor design for tissue engineering. In: Vacanti, R.L.L. (Ed.), Principles of Tissue Engineering, fourth ed. Academic Press, Boston.

Campbell, P.G., Weiss, L.E., 2007. Tissue engineering with the aid of inkjet printers. Expert Opinion on Biological Therapy 7, 1123–1127.

Cohen, D.L., Lipton, J.I., Bonassar, L.J., Lipson, H., 2010. Additive manufacturing for in situ repair of osteochondral defects. Biofabrication 2, 035004.

Cui, X., Breitenkamp, K., Finn, M.G., Lotz, M., D'lima, D.D., 2012. Direct human cartilage repair using three-dimensional bioprinting technology. Tissue Engineering Part A 18, 1304–1312.

Cvetkovic, C., Raman, R., Chan, V., Williams, B.J., Tolish, M., Bajaj, P., Sakar, M.S., Asada, H.H., Saif, M.T.A., Bashir, R., 2014. Three-dimensionally printed biological machines powered by skeletal muscle. Proceedings of the National Academy of Sciences of the United States of America 111, 10125–10130.

Dababneh, A.B., Ozbolat, I.T., 2014. Bioprinting technology: a current state-of-the-art review. Journal of Manufacturing Science and Engineering 136, 061016.

Du, V., Fayol, D., Reffay, M., Luciani, N., Bacri, J.C., Gay, C., Wilhelm, C., 2015. Magnetic engineering of stable rod-shaped stem cell aggregates: circumventing the pitfall of self-bending. Integrative Biology 7, 170–177.

Elangovan, S., D'mello, S.R., Hong, L., Ross, R.D., Allamargot, C., Dawson, D.V., Stanford, C.M., Johnson, G.K., Sumner, D.R., Salem, A.K., 2014. The enhancement of bone regeneration by gene activated matrix encoding for platelet derived growth factor. Biomaterials 35, 737–747.

Evans, C.H., Ghivizzani, S.C., Robbins, P.D., 2009. Progress and Prospects: genetic treatments for disorders of bones and joints. Gene Therapy 16, 944–952.

Evans, C.H., 2012. Gene delivery to bone. Advanced Drug Delivery Reviews 64, 1331–1340.

Fritzsch, B., 2014. Electric organs: history and potential. Science 345, 631–632.

Gallant, J.R., Traeger, L.L., Volkening, J.D., Moffett, H., Chen, P.-H., Novina, C.D., Phillips, G.N., Anand, R., Wells, G.B., Pinch, M., Güth, R., Unguez, G.A., Albert, J.S., Zakon, H.H., Samanta, M.P., Sussman, M.R., 2014. Genomic basis for the convergent evolution of electric organs. Science 344, 1522–1525.

Gerlach, J.C., Johnen, C., Mccoy, E., Bräutigam, K., Plettig, J., Corcos, A., 2011. Autologous skin cell spray-transplantation for a deep dermal burn patient in an ambulant treatment room setting. Burns 37, e19–e23.

Greggio, C., De Franceschi, F., Figueiredo-Larsen, M., Gobaa, S., Ranga, A., Semb, H., Lutolf, M., Grapin-Botton, A., 2013. Artificial three-dimensional niches deconstruct pancreas development in vitro. Development 140, 4452–4462.

Gudapati, H., Dey, M., Ozbolat, I.T., 2016. A comprehensive review on droplet-based bioprinting: past, present and future. Biomaterials 102, 20–42.

Hajdu, Z., Mironov, V., Mehesz, A.N., Norris, R.A., Markwald, R.R., Visconti, R.P., 2010. Tissue spheroid fusion-based in vitro screening assays for analysis of tissue maturation. Journal of Tissue Engineering and Regenerative Medicine 4, 659–664.

Hellman, K., 2008. Tissue engineering: translating science to product. In: Ashammakhi, N., Reis, R., Chiellini, F. (Eds.), Topics in Tissue Engineering. Clarksburg.

Hockaday, L.A., Kang, K.H., Colangelo, N.W., Cheung, P.Y.C., Duan, B., Malone, E., Wu, J., Girardi, L.N., Bonassar, L.J., Lipson, H., Chu, C.C., Butcher, J.T., 2012. Rapid 3D printing of anatomically accurate and mechanically heterogeneous aortic valve hydrogel scaffolds. Biofabrication 4, 035005.

Kay, M.A., 2011. State-of-the-art gene-based therapies: the road ahead. Nature Reviews Genetics 12, 316–328.

Keriquel, V., Guillemot, F., Arnault, I., Guillotin, B., Miraux, S., Amédée, J., Fricain, J.-C., Catros, S., 2010. In vivo bioprinting for computer- and robotic-assisted medical intervention: preliminary study in mice. Biofabrication 2, 014101.

Khatiwala, C., Law, R., Shepherd, B., Dorfman, S., Csete, M., 2012. 3D cell bioprinting for regenerative medicine research and therapies. Gene Therapy and Regulation 07, 1230004.

Krock, B.L., Skuli, N., Simon, M.C., 2011. Hypoxia-induced angiogenesis: good and evil. Genes & Cancer 2, 1117–1133.

Loozen, L.D., Wegman, F., Oner, F.C., Dhert, W.J.A., Alblas, J., 2013. Porous bioprinted constructs in BMP-2 non-viral gene therapy for bone tissue engineering. Journal of Materials Chemistry B 1, 6619–6626.

Malda, J., Visser, J., Melchels, F.P., Jungst, T., Hennink, W.E., Dhert, W.J.A., Groll, J., Hutmacher, D.W., 2013. 25th anniversary article: engineering hydrogels for biofabrication. Advanced Materials 25, 5011–5028.

Mannoor, M.S., Jiang, Z., James, T., Kong, Y.L., Malatesta, K.A., Soboyejo, W.O., Verma, N., Gracias, D.H., Mcalphine, M.C., 2013. 3D printed bionic ears. Nano Letters 13, 2634–2639.

Marcos, R., Monteiro, R.A.F., Rocha, E., 2006. Design-based stereological estimation of hepatocyte number, by combining the smooth optical fractionator and immunocytochemistry with anti-carcinoembryonic antigen polyclonal antibodies. Liver International 26, 116–124.

Mironov, V., Visconti, R.P., Kasyanov, V., Forgacs, G., Drake, C.J., Markwald, R.R., 2009. Organ printing: tissue spheroids as building blocks. Biomaterials 30, 2164–2174.

Mironov, V., Kasyanov, V., Markwald, R.R., 2011. Organ printing: from bioprinter to organ biofabrication line. Current Opinion in Biotechnology 22, 667–673.

Murphy, S.V., Atala, A., 2014. 3D bioprinting of tissues and organs. Nature Biotechnology 32, 773–785.

Norotte, C., Marga, F.S., Niklason, L.E., Forgacs, G., 2009. Scaffold-free vascular tissue engineering using bioprinting. Biomaterials 30, 5910–5917.

O'connell, C.D., Bella, C.D., Thompson, F., Augustine, C., Beirne, S., Cornock, R., Richards, C.J., Chung, J., Gambhir, S., Yue, Z., Bourke, J., Zhang, B., Taylor, A., Quigley, A., Kapsa, R., Choong, P., Wallace, G.G., 2016. Development of the Biopen: a handheld device for surgical printing of adipose stem cells at a chondol wound site. Biofabrication 8, 015019.

Olsen, T.R., Mattix, B., Casco, M., Herbst, A., Williams, C., Tarasidis, A., Simionescu, D., Visconti, R.P., Alexis, F., 2015. Manipulation of cellular spheroid composition and the effects on vascular tissue fusion. Acta Biomaterialia 13, 188–198.

Owens, C.M., Marga, F., Forgacs, G., Heesch, C.M., 2013. Biofabrication and testing of a fully cellular nerve graft. Biofabrication 5, 045007.

Ozbolat, I.T., Yin, Y., 2013. Bioprinting toward organ fabrication: challenges and future trends. IEEE Transactions on Biomedical Engineering 60, 691–699.

Ozbolat, I.T., Yu, Y., 2013. Bioprinting towards organ fabrication: challanges and future trends. IEEE Transactions on Biomedical Engineering 60, 691–699.

Ozbolat, I.T., Chen, H., Yu, Y., 2014. Development of 'Multi-arm Bioprinter' for hybrid biofabrication of tissue engineering constructs. Robotics and Computer-Integrated Manufacturing 30, 295–304.

Ozbolat, I., May 2015a. Scaffold-based or scaffold-free bioprinting: competing or complementing approaches? Journal of Nanotechnology in Engineering and Medicine 6 (2), 024701-5.

Ozbolat, I.T., 2015b. Bioprinting scale-up tissue and organ constructs for transplantation. Trends in Biotechnology 33, 395–400.

Pena-Francesch, A., Florez, S., Jung, H., Sebastian, A., Albert, I., Curtis, W., Demirel, M.C., 2014. Materials fabrication from native and recombinant thermoplastic squid proteins. Advanced Functional Materials 24, 7401–7409.

Peng, W., Unutmaz, D., Ozbolat, I.T., September 2016. Bioprinting towards physiologically relevant tissue models for pharmaceutics. Trends in Biotechnology 34 (9), 722–732. http://dx.doi.org/10.1016/j.tibtech.2016.05.013.

Rezende, R.A., Pereira, F.D.A.S., Kasyanov, V., Ovsianikov, A., Torgensen, J., Gruber, P., Stampfl, J., Brakke, K., Nogueira, J.A., Mironov, V., Da Silva, J.V.L., 2012. Design, physical prototyping and initial characterisation of 'lockyballs'. Virtual and Physical Prototyping 7, 287–301.

Root Analysis Private Ltd., 2014. 3D Bioprinting Market, pp. 2014–2030.

Skardal, A., Mack, D., Kapetanovic, E., Atala, A., Jackson, J.D., Yoo, J., Soker, S., 2012. Bioprinted amniotic fluid-derived stem cells accelerate healing of large skin wounds. Stem Cells Translational Medicine 1, 792–802.

Takebe, T., Sekine, K., Enomura, M., Koike, H., Kimura, M., Ogaeri, T., Zhang, R.-R., Ueno, Y., Zheng, Y.-W., Koike, N., Aoyama, S., Adachi, Y., Taniguchi, H., 2013. Vascularized and functional human liver from an iPSC-derived organ bud transplant. Nature 499, 481–484.

Tasoglu, S., Yu, C.H., Gungordu, H.I., Guven, S., Vural, T., Demirci, U., 2014. Guided and magnetic self-assembly of tunable magnetoceptive gels. Nature Communications 5.

Temple, J.P., Hutton, D.L., Hung, B.P., Huri, P.Y., Cook, C.A., Kondragunta, R., Jia, X., Grayson, W.L., 2014. Engineering anatomically shaped vascularized bone grafts with hASCs and 3D-printed PCL scaffolds. Journal of Biomedical Materials Research Part A 102, 4317–4325.

Xu, T., Rohozinski, J., Zhao, W., Moorefield, E.C., Atala, A., Yoo, J.J., 2008. Inkjet-mediated gene transfection into living cells combined with targeted delivery. Tissue Engineering Part A 15, 95–101.

Yu, Y., Brouillette, M.J., Seol, D., Zheng, H., Buckwalter, J.A., Martin, J.A., 2015. Use of recombinant human stromal cell–derived factor 1α–loaded fibrin/hyaluronic acid hydrogel networks to achieve functional repair of full-thickness bovine articular cartilage via homing of chondrogenic progenitor cells. Arthritis & Rheumatology 67, 1274–1285.

Zhang, Y., Yu, Y., Ozbolat, I.T., 2013. Direct bioprinting of vessel-like tubular microfluidic channels. Journal of Nanotechnology in Engineering and Medicine 4, 021001.

Index

'*Note:* Page numbers followed by "f" indicate figures, "b" indicate boxes and "t" indicate tables.'

9780128030103